Functional and Motility Disorders of the Gastrointestinal Tract

Brian E. Lacy • Michael D. Crowell
John K. DiBaise
Editors

Functional and Motility Disorders of the Gastrointestinal Tract

A Case Study Approach

Springer

Editors
Brian E. Lacy
Division of Gastroenterology
and Hepatology
Dartmouth-Hitchcock Medical Center
Lebanon, NH, USA

Geisel School of Medicine at Dartmouth
Lebanon, NH, USA

Michael D. Crowell
Division of Gastroenterology
and Hepatology
Mayo Clinic
Scottsdale, AZ, USA

John K. DiBaise
Division of Gastroenterology
and Hepatology
Mayo Clinic
Scottsdale, AZ, USA

ISBN 978-1-4939-1497-5 ISBN 978-1-4939-1498-2 (eBook)
DOI 10.1007/978-1-4939-1498-2
Springer New York Heidelberg Dordrecht London

Library of Congress Control Number: 2014949898

Printed on acid-free paper

Springer is part of Springer Science+Business Media (www.springer.com)

Preface

Functional gastrointestinal disorders (FGIDs) and motility disorders of the gastrointestinal tract are highly prevalent disorders routinely encountered by all healthcare providers, regardless of specialty. Conservative estimates are that, at any one time, at least 40 % of the United States population has symptoms of at least one of the FGIDs or motility disorders described in this book. These symptoms, which are frequently nonspecific, thus making the diagnosis difficult, include dysphagia, chest pain, heartburn, bloating, abdominal pain, constipation, diarrhea, nausea, and vomiting. The disorders reviewed in this book are "equal opportunity" diseases affecting all genders, races, age groups, and socioeconomic classes. A clear understanding of these common disorders is important for all healthcare providers as the symptoms of FGIDs and motility disorders cause significant patient distress, greatly reduce the quality of these patients' lives, and result in substantial health resource utilization leading to a significant negative economic impact on our healthcare system. As these disorders are often difficult to diagnose and treat, and because few comprehensive resources are available to guide busy clinicians, we hope that this book will be useful in the care of your patients.

Healthcare providers generally learn best when confronted with a patient and his or her symptoms. For that reason, this book was organized using a Case Study approach. Each chapter begins with an actual case, followed by a comprehensive, but succinct, review of the epidemiology, pathophysiology, diagnosis, and treatment of each disorder. Self-assessment questions are provided at the end of each chapter, with answers situated in an appendix at the end of the book. Each chapter also includes a list of key references for the reader who wants to further pursue a topic. Algorithms and summary tables are widely used to help summarize key information. An Index is located at the end of the book. You may want to read the book from the start, and work through each of the seven parts (esophagus, gastroduodenal, small intestine, gallbladder, colon, anorectal, and the functional patient) sequentially. Alternatively, each chapter is meant to stand alone, and can be read without reference to preceding or succeeding chapters.

We are fortunate to have gathered international experts in the field to contribute to this book. The authors are experienced clinician-researchers who have made significant contributions to the field of gastroenterology, and more specifically to the disciplines of functional gastrointestinal and motility disorders. We greatly appreciate their contribution to this textbook, and we hope that you find their collective expertise valuable.

Lebanon, NH, USA Brian E. Lacy
Scottsdale, AZ, USA Michael D. Crowell
Scottsdale, AZ, USA John K. DiBaise

Contents

Contributors

Sami R. Achem, M.D., FACG, FAGA, FASGE Division of Gastroenterology and Hepatology, Mayo Clinic, Jacksonville, FL, USA

Cristina Almansa, M.D., Ph.D. Division of Gastroenterology and Hepatology, Mayo Clinic, Jacksonville, FL, USA

Raul Badillo, M.D. Division of Gastroenterology, Mayo Clinic Florida, Jacksonville, FL, USA

Todd H. Baron, M.D., FASGE Division of Gastroenterology and Hepatology, Mayo Clinic, Rochester, MN, USA

Adil E. Bharucha, M.B.B.S., M.D., FAGA Division of Gastroenterology and Hepatology, Mayo Clinic, Rochester, MN, USA

Andrea Bollom, B.S. Division of Gastroenterology, Beth Israel Deaconess Medical Center, Boston, MA, USA

Ernest P. Bouras, M.D. Division of Gastroenterology, Mayo Clinic Florida, Jacksonville, FL, USA

Michael Camilleri, M.D. Division of Gastroenterology and Hepatology, Mayo Clinic, Rochester, MN, USA

Vanessa C. Costilla, M.D. Department of Internal Medicine, Mayo Clinic, Scottsdale, AZ, USA

Michael D. Crowell, Ph.D. Division of Gastroenterology and Hepatology, Mayo Clinic, Scottsdale, AZ, USA

Lincoln Eduardo Villela Vieira de Castro Ferreira, M.D. Universidade Federal de Juiz de Fora, Juiz de Fora, Brazil

Fábio Heleno de Lima Pace Hepatology Reference Center, Gastroenterology Department, Universidade Federal de Juiz de Fora, Juiz de Fora, Brazil

Kenneth R. DeVault, M.D. Department of Medicine, Mayo Clinic, Jacksonville, FL, USA

Division of Gastroenterology and Hepatology, Mayo Clinic, Jacksonville, FL, USA

John K. DiBaise, M.D. Division of Gastroenterology and Hepatology, Mayo Clinic, Scottsdale, AZ, USA

Kelly Everhart, B.A., M.S. Division of Gastroenterology and Hepatology, Dartmouth-Hitchcock Medical Center, Lebanon, NH, USA

Amy E. Foxx-Orenstein, D.O. Division of Gastroenterology and Hepatology, Mayo Clinic, Scottsdale, AZ, USA

Dawn Francis, M.D., M.H.S. Division of Gastroenterology and Hepatology, Mayo Clinic Florida, Jacksonville, FL, USA

Scott Gabbard, M.D. Division of Gastroenterology and Hepatology, Cleveland Clinic, Cleveland, OH, USA

Lucinda Harris, M.D. Division of Gastroenterology and Hepatology, Mayo Clinic, Scottsdale, AZ, USA

Stephanie L. Hansel, M.D., M.S. Division of Gastroenterology and Hepatology, Mayo Clinic, Rochester, MN, USA

Kimberly N. Harer, M.D. Division of Gastroenterology and Hepatology, Mayo Clinic, Rochester, MN, USA

Stefan D. Holubar, M.D., M.S., FACS, FASCRS Division of Colon & Rectal Surgery, Department of Surgery, Dartmouth-Hitchcock Medical Center, Lebanon, NH, USA

Lesley A. Houghton, Ph.D. Division of Gastroenterology and Hepatology, Mayo Clinic, Jacksonville, FL, USA

Zilla H. Hussain, M.D. Division of Gastroenterology and Hepatology, Dartmouth-Hitchcock Medical Center, Lebanon, NH, USA

David A. Katzka, M.D. Division of Gastroenterology and Hepatology, Mayo Clinic, Rochester, MN, USA

Robert T. Kavitt, M.D., M.P.H. Section of Gastroenterology, Department of Medicine, University of Chicago, Chicago, IL, USA

Kenneth L. Koch, M.D. Section of Gastroenterology, Wake Forest Baptist Medical Center, Winston-Salem, NC, USA

Brian E. Lacy, M.D., Ph.D. Division of Gastroenterology and Hepatology, Dartmouth-Hitchcock Medical Center, Lebanon, NH, USA

Geisel School of Medicine at Dartmouth, Lebanon, NH, USA

Anthony Lembo, M.D. Beth Israel Deaconess Medical Center, Boston, MA, USA

Kate E. Napthali, FRACP John Hunter Hospital, University of Newcastle, Newcastle, NSW, Australia

Amy S. Oxentenko, M.D. Department of Internal Medicine, Mayo Clinic, Rochester, MN, USA

Division of Gastroenterology and Hepatology, Mayo Clinic, Rochester, MN, USA

Darrell S. Pardi, M.D. Division of Gastroenterology and Hepatology, Mayo Clinic, Rochester, MN, USA

Mark Pimentel, M.D., FRCP(C) GI Motility Program, Division of Gastroenterology, Cedars-Sinai Medical Center, Los Angeles, CA, USA

Blake Scott, M.D. Wake Forest School of Medicine, Winston-Salem, NC, USA

Benjamin N. Stein, M.D., M.P.H. Division of Gastroenterology and Hepatology, Dartmouth-Hitchcock Medical Center, Lebanon, NH, USA

Nicholas J. Talley, M.D., Ph.D. Faculty of Health and Medicine, University of Newcastle, New Lambton, NSW, Australia

Konstantinos Triantafyllou, M.D., Ph.D. Hepatogastroenterology Unit, Second Department of Internal Medicine and Research Institute, Attikon University General Hospital, Haidari, Greece

Sarah Umar, M.D. Division of Gastroenterology and Hepatology, Mayo Clinic, Scottsdale, AZ, USA

Michael F. Vaezi, M.D., Ph.D., M.Sc. (Epi) Division of Gastroenterology, Hepatology, and Nutrition, Department of Medicine, Vanderbilt University Medical Center, Nashville, TN, USA

Maria I. Vazquez-Roque, M.D. Division of Gastroenterology, Mayo Clinic Florida, Jacksonville, FL, USA

Part I
Esophageal Disorders

Chapter 1
Globus

Robert T. Kavitt and Michael F. Vaezi

Case Study

A 33-year-old woman presents to her gastroenterologist with symptoms of a lump in her throat. These symptoms have been present continuously for the past 8 months. She does not describe dysphagia although she reports a near constant sensation as if a pill is stuck in her throat. She also reports infrequent heartburn for the past 15 years. A prior upper endoscopy noted mild erythema of the distal esophagus and a small hiatal hernia. The patient's past medical history is notable for asthma and hyperlipidemia. Her only surgery was an uncomplicated Cesarean section. She does not smoke and has 1–2 alcoholic drinks each week. Her current medications include atorvastatin and albuterol on a p.r.n. basis. Physical examination, including a careful examination of the neck and oropharynx, is unremarkable. She subsequently underwent otolaryngological examination which was unrevealing. A videofluoroscopic swallow study was also unremarkable.

R.T. Kavitt, M.D., M.P.H.
Department of Medicine, Section of Gastroenterology, University of Chicago, Chicago, IL, USA

M.F. Vaezi, M.D., Ph.D., M.Sc. (Epi) (✉)
Department of Medicine, Vanderbilt University Medical Center, Nashville, TN, USA

Division of Gastroenterology, Hepatology, and Nutrition, Vanderbilt University Medical Center, 1660 TVC, 1301-22nd Ave. South, Nashville, TN 37232-5280, USA
e-mail: Michael.Vaezi@vanderbilt.edu

B.E. Lacy et al. (eds.), *Functional and Motility Disorders of the Gastrointestinal Tract*, DOI 10.1007/978-1-4939-1498-2_1

Introduction

Globus refers to the non-painful sensation of a lump in the throat, usually in the region of the sternal notch. Patients with globus may describe their symptoms as a sensation of a lump, fullness, or a "tickle" in the throat. Globus is differentiated from dysphagia, as food transit is not limited in globus and globus is often described as a continuously persistent symptom. Globus is unrelated to swallowing and in some cases may improve with swallowing. Most patients with globus do not report dysphagia with food, although many describe the sensation of a pill or other obstruction in the throat when no such obstruction exists. The sensation may be related to inflammation of the larynx or hypopharynx in the setting of esophageal dysmotility, spasm of the cricopharyngeus, or incomplete relaxation of the upper esophageal sphincter. Globus may at times be a symptom of reflux laryngitis, although the relationship between globus and GERD is not strong.

The sensation of globus is often psychogenic in origin and may be related to increased visceral sensation, anxiety, depression, somatization, or other conditions. A detailed investigation of the larynx, pharynx, neck, and esophagus should be conducted in order to evaluate other potential etiologies.

This condition is also occasionally referred to as globus pharyngeus and globus hystericus. The symptom was once believed to occur primarily in women and was given the name "globus hystericus" to indicate a relationship between the uterus and this symptom. Reports from the early twentieth century emphasized a purported psychogenic etiology, including "materialization of a repressed idea" or manifestation of a nervous illness. Later studies suggested globus as a symptom of a somatization or conversion disorder.

Epidemiology

The incidence of globus peaks in middle age and may occur infrequently in healthy individuals, although it is unusual in those under the age of 20. Globus has a similar prevalence in men and women, although women are more likely to seek care regarding this symptom.

Pathophysiology

No quality evidence exists demonstrating that globus is related to an anatomic finding such as a cricopharyngeal bar. Some patients with globus have been shown to have hyperdynamic changes involving the upper esophageal sphincter pressure with elevated residual pressures in response to respiration (see Fig. 1.1). It is thought that an increased frequency of swallows may promote globus symptoms via entrapment

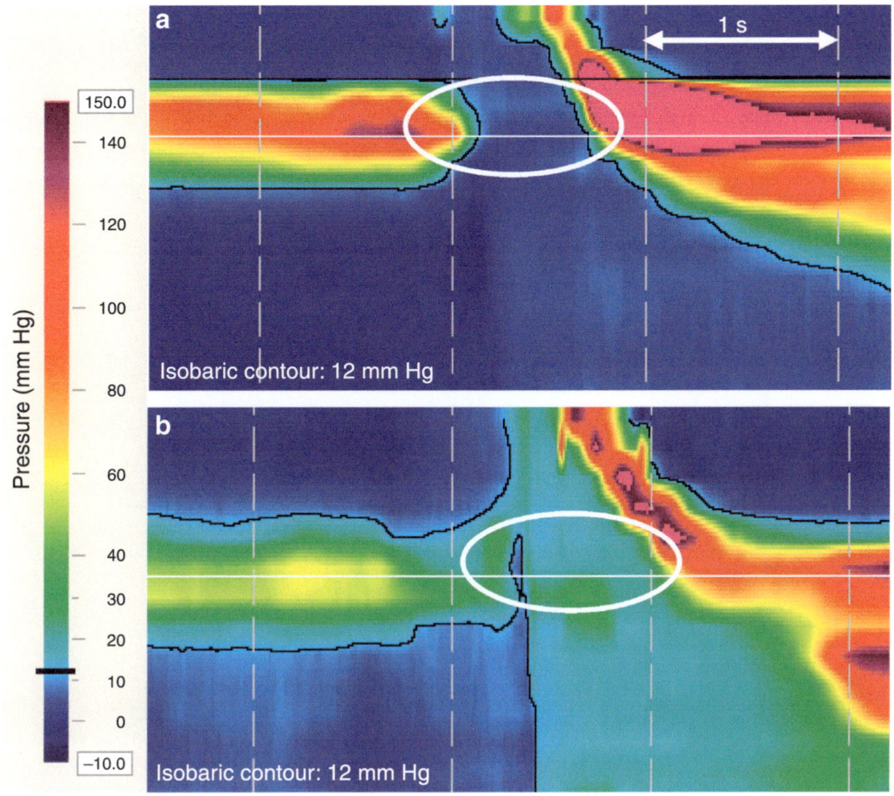

Fig. 1.1 Assessment of nadir upper esophageal sphincter relaxation pressure using high-resolution esophageal manometry isobaric contour tool. (**a**) depicts a patient with normal upper esophageal sphincter relaxation. (**b**) depicts a patient with abnormal upper esophageal sphincter relaxation with elevated residual pressure. (Adapted by permission from Nature Publishing Group: American Journal of Gastroenterology (Kwiatek MA, Mirza F, Kahrilas PJ, Pandolfino JE. Hyperdynamic upper esophageal sphincter pressure: a manometric observation in patients reporting globus sensation. Am J Gastroenterol 2009; 104(2):289–98), copyright 2009)

of air in the proximal esophagus. Esophageal hypersensitivity may also play a contributing role. As noted, a strong relationship between gastroesophageal reflux disease (GERD) and globus has not been found. Although some studies of small sample size have raised the possibility that GERD may be a contributing etiology to globus, other studies have found no such association. Esophageal motility disorders may include a globus sensation among their presenting symptoms, although these mechanisms are not thought to be a significant contributing factor in the pathophysiology of globus. The finding of a gastric inlet patch on endoscopy has been associated with globus (see Fig. 1.2). Endoscopic ablation of an inlet patch has been shown to improve globus symptoms in some patients; however, this practice is controversial and not recommended.

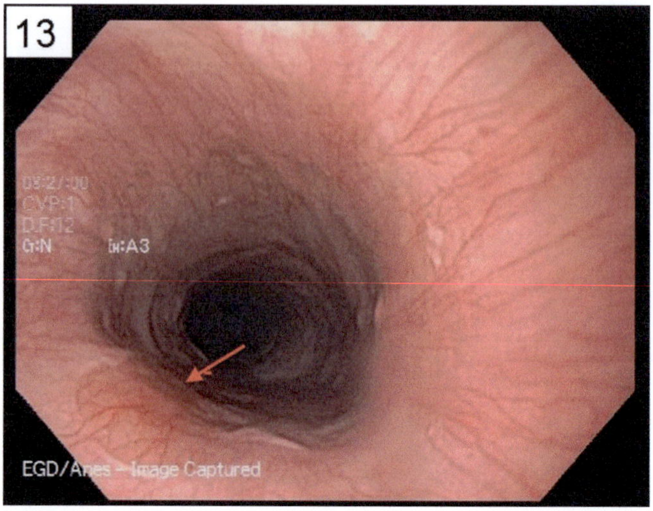

Fig. 1.2 Gastric inlet patch (see *arrow*) visualized during upper endoscopy which visually is salmon *pink* in color, reflecting columnar mucosa, with a smooth border and usually round or oval in shape

Several studies have found that patients with globus report an increase in stressful life events prior to the onset of symptoms. One study noted that nearly 96 % of globus patients reported an increase in their symptoms when experiencing strong emotion. This is a rationale for the use of tricyclic antidepressants in those with no structural or motility abnormalities who have not responded to an empiric trial of acid suppressive therapy.

Diagnosis and Evaluation

The Rome III diagnostic criteria for globus (see Table 1.1) require the presence of symptoms for the last 3 months with onset at least 6 months prior to diagnosis. It is important that conditions such as GERD, motility disorders of the esophagus, and structural lesions are ruled out. Table 1.2 highlights a broad differential diagnosis to consider in patients presenting with globus sensation.

Proper diagnosis of persistent globus requires a detailed clinical history and must ensure that dysphagia is not present. Alarm symptoms such as odynophagia, pain, hoarseness, or weight loss warrant additional assessment. Physical examination of the neck should be performed, as should referral to an otolaryngologist for nasolaryngoscopic examination of the pharynx if deemed appropriate. If classical reflux symptoms are present, either ambulatory pH monitoring or a therapeutic trial of a proton pump inhibitor should be considered. Table 1.3 highlights diagnostic tests to

Table 1.1 Rome III diagnostic criteria for globus

1.	Persistent or intermittent, non-painful sensation of a lump or foreign body in the throat
2.	Occurrence of the sensation between meals
3.	Absence of dysphagia or odynophagia
4.	Absence of evidence that gastroesophageal reflux is the cause of the symptom
5.	Absence of histopathology-based esophageal motility disorders

All criteria listed must be met. The criteria must be fulfilled for the last 3 months with symptom onset at least 6 months prior to diagnosis

Adapted from Galmiche JP, Clouse RE, Balint A, et al. Functional esophageal disorders. Gastroenterology 2006; 130:1459–65

Table 1.2 Differential diagnosis in the evaluation of suspected globus

Gastrointestinal disorders	Non-gastrointestinal disorders
Esophageal dysmotility	Head and neck (particularly tongue) cancer
Achalasia	Cervical lymphadenopathy
Gastric inlet patch	Goiter
GERD	Hyperplastic tonsils
Esophageal ring or obstructing esophageal lesions	Prior uvulopalatoplasty
Hiatal hernia	Paraesophageal mass
Hypertensive upper esophageal sphincter	Chronic tonsillitis or pharyngitis
Ring or web of cervical esophagus or postcricoid region	Thyroid disease
Zenker's diverticulum	Cervical spondylosis/cervical osteophytes
	Stress
	Psychologic/psychiatric disorders

Table 1.3 Diagnostic tools useful in the evaluation of patients with globus

Detailed history and physical examination
Otolaryngological examination
Videofluoroscopic swallow study
Esophagram
Esophageal manometry
Esophagogastroduodenoscopy (EGD)
Ambulatory pH monitoring
Esophageal multichannel intraluminal impedance study
Gastric emptying study
Psychiatric interview

consider in patients presenting with globus sensation. They should be directed to an individual patient's associated symptoms and underlying illnesses. The role of diagnostic testing in patients with globus is to ensure that there are no anatomic or physiologic causes for the symptom.

Treatment

A prospective trial observed that globus symptoms persist in up to 75 % of patients after 3 years. Limited treatment options for this condition are available, and although the symptom can be frustrating for patients, after excluding certain etiologies, the symptom itself is benign. Supportive care with explanation and reassurance are important elements in the care of patients with globus. A trial of an anti-reflux medication is reasonable, especially among those who also have typical reflux symptoms. Empiric dilation may also be reasonable during the endoscopic evaluation even if no stricture is identified.

For patients with persistent symptoms, a psychiatric consultation should be considered. The use of imipramine may benefit patients with coexistent psychiatric disorders or those whose symptoms may be anxiety related. Relaxation therapy may also aid patients with globus.

Case Resolution

An empiric trial of omeprazole 20 mg daily was initiated. In follow-up after one month, her globus had improved significantly although she still noted symptoms approximately three times each week. Subsequent esophageal dilation and reassurance provided further relief. She was educated about the role of stress in her symptomatology.

Key Clinical Teaching Points

- The Rome III diagnostic criteria (see Table 1.1) should be used to define globus.
- It is important to rule out a variety of contributing etiologies that may be the true source of the presenting symptom, although most globus is ultimately idiopathic in nature and persists despite therapeutic intervention.
- Diagnostic testing should be directed based on symptom severity, duration, and presence or absence of alarm symptoms (e.g., dysphagia, odynophagia, weight loss, anemia) and other associated symptoms.
- Patient education and reassurance are critical elements of management and cannot be overemphasized.

Teaching Questions

1. Which one of the following is not part of the Rome III diagnostic criteria for globus?
   (A) Sensation of a lump or foreign body in the throat
   (B) Presence of dysphagia and/or odynophagia
   (C) Absence of evidence that gastroesophageal reflux is the cause of the symptom
   (D) Absence of histopathology-based esophageal motility disorders
2. Which one of the following is not considered a reasonable treatment option for globus?
   (A) Proton pump inhibitors
   (B) Relaxation therapy
   (C) Tricyclic antidepressants
   (D) Baclofen
3. Which one of the following is not considered a reasonable diagnostic test in the evaluation of globus?
   (A) Esophageal manometry
   (B) Barium esophagram
   (C) Ambulatory esophageal pH testing
   (D) Endoscopic ultrasound

Key References

1. Gale CR, Wilson JA, Deary IJ. Globus sensation and psychopathology in men: the Vietnam experience study. Psychosom Med. 2009;71:1026–31. This article assessed the prevalence of globus in U.S. male veterans and examined the correlation of this symptom with psychopathology.
2. Galmiche JP, Clouse RE, Balint A, Cook IJ, Kahrilas PJ, Paterson WG, Smout AJ. Functional esophageal disorders. Gastroenterology. 2006;130:1459–65. This article describes the Rome III diagnostic criteria for globus.
3. Harar RP, Kumar S, Saeed MA, Gatland DJ. Management of globus pharyngeus: Review of 699 cases. J Laryngol Otol. 2004;118:522–7. This article involved a retrospective study of a large patient population with globus.
4. Hill J, Stuart RC, Fung HK, Ng EK, Cheung FM, Chung CS, van Hasselt CA. Gastroesophageal reflux, motility disorders, and psychological profiles in the etiology of globus pharyngis. Laryngoscope. 1997;107:1373–7. This article assessed 26 patients with globus and found an association between GERD and globus.
5. Moser G, Wenzel-Abatzi TA, Stelzeneder M, Wenzel T, Weber U, Wiesnagrotski S, et al. Globus sensation: Pharyngoesophageal function, psychometric and psychiatric findings, and follow-up in 88 patients. Arch Intern Med. 1998;158:1365–73. This article involved the study of 88 patients referred for evaluation of globus by investigating potential structural, functional, and psychiatric etiologies.

Chapter 2
Dysphagia

Kimberly N. Harer and David A. Katzka

Case Study 1

A 32-year-old man with a history of asthma presents to the emergency department with acute difficulty swallowing after taking the first bite of his chicken nugget. He complains of a 6-month history of solid food intermittently getting "stuck" while swallowing. He also notes that for "years" he had been a slow eater and avoids steak. He denies heartburn, regurgitation, or odynophagia. On physical exam, he is noted to be drooling and appeared uncomfortable. Emergent endoscopy was performed and demonstrated a food impaction which was removed. Esophageal rings and linear furrows were noted on endoscopy (see Fig. 2.1). There was no evidence of erosive esophagitis. Esophageal mucosal biopsy demonstrated a maximum of 50 eosinophils/high-power field.

K.N. Harer, M.D. • D.A. Katzka, M.D. (✉)
Division of Gastroenterology and Hepatology, Mayo Clinic, Rochester, MN, USA
e-mail: Katzka.David@mayo.edu

B.E. Lacy et al. (eds.), *Functional and Motility Disorders of the Gastrointestinal Tract*, DOI 10.1007/978-1-4939-1498-2_2

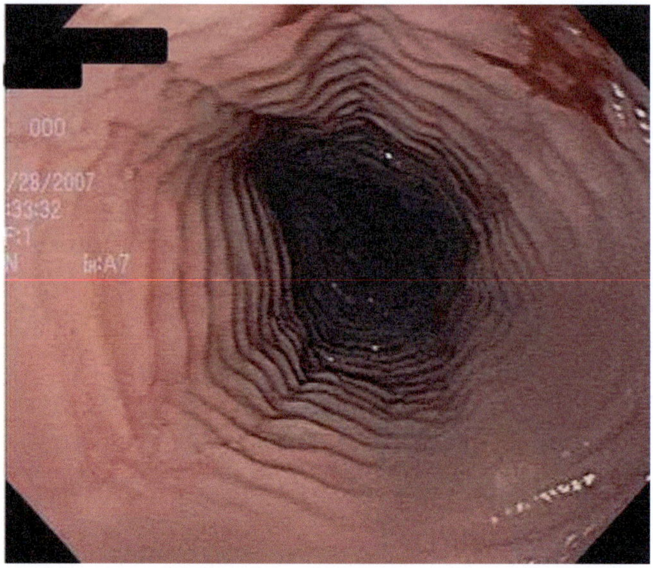

Fig. 2.1 Endoscopic image of eosinophilic esophagitis. From Moawad FJ, Beerappan GR, Wong RK. Eosinophilic esophagitis. 2009;54(9):1818–28; with permission

Case Study 2

A 76-year-old woman with a history of stroke, diabetes mellitus, and hypertension is seen in the outpatient clinic for evaluation of recurrent pneumonia. Over the past 6 months, she has been hospitalized three times for pneumonia treated with broad-spectrum antibiotics. She admits to coughing during meals and intermittent nasal regurgitation while drinking fluids. On physical exam, she appears thin and is noted to have a residual left facial droop from her prior cerebrovascular accident (CVA). She is given a glass of water to drink and takes small sips and tucks her chin when swallowing. Her voice after drinking is wet sounding. She swallows a bite of pudding without noticeable difficulty.

Introduction

Dysphagia (see Table 2.1) is a symptom that results from the slowing or cessation of a food or liquid bolus as it passes from the oral cavity through the esophagus and into the stomach. An estimated 10 million Americans are evaluated each year with swallowing difficulties in inpatient and outpatient settings. Dysphagia is also associated with significant morbidity, mortality, and healthcare cost. In one study, the average hospital length of stay was almost double for patients with dysphagia when compared with dysphagia-free patients, an estimated cost difference of approximately $547 billion. Aspiration pneumonia, malnutrition, and social embarrassment

Table 2.1 Definitions

Dysphagia
Sense of solid and/or liquid foods sticking, lodging, or passing abnormally through the esophagus
Functional dysphagia
Diagnostic criteria[a] *must include* ***all*** *of the following:* Sense of solid and/or liquid foods sticking, lodging, or passing abnormally through the esophagus Absence of evidence that gastroesophageal reflux is the cause of the symptom Absence of histopathology-based esophageal motility disorders[a]

[a]Criteria fulfilled for the last 3 months with symptom onset at least 6 months prior to diagnosis

Table 2.2 Differential diagnosis of dysphagia

Oropharyngeal dysmotility	Oropharyngeal mechanical	Esophageal dysmotility	Esophageal mechanical
• **Central nervous system** CVA Head trauma Alzheimer's disease Multiple sclerosis Cerebral palsy ALS Drugs • **Peripheral nervous system** Spinal muscular atrophy Guillain-Barre Post polio syndrome Diphtheria • **Myogenic** Myasthenia gravis Botulism Dermatomyositis Sarcoid Hypothyroidism Paraneoplastic Muscular dystrophy Radiation	• Zenker's diverticulum • Cricopharyngeal bar • Tonsillar or pharyngeal cancer • Thyroid goiter or cancer • Thyroglossal cyst • Cervical osteophytes • Aberrant subclavian artery (dysphagia lusoria)	• Achalasia • Diffuses esophageal spasm • Hypertensive LES • Eosinophilic esophagitis • Scleroderma • Amyloidosis • Status-post fundoplication • Diabetes mellitus • GERD	• Strictures (GERD, medication induced, radiation, skin disease) • Rings and webs • Eosinophilic esophagitis (rings) • Malignancy • Extrinsic compression (mass, vascular, lung cancer) • Esophageal diverticula

LES lower esophageal sphincter, *CVA* cerebral vascular accident, *ALS* Amyotrophic lateral sclerosis, *GERD* gastroesophageal reflux disease

are common complications of dysphagia and have a significant impact on patients' overall health and quality of life.

There are numerous potential etiologies of dysphagia to consider in the differential diagnosis (see Table 2.2). During the initial evaluation it is necessary to differentiate dysphagia from a globus sensation, odynophagia, and esophageal hypersensitivity (functional dysphagia); however, distinguishing these disorders can be challenging.

Epidemiology

There is limited published data regarding the incidence and prevalence of dysphagia in the population. Dysphagia becomes more common with aging and one study of patients in a primary care setting aged 62 years and older found that 7 % complained of solid food dysphagia. The incidence of dysphagia has been estimated to be as high as 33 % in acute care clinics and 30–40 % in nursing homes. The prevalence of achalasia, a primary motility disorder of the esophagus, has been estimated at 7.9–12.6 per 100,000 population with an incidence rate of 1 in 100,000 people.

The natural history of dysphagia differs based on the underlying etiology. For example, malignant causes of dysphagia will progress as will benign disorders such as achalasia and eosinophilic esophagitis. In contrast, anatomical disorders such as a Schatzki's ring or a stricture due to gastroesophageal reflux may remain static for years until treatment is initiated.

Pathophysiology

Swallowing is a complex process of synchronized neuromuscular activity that is composed of two phases—the oropharyngeal phase and the esophageal phase. Dysphagia occurs when a mechanical (anatomic) or a motility (motor) disorder affects the coordinated swallowing mechanism required to transport a food bolus from the oral cavity to the stomach.

The oropharyngeal phase of swallowing consists of synchronized neuromuscular actions which move the food bolus from the oral cavity into the esophagus. The initial phase is voluntary and includes closure of the lips and elevation of the tongue against the palate to push the food bolus posteriorly into the pharynx. The soft palate then elevates to seal the nasopharynx, the hyoid moves anteriorly and forward, and the bolus passes from the oral cavity into the pharynx. This stimulates involuntary pharyngeal muscle peristalsis which causes elevation of the pharynx. As the pharynx elevates, the cricopharyngeus relaxes which results in the opening of the upper esophageal sphincter (UES), thus allowing passage of the food bolus into the esophagus. The cerebral cortex and cranial nerves V and IX–XII are vital in coordinating and controlling these actions both from a voluntary and involuntary level. It is also important to note that these same actions not only facilitate bolus passage through the oropharynx but also provide protective mechanisms against aspiration including epiglottic closure over the laryngeal vestibule and elevation of the larynx away from the bolus.

The esophageal phase is involuntary and commences after relaxation of the UES with passage of the bolus into the proximal esophagus. Peristalsis is initiated in the striated upper third of the proximal esophagus under brainstem control and sustained in the distal smooth muscle esophagus under the control of the myenteric plexus. The food bolus then passes through the lower esophageal sphincter (LES), which relaxes primarily via nitric oxide release from the myenteric neurons, and into the stomach.

Diagnosis and Evaluation

The first step in the evaluation of dysphagia is to distinguish between oropharyngeal and esophageal dysphagia (see Table 2.2 and 2.3). A thorough history and physical exam will differentiate these two processes and help guide the selection of appropriate diagnostic testing. The Mayo Dysphagia Questionnaire has been shown to be useful in both clinical practice and research studies in this regard.

Symptoms suggestive of oropharyngeal dysphagia include trouble initiating a swallow, coughing or nasal regurgitation during swallowing, double swallowing,

Table 2.3 Dysphagia questionnaire

Question	Comments
How long have you been experiencing swallowing difficulties?	Need to define acute versus chronic dysphagia
Do you have trouble initiating a swallow?	Trouble initiating a swallow is consistent with an oropharyngeal etiology
Do you feel the food "sticks"? Where?	Cervical region consistent with an oropharyngeal etiology. Location is less specific for esophageal etiologies, but usually inferior to the sternoclavicular notch
Do you have trouble swallowing solid food, liquids, or both?	Helps differentiate motor from mechanical causes of esophageal dysphagia
Are your symptoms progressive or intermittent?	Useful in further defining the etiology of esophageal dysphagia
Have you lost weight?	Weight loss most commonly due to malignancy, achalasia, or severe neuromuscular dysphagia
Do you experience nausea, vomiting, or regurgitation of food?	Regurgitation of old food common with achalasia or Zenker's diverticulum. Recently swallowed food regurgitation seen with strictures or eosinophilic esophagitis
Do you have heartburn?	Chronic GERD can cause strictures. Heartburn also seen in scleroderma
Have you experienced voice changes, cough, nasal regurgitation, or pneumonia?	Consistent with an oropharyngeal etiology
Do you have a history of stroke, Parkinson's disease, Alzheimer's disease, ALS, multiple sclerosis, or another neuromuscular disorder?	Consistent with an oropharyngeal etiology
Do you have a history of cancer?	Think recurrence or metastatic disease. Prior radiation therapy can also cause strictures
Have you ever had surgery involving your mouth, throat, esophagus, stomach, or spine?	Prior surgery can cause scarring or nerve damage
What medications are you taking?	Medications can cause pill esophagitis and stricturing (e.g., doxycycline, potassium, NSAID's, biphosphonates) Neuromodulators can affect swallowing mechanism

drooling, sensation that food is getting stuck in the cervical region, or the sensation of not being able to breathe during the episode. It is important to note that because the cranial nerves that control the muscles responsible for swallowing also contribute to structures responsible for other functions such as speaking, patients may also have dysarthria and changes to the quality of their voice. A history of stroke or neuromuscular disease is also strongly associated with oropharyngeal dysphagia compared with esophageal dysphagia.

Symptoms of esophageal dysphagia are generally more nonspecific. Although patients may point to an anatomical location where food is getting "stuck," this localization of a structural lesion is not generally accurate. Retching and vomiting may occur if the bolus obstruction persists and regurgitation of food often consists of more than a single bolus. Patients are also less panicked about esophageal dysphagia due to the lack of airway symptoms and decreased concern for aspiration. There are two broad etiologies of esophageal dysphagia—mechanical obstruction and dysmotility. Each presents differently and will be discussed below.

Mechanical esophageal dysphagia often presents with episodic trouble swallowing solid food, pills, or large boluses, and often the patient can feel the individual bite of food getting stuck. Patients will often "wash down" the bolus with liquid to alleviate the symptom and then resume eating after the bolus passes or they regurgitate it. The frequency may increase if the patient is in a setting in which they are not concentrating on their chewing, such as at a party or during the first bites of a meal when they are rapidly eating. In contrast, dysmotility-induced esophageal dysphagia often presents with difficulty swallowing both liquid and solid food. As opposed to mechanical causes, the dysphagia can occur anytime during a meal, regurgitation is more common, and the patient often stops eating after the episode.

It is also important to keep in mind, particularly with benign causes of dysphagia, that patients commonly compensate with accommodating mechanisms prior to seeking medical attention. These may include chewing carefully, eating slowly, avoiding certain foods or beverages, adjusting their eating posture such as sitting up straight (as in achalasia) or tucking their chin when they swallow, and even changing their diet to mostly soft foods or liquids.

When performing the physical exam, pay close attention to the patient's dentition and swallowing mechanism. Have the patient chew and swallow in the exam room and observe for coughing, a "wet" voice, or compensating techniques such as chin tucking, double swallowing, taking abnormally small sips, or prolonged chewing. The neck should be examined for enlarged lymph nodes, thyroid enlargement or masses, or tracheal deviation. Cranial nerve exam should be performed to evaluate for a central nervous system etiology.

The initial investigative study to evaluate dysphagia is driven by whether the etiology is thought to be oropharyngeal or esophageal, mechanical, or dysmotility. An evaluation algorithm is outlined in Fig. 2.2. If an oropharyngeal dysmotility etiology is suspected, the best initial evaluation is the videofluoroscopic swallow study performed with the assistance of a trained speech pathologist or occupational therapist. Conversely, nasopharyngeal laryngoscopy should be performed if an oropharyngeal malignancy is suspected (see Fig. 2.3). For patients with a suspected

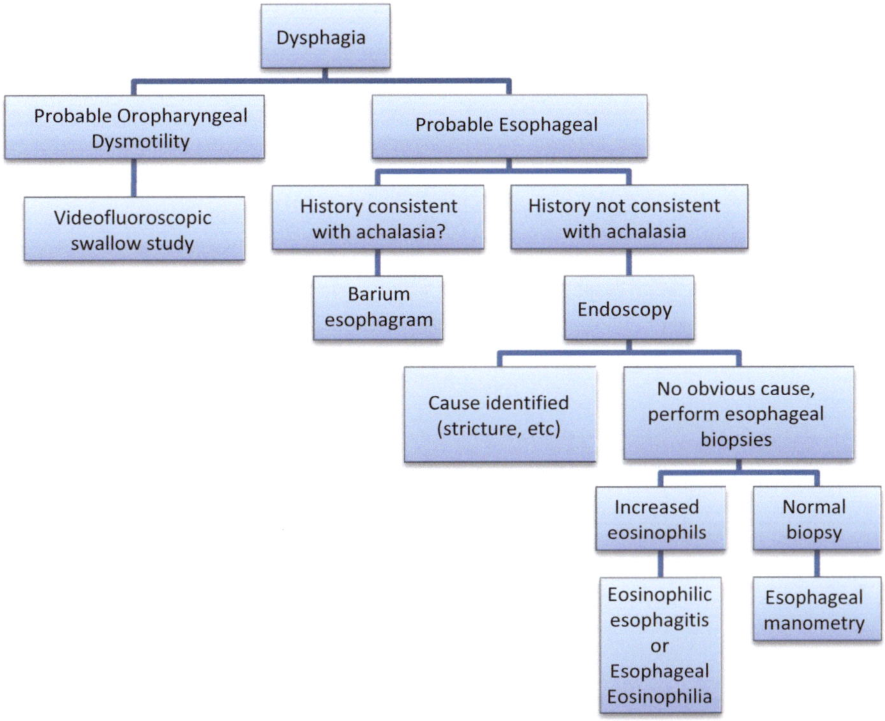

Fig. 2.2 Approach to the evaluation of dysphagia

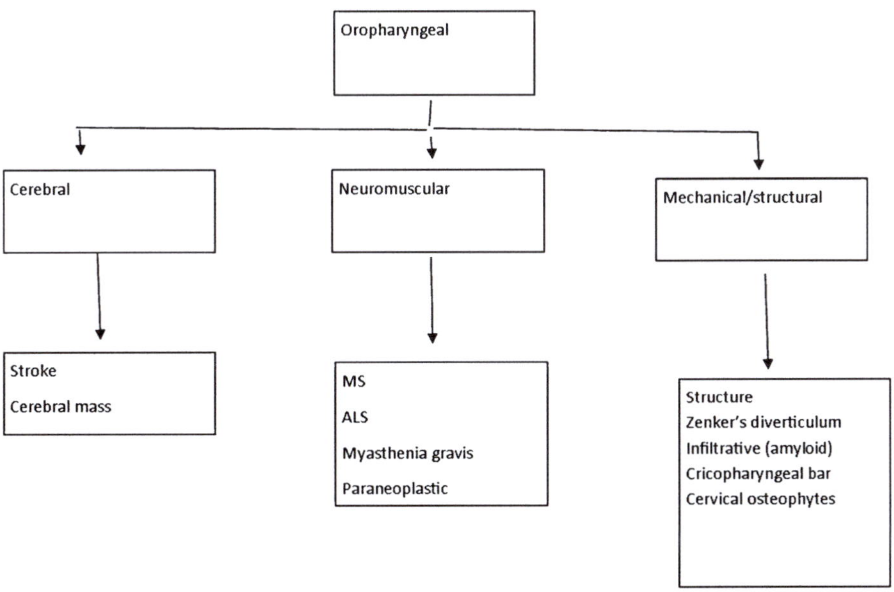

Fig. 2.3 Diagnostic algorithm for dysphagia

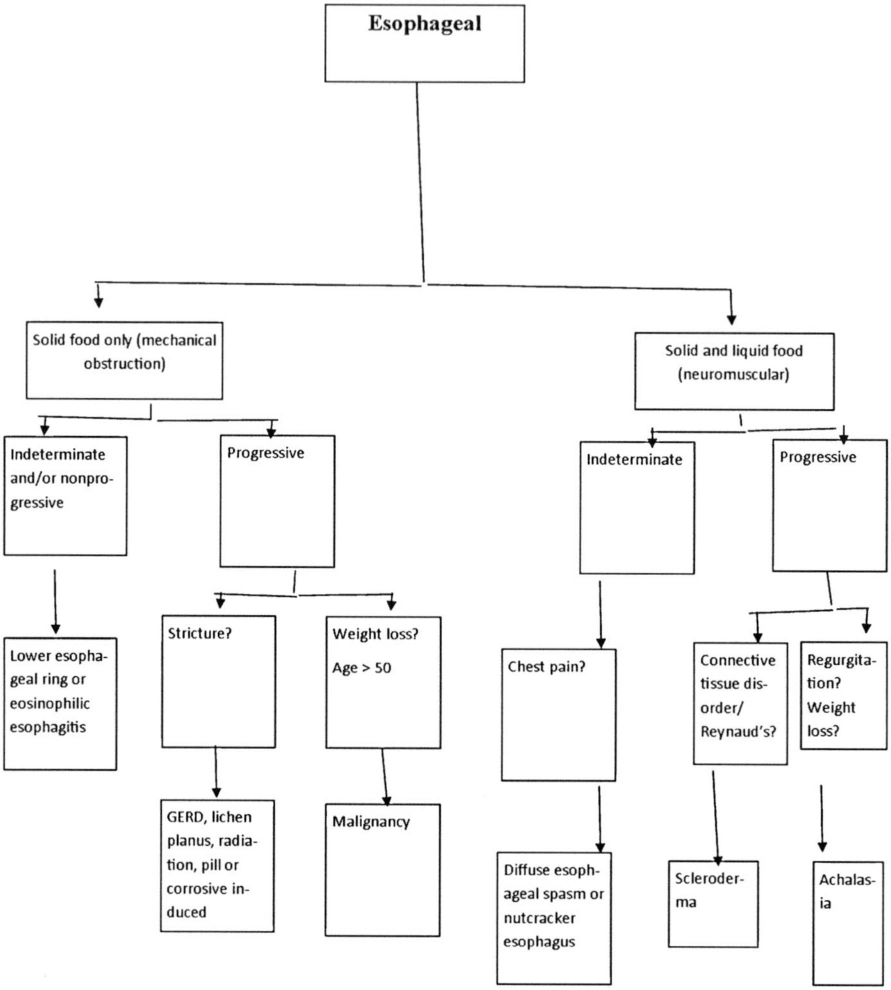

Fig. 2.3 (continued)

esophageal mechanical cause of dysphagia, upper endoscopy is generally preferred as the initial test, as biopsies are likely to be necessary and a therapeutic maneuver may need to be performed during the procedure. When esophageal dysmotility is suspected, a barium esophagogram may be performed to better aid in diagnosis and plan therapy. There is no absolute correct approach to dysphagia, however, and the choice of diagnostic test frequently depends on the local expertise in endoscopy and radiography. These tests often complement each other in the evaluation of dysphagia. Finally, esophageal manometry is useful to confirm a diagnosis of achalasia or for suspected esophageal motility disorders, once a mechanical cause has been ruled out.

Treatment

Treatment options for oropharyngeal dysphagia are variable and depend on the underlying etiology (see Table 2.4). Interventions should address the underlying pathophysiology whenever possible. Speech therapy and/or swallowing maneuvers may be the treatments of choice for many neuromuscular disorders causing

Table 2.4 Treatment options for disorders of dysphagia

Disorder	Pathogenesis	Treatment
Oropharyngeal etiologies		
Neuromuscular disorders	Variable	– Treatment of underlying disease – Speech therapy – Swallowing maneuvers
Zenker's diverticulum	Poorly compliant UES resulting in esophageal outpouching	– Diverticulectomy with UES myomectomy – UES botulinum toxin injection
Cricopharyngeal bar	Enlargement of the cricopharyngeus muscle resulting in protrusion of the posterior esophageal wall into the lumen	– Cricopharyngeal myotomy – Botulinum toxin injection
Esophageal etiologies		
Achalasia	Loss of distal esophageal peristalsis and hypertonic LES	– LES botulinum toxin injection—pneumatic dilation – Surgical myotomy – Calcium channel blocker, nitrates, and sildenafil can be tried but usually of minimal benefit
Diffuse esophageal spasm (DES)	Uncoordinated, prolonged esophageal contractions	– Calcium channel blocker, nitrates, sildenafil – Botulinum toxin injection – Long esophagomyotomy in refractory, severe cases with dysphagia
Eosinophilic esophagitis (EoE)	Incompletely understood, increased eosinophilic infiltration due to environmental or allergic factors	Swallowed corticosteroid, avoidance of food triggers
Esophageal cancer	Adenocarcinoma—smoking, GERD, central obesity Squamous cell carcinoma—smoking	Chemoradiotherapy, surgery, endoscopic resection, stenting
Nutcracker esophagus	Prolonged, high-amplitude esophageal contractions	– Calcium channel blockers – Possibly nitrates, sildenafil – Tricyclic antidepressants – Bougie dilatation – Control of GERD

(continued)

Table 2.4 (continued)

Disorder	Pathogenesis	Treatment
Ring or web	Ring—ring of tissue or muscle causing luminal narrowing in the lower esophagus Web—thin mucosal membrane causing luminal narrowing in the upper/mid-esophagus	Savary or balloon dilation
Scleroderma	Low/absent LES pressure and peristalsis	– No definitive treatment – Important to treat GERD
Stricture	Usually caused by chronic mucosal injury due to untreated GERD, eosinophilic esophagitis, skin diseases, radiation, medications	– Savary or balloon dilation – Treatment of underlying disease

oropharyngeal dysphagia. For esophageal dysphagia, there is a broader range of therapeutic options, and the treatment of choice is based on the identified etiology. Motility disorders with LES, and sometimes esophageal body dysfunction (e.g., achalasia, diffuse esophageal spasm, nutcracker esophagus, hypertensive LES), can be treated with smooth muscle relaxants such as calcium channel blockers, nitrates, sildenafil, or botulinum toxin injection. Pneumatic dilation and myotomy of the LES are the preferred treatments for achalasia. Smooth muscle relaxants have also been used to treat achalasia but are often of limited benefit. Mechanical causes of esophageal dysphagia such as strictures, rings, and webs are best treated with bougie or balloon dilation. To prevent recurrence of strictures, it is important to appropriately manage the underlying disorders. Gastroesophageal reflux should be controlled with proton pump inhibitors or fundoplication. Eosinophilic esophagitis should be treated with topical steroid therapy and, occasionally, dietary intervention. Esophageal malignancies will require oncologic therapy but may also require mechanical treatments such as dilation and/or stent placement.

Case 1 Resolution

This patient has esophageal eosinophilia. Whether the etiology of this finding is due to gastroesophageal reflux disease and/or eosinophilic esophagitis remains to be determined. The first step in managing this patient is to perform esophageal dilation to help prevent another recurrence of food impaction. Concurrently, per consensus guidelines, treatment with 8 weeks of a twice daily proton pump inhibitor followed by repeat endoscopy and esophageal biopsies is recommended as esophageal eosinophilia may respond to proton pump inhibitors even without evidence of reflux disease. If esophageal eosinophilia persists, a topical swallowed steroid preparation, such as fluticasone or budesonide, is recommended.

Case 2 Resolution

The patient underwent videoesophagography which demonstrated marked pharyngeal weakness, poor epiglottic tilt over the larynx with penetration, and pooling of barium in the vallecular and pyriform sinuses. There was no evidence of myasthenia gravis on examination. Muscle enzymes were not elevated in the serum in evaluation for myositis, and electromyography was negative for any evidence of a neurodegenerative disorder such as amyotrophic lateral sclerosis. MRI of the brain revealed a new area of ischemic focus in the brain stem. The patient was instructed to thicken all thin liquids. A chin-tuck maneuver was trialed during the videofluoroscopic swallow study and demonstrated reduction in laryngeal penetration. Finally, she received instructions on practicing effortful swallow and exercises to strengthen her pharyngeal musculature.

Key Clinical Teaching Points

- Patients commonly accommodate to their dysphagia using self-learned techniques to avoid symptoms such as avoidance of certain foods and slow eating.
- Following esophageal disimpaction, patients who present with food impaction should be treated with dilation, when possible, to prevent further impaction and potential complications of perforation and aspiration.
- Esophageal eosinophilia is not the equivalent of eosinophilic esophagitis as eosinophils can also be a marker of gastroesophageal reflux. Thus, an evaluation for GERD (i.e., a wireless pH capsule or transnasal probe) and/or a trial of proton pump inhibitors should be tried prior to the initiation of topical steroids or diet therapy for presumed eosinophilic esophagitis.
- In patients with suspected dysmotility in the oropharynx, a videoesophagram should be performed first. This provides important diagnostic information and potentially therapeutic input from a speech and swallowing therapist.
- A cerebrovascular accident is the most common cause of acute onset dysphagia in the elderly but other neuromuscular diseases need to be considered. Consultation with a neurologist is common in these patients.

Teaching Questions

1. A 74-year-old man is evaluated for intermittent solid food dysphagia. The dysphagia is associated with halitosis and a "gurgling" sensation in his throat after eating. A Zenker's diverticulum is suspected. Which one of the following is the best initial diagnostic test?

(A) Upper endoscopy
(B) Esophageal manometry
(C) CT scan of the neck
(D) Barium esophagography

2. A 54-year-old man with uncontrolled hypertension is evaluated in the outpatient setting after presenting to the emergency department twice in the past month with substernal chest pain. Both times, electrocardiograms and troponin levels were normal. He also underwent an exercise stress test which was negative for ischemia. The pain was not reproducible with firm sternal pressure. He states both episodes occurred during dinner and were associated with mild dysphagia. Upper endoscopy was subsequently performed and was normal. Due to a suspicion for a hypercontractile esophageal motility disorder, esophageal manometry was performed and demonstrated simultaneous, high-amplitude, and prolonged esophageal contractions consistent with diffuse esophageal spasm. Which one of the following would be the initial treatment of choice?

   (A) Long esophagomyotomy
   (B) Diltiazem
   (C) Botulinum toxin injection
   (D) Pneumatic dilatation

3. A 27-year-old man with a history of asthma is evaluated for a 6-month history of intermittent solid food dysphagia which is worsened by eating meat and bread. Upper endoscopy demonstrates a "ringed" esophagus, and esophageal biopsies demonstrate 40 eosinophils per high-power field. Ambulatory 24-h combined esophageal pH-impedance testing was negative for gastroesophageal reflux. A diagnosis of eosinophilic esophagitis is made. Which one of the following would be the best choice for initial management?

   (A) Proton pump inhibitor for 8 weeks followed by repeat endoscopy with biopsies
   (B) Skin-prick allergy testing with subsequent avoidance of positive reacting food antigens
   (C) Swallowed topical steroid for 8 weeks
   (D) Esophageal dilation

4. True or false: If a barium esophagram is suggestive of achalasia and the patient is able to maintain their weight and control their symptoms with lifestyle modification, no further evaluation is required.

   (A) True
   (B) False

5. A 64-year-old woman with a history of gastroesophageal reflux presents to her primary care clinic for evaluation of a 1-year history of episodic solid food dysphagia. She points to the xiphoid area where she feels the food getting "stuck." The sensation usually abates after taking a few drinks of water; however, she

occasionally has to regurgitate the food bolus. Following the episode, she is able to continue eating normally. She denies odynophagia, weight loss, nasal regurgitation, or cough. Which one of the following is the most likely cause of her dysphagia?

(A) Peptic stricture
(B) Eosinophilic esophagitis
(C) Achalasia
(D) Zenker's diverticulum

Key References

1. Levine MS, Rubesin SE, Laufer I. Barium esophagography: A study for all seasons. Clin Gastroenterol Hepatol. 2008;6:11–25. A superb review of the capabilities of radiography in the diagnosis of esophageal disorders by, arguably, the finest barium esophagography unit in the world.
2. Logeman JA. Swallowing disorders. Best Pract Res Clin Gastroenterol. 2008;21:563–73. A superb review of pathophysiology, diagnosis and treatment of oropharyngeal dysmotility disorders. It is a must read for all gastroenterologists.
3. Pandolfino JE, Fox MR, Bredenoord J, Kahrilas PJ. High-resolution manometry in clinical practice: utilizing pressure topography to classify oesophageal motility abnormalities. Neurogastroenterol Motil. 2009;21:796–806. A nice review of the use of a technology that will likely become the future "gold standard" for evaluating neuromuscular function of the LES and esophageal body.

Recommended Reading

Francis DL, Katzka DA. Achalasia: Update on the disease and its treatment. Gastroenterology. 2010;139:369–74.
Liacouras CA, Furuta GT, Hirano I, et al. Eosinophilic esophagitis: Updated consensus recommendations for children and adults. J Allergy Clin Immunol. 2011;128:3–20.
Mold JW, Reed LE, Davis AB, Allen ML, Decktor DL, Robinson M. Prevalence of gastroesophageal reflux in elderly patients in a primary care setting. Am J Gastroenterol. 1991;86:965–70.
Siersema PD, de Wijkerslooth LR. Dilation of refractory benign esophageal strictures. Gastrointest Endosc. 2009;70:1000–12.

Chapter 3
Noncardiac Chest Pain

Sami R. Achem

Case Study

A 43-year-old woman, previously healthy except for mild hypertension, presents for the evaluation of chest pain. She reports a 9-month history of intermittent episodes of midline/substernal chest pressure with radiation to the left arm. The pain typically lasts 30–40 min, is unrelated to exercise, but may be worsened by stress. She denies any other symptoms. One week prior to her consultation, she was admitted to the hospital for an episode of severe chest pain that led to a cardiac catheterization that was normal. Her physical examination is unremarkable. Chest pain cannot be reproduced by palpating the chest wall. A chest X-ray, abdominal ultrasound, barium swallow, and upper endoscopy were subsequently performed and were unremarkable. Laboratory studies including complete blood count, liver chemistries, amylase, and lipase were also normal.

Introduction

Noncardiac chest pain (NCCP) may be defined as recurrent episodes of angina-like pain without evidence of either functional or obstructive coronary artery disease. The Rome III diagnostic criteria for functional chest pain are summarized in Table 3.1. NCCP represents a diagnostic challenge since the chest pain is often indistinguishable from ischemic heart disease.

NCCP is a major source of healthcare expenditure and disability. Recent data indicate that 5.5 million patients visited emergency departments in the United

S.R. Achem, M.D., FACG, FAGA, FASGE (✉)
Division of Gastroenterology and Hepatology, Mayo Clinic, Jacksonville, FL, USA
e-mail: Achem.Sami@Mayo.edu

B.E. Lacy et al. (eds.), *Functional and Motility Disorders of the Gastrointestinal Tract*, DOI 10.1007/978-1-4939-1498-2_3

Table 3.1 Rome III criteria: functional chest pain of presumed esophageal origin

Midline chest pain or discomfort that is not burning in quality
Absent evidence that GERD is the cause of the symptom
Absence of histopathology-based esophageal motility disorders
Criteria fulfilled for at least 3 months with symptom onset at least 6 months prior to diagnosis

States with the chief complaint of chest pain during 2007–2008. Chest pain is the second most common cause for emergency room visits after abdominal pain. NCCP is one of the most frequent causes of hospital admission in the Western world. In England and Wales, acute chest pain is responsible for approximately 700,000 patient visits annually at emergency departments and 20–30 % of emergency medical admissions.

A recent study of elective coronary angiograms performed in the United States found that as many as 44 % of patients with atypical chest pain and 27 % of those with angina-like pain had no evidence of obstructive coronary artery disease. Extrapolating these data to current US demographics, an estimated 90 million patients may suffer from NCCP.

The evaluation of chest pain is expensive and varies considerably depending on the geographic location. For instance, according to a recent report, being hospitalized for chest pain costs an average of $2,459 when treated at Lake Whitney Medical Center in Whitney, Texas, but $81,083 at Bayonne Hospital Center in Bayonne, New Jersey. These costs do not reflect additional expenditures such as work loss, wages, and other indirect costs. Patients with NCCP in the United States lose an average of 13 days of work yearly. An Australian study reported work-related absenteeism rates of 29 % and interruptions to daily activities in 63 % of patients. Thus, by all accounts patients with chest pain represent a very common medical condition, a major diagnostic challenge, and a major source of healthcare expenditure and disability.

Epidemiology

Population-based studies indicate that in the United States, an estimated 23 % of the population suffer from NCCP. Studies from other nations (e.g., Australia, Spain, Argentina, and China) also describe a high prevalence ranging from 8 to 33 %. The prevalence of chest pain seems to be equal between genders and appears to decrease with aging. Women under 25 years of age and men and women between 45 and 55 years of age have the highest prevalence rates of NCCP. Compared to patients with ischemic heart disease, those with NCCP tend to consume more alcohol and tobacco and have higher degrees of anxiety.

Pathophysiology

The pathophysiology of NCCP is complex and incompletely understood. Several mechanisms have been identified as possible sources of the pain, including gastroesophageal reflux (GER), esophageal dysmotility, visceral hyperalgesia, abnormal biomechanical properties of the esophageal wall, sustained esophageal contractions, abnormal cerebral processing of visceral stimulation, disrupted autonomic activity, and psychiatric illness. GERD is the most common cause of NCCP.

Gastroesophageal Reflux Disease

Evidence supporting the role of GERD in NCCP comes from several sources. NCCP is more common in patients who experience heartburn weekly as opposed to those having heartburn less than once a week. Ambulatory pH testing in large numbers of patients with NCCP reveals that approximately 50 % have abnormal reflux. More convincingly, therapeutic trials aimed at acid inhibition have shown approximately an 80 % response to proton pump inhibitors (PPIs).

Esophageal Motility Disorders

Esophageal motility disorders were previously considered the most common cause of NCCP. With the advent of ambulatory pH testing in the 1980s, it became apparent that GERD is a more common cause of NCCP than abnormal esophageal motility. Indeed, only about 30 % of patients with non-GERD-related NCCP have esophageal dysmotility. Furthermore, in those patients with abnormal esophageal motility, a spectrum of esophageal motility disorders can be observed including esophageal spasm (now termed "distal" esophageal spasm to emphasize the distal location of abnormal motility findings), nutcracker esophagus, hypertensive lower esophageal sphincter (LES), nonspecific motility disorders (now described mostly as "ineffective motility"), and, rarely, achalasia. The recent introduction of high-resolution esophageal manometry has uncovered other motility disorders such as "jackhammer esophagus" that may be seen in patients with NCCP. Despite the recognition that some patients with NCCP have abnormal esophageal motility, it has been difficult to prove that these disorders cause NCCP. Many patients have abnormal motility, yet, at the time of testing, they do not experience chest pain. In addition, therapeutic trials aimed at reducing or normalizing the spastic motility have not resulted in consistent improvement of chest pain. These observations have led investigators to consider that these motility abnormalities represent a "marker" associated with NCCP, but not the cause.

Sustained Esophageal Contractions

Using high-frequency intraluminal ultrasonography (a research tool that allows for evaluation of smooth muscle esophageal contractions), investigators have identified a unique pattern of esophageal muscle contractions in patients with NCCP termed "sustained esophageal contractions." These esophageal muscle contractions appear to arise from the longitudinal muscle layer. As such, they are not detectable by conventional esophageal motility which measures circular esophageal muscle contraction primarily. These contractions occur either spontaneously or can be induced by edrophonium and generally precede episodes of chest pain. Interestingly, while the duration of swallow-induced contractions lasts about 6.4 s, those associated with chest pain last 68 s. Shorter duration of contractions is also more commonly linked to heartburn. Further studies, particularly therapeutic trials, are needed to determine whether the correction of this contractile pattern results in symptom improvement.

Visceral Hypersensitivity

Visceral hypersensitivity has been repeatedly demonstrated using various techniques in NCCP. Using intra-esophageal balloon distension, NCCP patients perceive chest pain at lower volumes of esophageal balloon distension compared to healthy controls. Perceptual responses to intraluminal esophageal balloon distension using an electronic barostat showed that, when compared with saline, acid perfusion reduces the perception threshold (innocuous sensation) and tended to reduce the pain threshold (aversive sensation). This study demonstrated short-term sensitization of mechanosensitive afferent pathways by transient exposure to acid and led the investigators to suggest that in NCCP, acid reflux induces sensitization of the esophagus, which may subsequently alter the way the esophagus perceives otherwise normal esophageal distention. Patients with NCCP also experience visceral hypersensitivity to an innocuous stimulus in normal tissue proximal to a site of injury (allodynia) as well as in the somatic area (chest wall). These findings suggest that in NCCP there are both visceral hypersensitivity and amplified secondary allodynia. Recent studies have shown that in patients with GERD-related NCCP, there is a lower esophageal threshold for chest pain than controls and that PPI therapy reduces this hypersensitivity. It is likely that the visceral (esophageal) hypersensitivity noted in patients with NCCP may be triggered by noxious stimulus, such as acid, bile, or the release of local irritants or neuropeptides. These agents in turn stimulate afferent sensory visceral nerves whose impulses travel to the spinal cord via sensory neurons into the sensory cerebral cortex. A better understanding of the origin of esophageal pain, putative neurotransmitters, neurosensory transmission, and perception will lead to more selective pharmacologic intervention in the management of NCCP.

Disturbed Central Processing

Other investigations have identified a number of differences in central nervous processing of esophageal stimuli between NCCP patients and controls suggesting that the perception of chest pain in patients is unique and may be modulated at the central level. Again, these observations open new avenues for future treatment interventions capable of altering central perception of pain.

Psychological Abnormalities

Psychological disorders have been reported in 17–43 %, and as high as 75 % of patients, in some studies of NCCP. The most common disorders observed in NCCP include anxiety, panic disorders, depression, neuroticism, and hypochondriac behavior. When NCCP patients are compared to coronary artery disease controls, the prevalence of psychological disorders is not uniformly higher in NCCP. The high association between psychological disorders and NCCP raises several questions: which came first, the psychological problem or chest pain, and how does the psychological disorder influence NCCP and vice versa?

Natural History

A main concern for patients with NCCP is whether the diagnostic label of NCCP confers these patients a good prognosis. Will their chest pain resolve over time? Will long-term follow-up reveal diagnostic pitfalls? A number of studies of variable sample size and design have examined the natural history of NCCP. For the most part, the available data indicate that overall mortality is low and, specifically, deaths from coronary artery disease are rare. One study of 176 patients with an initial negative coronary angiogram followed for a mean period of 12.8 years reported an incidence of coronary events of 8 % (0.65 %/year) after an average of 9.3 years (median 9.2). Patients with a coronary event had significantly more coronary risk factors (hypercholesterolemia, hypertension, cigarette smoking, diabetes type II) than did those without an event (average 2.4/patient vs. 1.3/patient, $p<0.01$).

Most patients with NCCP (between 67 and 74 %, depending on the studies) continue to experience recurrent chest pain, debilitating symptoms, impaired functional status, chronic use of a variety of medications (e.g., GI, cardiac, and psychiatric), repeated admissions to the hospital, and repeated cardiac and noncardiac diagnostic testing. Additional contemporary studies are required to better understand the longitudinal course of these patients, especially in the current era of PPI therapy and high-resolution manometry.

Diagnosis

Exclude Cardiac and Other Non-esophageal Sources of Pain

An important priority in the initial approach to the patient with chest pain is to ensure that life-threatening conditions such as coronary artery disease and other cardiac causes of chest pain are excluded. This typically requires cardiac consultation and objective testing. Once this has been done, it is also important that other non-esophageal sources of pain are excluded. The differential diagnosis of chest pain is broad (see Table 3.2). Thus, a careful history and physical exam are imperative to secure an accurate diagnosis. Once cardiac, pericardial, vascular, pulmonary, gastrointestinal, and musculoskeletal sources of chest pain have been excluded, esophageal sources must be considered.

Consider GERD

Since GERD is the most common esophageal cause of NCCP, the initial diagnostic approach should include an evaluation of this condition. Evaluation may include an ambulatory esophageal pH study (using either a conventional transnasal catheter or a catheter-free system) or an "empirical PPI trial." A cost-effective approach involves an empirical course of a high-dose PPI trial, equivalent to omeprazole

Table 3.2 Differential diagnosis of noncardiac chest pain

Cardiac/vascular
– Angina, myocardial infarction – Syndrome X – Pericardial disease – Thoracic aortic aneurysm – Thoracic outlet syndrome
Pulmonary
– Pulmonary embolism/infarct – Pleurisy/pleural effusion – Pneumonia – Lung neoplasms
Musculoskeletal
– Tietze syndrome – Pectoral muscle syndromes – Cervical spine disorders
Gastrointestinal
– Boerhaave syndrome (rare) – Esophageal and gastric neoplasm (rare) – Peptic ulcer – Cholecystitis – Pancreatitis, pancreatic pseudocysts (uncommon)

40 mg taken 30 min before breakfast and 20 mg before dinner for 8–10 days. A positive response to this treatment trial suggests that GERD may be the source of pain and the patient can then be offered a reduced dose of PPI twice daily (30 min before breakfast and dinner) for an additional 8 weeks. After 8 weeks, the patient may be gradually weaned from the double dose PPI to a single dose with a future visit planned to assess whether the medication can eventually be discontinued. If the patient fails to respond to a high-dose PPI trial or initial pH testing is negative, then GERD is likely not the source of chest pain and additional testing should be considered.

Additional Testing

Barium Swallow

A barium swallow has modest diagnostic sensitivity in patients with NCCP, but in patients complaining of additional symptoms like dysphagia, it may help detect features of achalasia, a "corkscrew" appearance suggestive of esophageal spasm, or structural esophageal disorders (e.g., tumors, extrinsic compression) that may occasionally present with chest pain.

Esophagogastroduodenoscopy

Upper endoscopy is useful to recognize mucosal abnormalities such as benign or malignant tumors, ulcerations, or strictures. The diagnostic yield of esophagogastroduodenoscopy (EGD) in NCCP is approximately 29 %. Most findings tend to be GERD related (e.g., hiatal hernia, erosive esophagitis, Barrett's esophagus). Esophageal tumors are rarely found, but must be excluded, especially in patients >45 years of age and those with dysphagia, unexplained anemia, and/or weight loss.

Esophageal Manometry

Esophageal motility testing with either conventional (solid state or water perfused) or, ideally, high-resolution manometry should be considered. The most important diagnosis to exclude is achalasia since recognition of this condition requires specific therapy. Although the typical symptom presentation of achalasia is dysphagia, approximately 15 % of patients may present with chest pain. Other esophageal motility disorders can also be recognized by esophageal manometry (see Table 3.3) although the relationship between these disorders and chest pain remains to be fully established.

Table 3.3 Esophageal motility disorders associated with NCCP

Distal esophageal spasm (DES)
Nutcracker esophagus (NE)
"Jackhammer esophagus"
Hypertensive lower esophageal sphincter (HLES)
Hypotensive lower esophageal sphincter
Achalasia
Nonspecific esophageal motility disorders/ineffective body motility

Provocative Testing

A number of pharmacologic tests have been developed in an attempt to elicit chest pain including the acid perfusion test (Bernstein test) and stimulation tests using edrophonium, bethanechol, ergonovine, and pentagastrin. Unfortunately, these tests add additional time and cost to the esophageal motility study and provide a low diagnostic yield (approximately 30 % reproduction of chest pain). More importantly, the information gained from a positive test has not been shown to change the therapeutic approach or facilitate the selection of a specific treatment program.

Esophageal balloon distension may also be used as provocative test. A recent study suggested that it may reveal the source of chest pain in 86 % of patients with NCCP, 42 % of whom may actually have GERD. This is useful information; however, the lack of standardization of the test and the invasive nature has tempered the popularity of this study. Future studies should be done to address these concerns.

Treatment

GERD-Related NCCP

As mentioned, GERD is the most common cause of NCCP. Thus, for patients with GERD documented by an abnormal pH test or for those who respond to an initial high-dose PPI therapy for 8–10 days, a double dose PPI course for 8 additional weeks has been shown effective in reducing chest pain in approximately 80 % of the patients. Patients should be advised to take PPIs 30 min before breakfast and dinner for better pharmacologic efficacy instead of single daily dose, although published comparative trials are lacking. There is also no published guidelines or data regarding therapy beyond 8 weeks in this setting. Thus, the author's personal approach is to attempt to gradually wean patients from PPI over the ensuing weeks in an attempt to reduce or discontinue therapy if there is no chest pain recurrence. However, this approach has not been critically appraised.

Non-GERD-Related NCCP

For patients without GERD or evidence of achalasia, visceral pain modulation therapy and cognitive behavioral therapy are appropriate options.

Visceral Pain Modulation

Visceral pain modulation with low-dose antidepressant therapy has been shown to be effective in pain perception. Several agents have been evaluated for the treatment of NCCP (see Table 3.4). Tricyclic antidepressants and/or serotonin regulators have been found to have beneficial effects in several studies when comparing these medications to placebo, although treatment trial duration, sample size, dose of medication, and outcome have been variable. The suggested approach is to use a medication with the best side effect profile and start at a low dose, such as an equivalent of 10 mg at bedtime of nortriptyline. The dose can be gradually increased by 10 mg every 7–10 days to reach approximately 40–50 mg depending upon tolerance and effectiveness. Patients should be told not to expect an immediate response since the

Table 3.4 Visceral analgesic therapy in NCCP

Medication	Suggested starting dose	Maximum suggested dose[a]	Possible side effects[c]
Tricyclics			
Trazodone	10 mg HS	150 mg HS	Priapism, anticholinergic, dizziness, drowsiness, fatigue
Imipramine	10 mg HS	50–75 mg HS	Anticholinergic/Q-T prolongation
Nortriptyline[b]	10 mg HS	50–75 mg HS	Anticholinergic, drowsiness, fatigue
Serotonin modulators SSRIs			
Sertraline	10 mg HS	50–200 mg HS	Restlessness, nausea, decreased libido, and delayed ejaculation
Paroxetine	10 mg HS	30–50 mg HS	Headache, somnolence, insomnia, dry mouth, nausea, constipation, joint/muscle pain, pharyngitis, rhinitis, and abnormal ejaculation
Fluoxetine	10 mg HS	20 mg HS	Diarrhea, nausea, indigestion, anorexia, xerostomia, asthenia, insomnia, anxiety, pharyngitis, rhinitis, influenza-like symptoms
Serotonin and noradrenaline modulators, SSNRI			
Venlafaxine	10 mg HS	75 mg HS	Sleep disturbance, nausea, dizziness, loss of appetite, fatigue, and constipation

[a]Suggested dose originates from original publication. However, critical dose response studies need to be done since individual responses may vary

[b]No comparative placebo-controlled publications are available with nortriptyline

[c]Most side effects were "tolerated" and rarely resulted in drug discontinuation

medication may take a few days to reach steady blood levels. Potential side effects should also be reviewed as well as the presumed mechanism of action of these compounds since patients may erroneously believe they are being treated for depression rather than visceral analgesia.

Cognitive Behavioral Therapy

Psychological disorders are common in NCCP. Nine controlled studies have shown that when compared to a "waiting list of control patients," cognitive behavioral therapy and pain coping skills afford significant improvement. Although the study design, sample size, and outcomes are variable, studies have reported improvement in chest pain scores and decrease in anxiety and depression scales. There is a need for trained therapists to make this valuable therapeutic program more widely available.

Smooth Muscle Relaxants

For patients with non-GERD, non-achalasia NCCP with documented spastic esophageal motility disorders, smooth muscle relaxants such as nitrates, anticholinergic agents, and calcium blockers may be used. Unfortunately, therapeutic trials with these compounds are limited to mostly open-label studies of small sample size. Nevertheless, clinical observation suggests that a proportion of NCCP patients may respond to this approach.

There is also limited favorable available experience with selective inhibitors of cyclic guanosine monophosphate (cGMP)-specific phosphodiesterase-5 (PDE-5) such as sildenafil and other related compounds. These agents potentiate nitric oxide and induce esophageal smooth muscle relaxation. Large placebo-controlled trials are still needed to confirm the utility of this approach.

Distal esophageal botulinum toxin injection has been used in several open-label studies with an approximately 72 % response rate. Relapse is common, however, and repeat injections maybe required. A most recent study from Belgium in 22 patients with distal esophageal spasm and/or nutcracker esophagus compared botulinum toxin to placebo. Patients received injections of botulinum toxin or saline in 4 quadrants at 2 and 7 cm above the esophagogastric junction. After 1 month, patients crossed over between groups and received additional endoscopic injections. Botulinum toxin was found to induce significantly more clinical improvement (chest pain and dysphagia) than placebo. Larger controlled trials are required as are long-term outcome follow-up studies.

Other Therapies

Newer treatment strategies are being investigated. Favorable initial results have been found with adenosine antagonists, and two small studies using hypnosis and complementary and alternative medicine showed beneficial outcomes. Larger studies using these strategies are eagerly awaited.

Case Resolution

The patient was initially treated with nortriptyline starting at 10 mg at bedtime. The dose was gradually increased over 4 weeks to 40 mg p.o. at bedtime at which point she reported improvement. She has remained chest pain-free during a 9-month follow-up period.

Key Teaching Points

- NCCP is a common, recurrent, debilitating, and expensive condition.
- Prior to establishing the diagnosis of NCCP, several other disorders must be excluded, especially cardiac disease and other life-threatening disorders.
- The pathogenesis of NCCP is incompletely understood and probably multifactorial.
- GERD is the most common mechanism involved in NCCP, and PPI therapy results in significant improvement in approximately 80 % of NCCP patients.
- The esophageal diagnostic evaluation, after excluding cardiac and non-esophageal sources of pain, is typically aimed first at determining if GERD is present via an empirical trial of high-dose PPI for 8–10 days or ambulatory esophageal pH testing.
- For non-GERD-related NCCP, exclusion of treatable conditions such as achalasia with high-resolution esophageal manometry is important.
- Once achalasia is excluded in the patient with non-GERD-related NCCP, treatment with visceral analgesics and/or cognitive behavioral therapy should be considered.
- In patients with NCCP and a spastic motility disorder without GERD, limited available information suggests that smooth muscle relaxants and botulinum toxin injection into the distal esophagus should be considered.

Teaching Questions

1. After reviewing the case study presentation, which one of the following would you recommend as the initial therapy or test?

   (A) Reassurance
   (B) Esophageal manometry
   (C) Nitrates
   (D) High-dose proton pump inhibitor trial for 8–10 days

2. This patient was treated with omeprazole 20 mg 30 min before breakfast and dinner for 8 weeks without significant chest pain improvement. At this time, which one of the following would you recommend?

   (A) Switch to another PPI
   (B) Esophageal pH testing while off acid suppressive medication
   (C) High-resolution esophageal manometry
   (D) Botulinum toxin injection into the distal esophagus

3. A high-resolution esophageal motility test is completely normal. The patient continues to experience recurrent chest pain. Which one of the following would you suggest next?

   (A) Psychiatric referral
   (B) Calcium blockers
   (C) Hypnosis
   (D) Visceral analgesic therapy

Key References

1. Achem SR. Noncardiac chest pain-treatment approaches. Gastroenterol Clin North Am. 2008;37:859–78. Comprehensive review of available therapeutic options.
2. Fass R, Achem SR. Noncardiac chest pain: Diagnostic evaluation. Dis Esophagus. 2012;25: 89–101. Informative review of diagnostic tests available to the practicing clinician to assess patients with NCCP.
3. Fass R, Achem SR. Noncardiac chest pain: epidemiology, natural course and pathogenesis. J Neurogastroenterol Motil. 2011;17:110–23. Comprehensive review of available literature coving NCCP epidemiology, natural history, and pathogenesis.
4. Fass R, Hyun JG, Sewel JL, et al. Pathophysiology of noncardiac chest pain. In: Fass R, Eslick G, editors. Noncardiac chest pain: A growing problem. San Diego, CA: Plural Publishing; 2007. p. 29–37. Excellent comprehensive book covering most important areas of NCCP.
5. Hershcovici T, Achem SR, Jha LK, Fass R. Systematic review: The treatment of noncardiac chest pain. Aliment Pharmacol Ther. 2012;35:5–14. An excellent systematic review of the currently available therapeutic options for NCCP.
6. Nguyen TM, Eslick GD. Systematic review: The treatment of noncardiac chest pain with antidepressants. Aliment Pharmacol Ther. 2012;35:493–500. Critical review of visceral analgesics for NCCP.
7. Wang W, Sun YH, Wang YY, Wang YT, Wang W, Li YQ, Wu SX. Treatment of functional chest pain with antidepressants: A meta-analysis. Pain Physician. 2012;15:E131–42. Well done study on available therapies.

Chapter 4
Gastroesophageal Reflux Disease

Dawn Francis and Raul Badillo

Case Study

A 38-year-old overweight male with obstructive sleep apnea, systemic hypertension, and impaired fasting glucose presents to his internist for evaluation of heartburn. For the past 10 years, he has suffered from retrosternal chest burning and acid regurgitation into the back of his throat. He has managed his reflux symptoms with as-needed antacids but more recently began taking an over-the-counter proton pump inhibitor (PPI) daily, which has resulted in better control of his symptoms. Given the chronicity of his symptoms and partial response to therapy, his internist referred him to a gastroenterologist for further evaluation. An upper endoscopy is performed and reveals Los Angeles classification Grade C esophagitis with no evidence of Barrett's esophagus. The patient is concerned about the possibility of lifelong need for medical therapy and requests a surgical consultation to discuss anti-reflux surgery. He is placed on a twice daily PPI with instructions on proper use and referred to a surgeon. By the time of his consultation, he has been on a twice daily PPI for 8 weeks with modest improvement in symptoms. After discussing with the surgeon his ongoing reflux symptoms in the setting of LA Grade C esophagitis and morbid obesity, his surgeon recommends proceeding with bariatric surgery in the form of a laparoscopic Roux-en-Y gastric bypass.

D. Francis, M.D., M.H.S. (✉)
Division of Gastroenterology and Hepatology, Mayo Clinic Florida, Jacksonville, FL, USA
e-mail: Francis.Dawn@mayo.edu

R. Badillo, M.D.
Division of Gastroenterology, Mayo Clinic Florida, Jacksonville, FL, USA

B.E. Lacy et al. (eds.), *Functional and Motility Disorders of the Gastrointestinal Tract*, DOI 10.1007/978-1-4939-1498-2_4

Introduction

Gastroesophageal reflux disease (GERD) is one of the most common diseases encountered by both primary care physicians and gastroenterologists. GERD is defined as a condition that develops when the reflux of stomach contents causes troublesome symptoms and/or complications. Generally speaking, the term GERD is applied to patients with symptoms suggestive of reflux such as heartburn or regurgitation, whereas reflux esophagitis describes a subgroup of patients with symptoms of GERD who also have endoscopic or histologic evidence of esophageal inflammation (see Table 4.1).

GERD can manifest in a wide array of symptoms. Typical symptoms include heartburn (retrosternal burning) and acid regurgitation (feeling of acidic gastric contents reaching the pharynx). Atypical symptoms such as epigastric fullness or pressure, epigastric pain, nausea, bloating, and belching may be indicative of GERD but may overlap with other conditions in the differential diagnosis such as peptic ulcer disease, achalasia, gastritis, dyspepsia, and gastroparesis (see Table 4.2). Lastly, there are a variety of extraesophageal symptoms that have been attributed to GERD including cough, wheezing, hoarseness, and sore throat; however, these are not specific to GERD. In general, symptoms tend to be more common after meals and while lying in the right lateral decubitus position.

Table 4.1 Definitions

Condition	Definition
Gastroesophageal reflux disease	A condition that develops when the reflux of stomach contents causes troublesome symptoms and/or complications
Reflux esophagitis	Symptoms of gastroesophageal reflux disease with endoscopic or histopathologic evidence of esophageal inflammation
Functional heartburn	According to Rome III diagnostic criteria, a burning retrosternal discomfort or pain + absence of evidence that gastroesophageal acid reflux is the cause of the symptoms + absence of histopathology-based esophageal motility disorders with criteria fulfilled for the last 3 months with symptom onset at least 6 months prior to diagnosis

Table 4.2 Differential diagnosis for GERD

• Peptic ulcer disease
• Non-ulcer dyspepsia
• Esophageal motor disorders
• Infectious esophagitis
• Pill esophagitis
• Eosinophilic esophagitis
• Cardiac disease
• Biliary tract disease
• Esophageal cancer

The socioeconomic burden of GERD is considerable. From a health economic standpoint, the high prevalence of GERD combined with the cost of acid-lowering medications results in high healthcare costs. Furthermore, it is associated with a dramatic impact on quality of life. Several studies have demonstrated that health-related quality of life in reflux disease patients is significantly impaired in comparison to the general population. A recent systematic review concluded that patients with persistent reflux symptoms despite PPI therapy have clinically relevant impairments in physical and mental well-being that are comparable to those of untreated patients with GERD.

Epidemiology

Epidemiologic estimates of the prevalence of GERD are based primarily on the typical symptoms of heartburn and regurgitation. This approach introduces certain limitations to the actual prevalence calculation because there are patients with endoscopic evidence of GERD (e.g., esophagitis or Barrett's esophagus) who do not present with heartburn or regurgitation. Furthermore, there are patients with these symptoms who do not have GERD.

Symptoms suggestive of GERD are common and become even more common with advancing age. In 2005, a systematic review found the prevalence of GERD to be 10–20 %, defined by at least weekly heartburn and/or acid regurgitation in the Western world, while in Asia it was lower, at less than 5 %. The incidence in the Western world was approximately 5 per 1,000 person-years, which appears low relative to the prevalence but is consistent with the disease's chronicity.

Without treatment, this prevalent disease can result in numerous esophageal complications including erosive esophagitis, peptic stricture, Barrett's esophagus, and esophageal adenocarcinoma. Complications of GERD are thought to be more common in males, Caucasians, and persons of advancing age. Of those with classical GERD symptoms who undergo an endoscopy, approximately one-third have erosive esophagitis, 10 % have benign strictures, and up to 20 % have Barrett's esophagus. Fortunately, only an extremely small number are found to have esophageal adenocarcinoma.

Pathophysiology

The principal event in the pathogenesis of GERD is movement of gastric contents from the stomach into the esophagus. Normally, there are several mechanical barriers and mechanisms in place to prevent this potential insult to the esophageal lining.

The key barrier to reflux is the lower esophageal sphincter (LES), a segment of tonically contracted smooth muscle at the distal esophagus. The LES relaxes with swallowing and also with gastric distension, allowing for venting of air. The LES may also relax at times not associated with swallowing; these relaxations are termed transient lower esophageal sphincter relaxations (tLESRs) and are of longer duration than swallow-related LES relaxation. In patients with GERD, tLESRs allow for venting of gastric liquid contents instead of air alone, resulting in acid reflux. An increased frequency of tLESRs is considered to be the major mechanism in most GERD patients, and this appears to be even more common in obese patients, although why this occurs is not completely understood.

Another mechanism that can render the gastroesophageal junction incompetent is a hypotensive lower esophageal sphincter. Although only a minority of patients with GERD have a grossly hypotensive LES, there are multiple factors that result in a reduction of LES pressure. These include gastric distension; certain foods such as fat, chocolate, caffeine, and alcohol; smoking; and a multitude of medications including calcium channel blockers, nitrates, and albuterol.

A third mechanism is the presence of a hiatal hernia. There are two primary ways a hiatal hernia may lead to GERD. The first relates to the loss of the crural diaphragm and the augmentation it normally provides the LES. The second occurs via a lowering of the threshold for eliciting tLESRs in response to gastric distension.

Other important mechanisms to consider that normally protect the esophageal mucosa from acid reflux include intrinsic mucosal factors (e.g., surface mucous and bicarbonate, stratified squamous epithelium, intercellular tight junctions, blood flow), esophageal peristalsis, and neutralization of the residual acid by bicarbonate-rich saliva. Any defect in these mechanisms including esophageal dysmotility or decreased salivary flow can lead to GERD.

With respect to extraesophageal symptoms, the mechanism likely involves direct aspiration with damage to the respiratory mucosa and/or a vagally mediated reflex triggered by pathologic acid reflux of the distal esophageal mucosa.

Diagnosis and Evaluation

A diagnosis of GERD is made using some combination of patient symptomatology, objective testing with endoscopy and/or ambulatory esophageal pH monitoring, and response to antisecretory therapy (see Table 4.3). The symptoms of heartburn

Table 4.3 Diagnostic testing for gastroesophageal reflux disease

Diagnostic test	Indication
• Proton pump inhibitor trial	Classic symptoms without alarm symptoms
• Esophageal pH monitoring	Refractory GERD symptoms, preoperative evaluation, GERD diagnosis in question
• Upper endoscopy	Noncardiac chest pain, alarm symptoms
• Barium radiographs	Evaluation of dysphagia, otherwise not a recommended test for GERD
• Esophageal manometry	Evaluation for a motility disorder prior to planned anti-reflux surgery, otherwise not a recommended test for GERD

and regurgitation are the most reliable for making a presumptive diagnosis based on history alone. It is neither necessary nor practical to perform a comprehensive evaluation in every patient with heartburn or regurgitation.

When GERD is suspected in those with typical symptoms and no alarm signs (see below), empiric medical therapy with a PPI is the recommended next step. A response can help support the diagnosis, although this is not a diagnostic criterion. There are some patients, however, who warrant further evaluation. Indications to proceed with further testing include: (1) confirming the diagnosis of GERD in those refractory to medical therapy, (2) assessing for complications of GERD, (3) assessing for alternative diagnoses, and (4) as part of a preoperative evaluation.

Upper endoscopy can aid in the diagnosis especially if evidence of erosive esophagitis, peptic strictures, or Barrett's esophagus is found. The majority of patients (approximately 70 %) with typical symptoms of GERD, however, will not have these findings. An upper endoscopy should always be considered in patients with alarm symptoms such as dysphagia, anemia, melena, or weight loss, in order to rule out complications from GERD such as a peptic stricture or an esophageal malignancy.

Ambulatory reflux monitoring is the only test that allows measurement of esophageal acid exposure, reflux episode frequency, and association between symptoms and reflux episodes (see Fig. 4.1). There are two types of ambulatory reflux monitoring, a telemetry capsule (aka wireless pH capsule) affixed to the distal esophagus or a transnasal catheter-based pH or combined impedance-pH probe. The telemetry capsule is typically applied during upper endoscopy to the mucosa of the lower esophagus and has the advantage of recording for 48 h (or even 96 h if necessary). Catheter-based monitoring will provide information during a 24-h period and with the addition of impedance testing allows for the detection of weakly acidic or non-acidic reflux. Both methods can be performed on or off medical therapy, and there is debate over which method is optimal.

Though commonly used, there are other tests that are not recommended routinely for the evaluation of GERD alone. For instance, a barium radiograph of the esophagus can be considered in the presence of dysphagia to evaluate for strictures or rings but otherwise is not recommended as a diagnostic test for reflux disease. Esophageal manometry is likewise not recommended as a sole diagnostic test for GERD as neither a decreased lower esophageal sphincter pressure nor the presence of a motility abnormality is specific of GERD. The primary role of esophageal manometry in the setting of GERD is to exclude the presence of achalasia or a scleroderma-like esophagus prior to an anti-reflux surgery, as these conditions are considered contraindications to such a procedure.

Treatment

The treatment of GERD includes lifestyle and diet modification, medical therapy, and, for a subset of properly selected patients, surgical therapy (see Table 4.4). A step-up or step-down approach may be used based on the severity of disease.

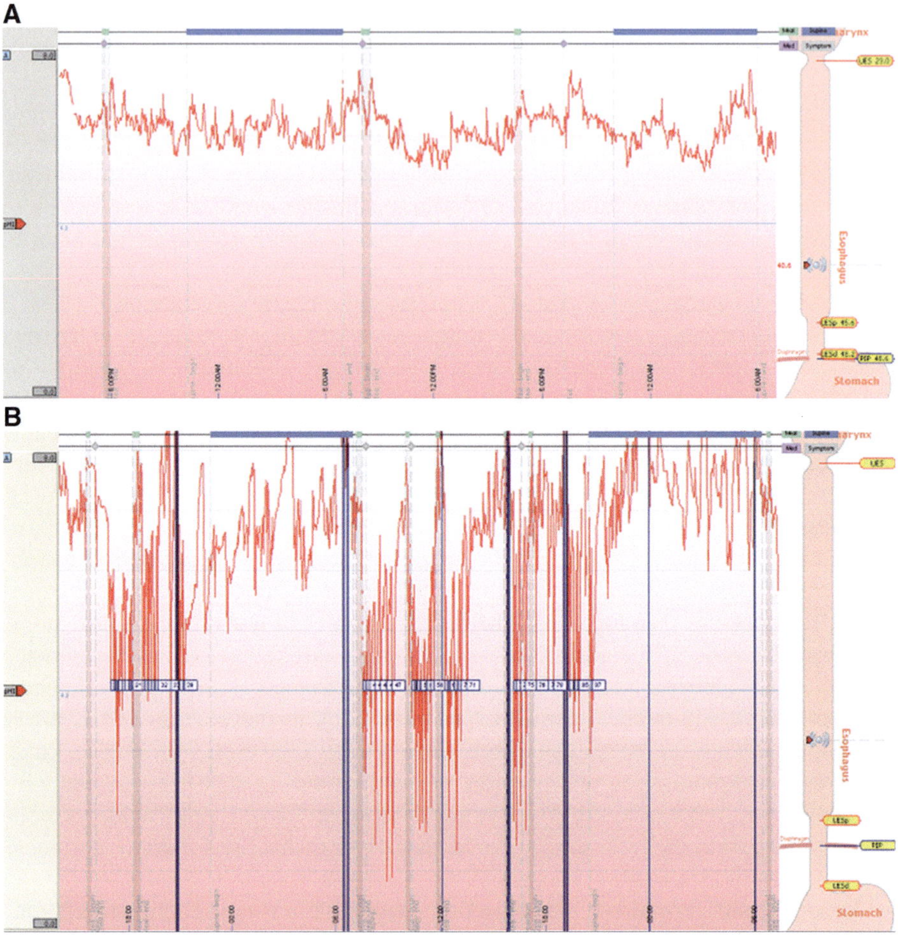

Fig. 4.1 Results of normal (A) and abnormal (B) ambulatory pH monitoring. An acid reflux episode is defined as an esophageal pH less than 4

Table 4.4 Treatment options for GERD

Therapy	Examples
Lifestyle modification	• Weight loss
	• Head of bed elevation
	• Avoidance of trigger foods
Medical therapy	• Antacids
	• Histamine 2 receptor antagonists
	• Proton pump inhibitors
Surgical therapy	• Nissen fundoplication
	• Sphincter augmentation
	• Bariatric surgery in morbidly obese
	• Endoscopic therapies (under investigation)

For example, a step-up approach starting with lifestyle modification and histamine type 2 receptor antagonists may be appropriate for a patient with mild symptoms and no evidence of erosive esophagitis on endoscopy. In contrast, a step-down approach starting with a PPI may be more appropriate for a patient with moderate to severe symptoms and erosive esophagitis.

Lifestyle and diet modification traditionally have included weight loss, head of bed elevation, avoidance of nighttime meals, and elimination of trigger foods such as chocolate, caffeine, and alcohol. A 2006 systematic review of 16 randomized trials that evaluated the impact of lifestyle measures on GERD concluded that only weight loss and elevation of the head of the bed improved esophageal pH and/or GERD symptoms.

The cornerstone of the medical treatment of GERD is acid suppression, which generally provides excellent healing of esophagitis and relief of symptoms. Histamine type 2 receptor blockers (H2RBs) act by blocking the histamine-induced stimulation of gastric parietal cells. They tend to provide a moderate benefit and are sometimes used to augment PPI therapy by giving the dose before bedtime to block nocturnal acid reflux. Unfortunately, tachyphylaxis is common and limits the long-term effectiveness of this approach. PPIs are more potent acid suppressors and result in faster healing of esophagitis and decreased relapse rates compared to H2RBs. They work by irreversibly inhibiting the H+-K+-ATPase pump, the final step in acid production. There are currently seven available PPIs with no proven clinically significant difference between them. It is essential, however, that providers take the time to discuss proper dosing of the PPI, which will allow for an optimal response. In this regard, PPI therapy should be initiated at once daily dosing and 30–60 min prior to breakfast. If only a partial response is obtained, twice daily dosing or, occasionally, switching to a different PPI may be required to further suppress GERD symptoms. Long-term maintenance therapy should be recommended for GERD patients who continue to have symptoms after discontinuation of PPI and in symptomatic patients with complications, including erosive esophagitis and Barrett's esophagus. In contrast, some studies have demonstrated that those with non-erosive esophageal reflux disease and otherwise noncomplicated GERD can be managed successfully with as-needed PPI therapy, despite lack of pharmacokinetic support for this regimen.

Finally, there are those patients with GERD-like symptoms that fail to respond to optimal medical therapy. It is important to further evaluate this group of patients with the goal of differentiating those patients with persistent acid reflux despite PPI from those with non-GERD etiologies (see Fig. 4.2). The first step is to ensure optimal PPI dosing and compliance. After this, it is reasonable to increase dosing to twice daily or switch to an alternative PPI. If symptoms persist, an upper endoscopy should be performed to rule out other non-GERD etiologies for the symptoms. If endoscopy is negative, the patient should be further evaluated with pH monitoring (either a wireless capsule or a transnasal probe) to confirm the diagnosis of GERD. Confirmation via pH testing would indicate PPI failure and need for escalation of therapy, such as a trial of nighttime H2RB; a trial of the $GABA_b$ agonist, baclofen, which acts by decreasing tLESRs and thereby reflux episodes; or consideration of

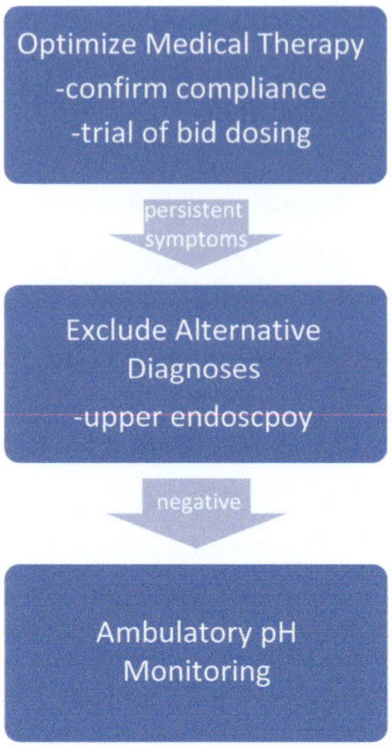

Fig. 4.2 Approach to the patient with typical GERD symptoms refractory to medical therapy. Ambulatory pH monitoring off medications should be performed when the diagnosis of GERD is in question

surgical options. Confirming the absence of GERD in a patient with typical heartburn symptoms would suggest a diagnosis of "functional heartburn."

Per Rome III criteria, all of the following must be met in order to make the diagnosis of functional heartburn: burning retrosternal discomfort or pain, absence of evidence that gastroesophageal acid reflux is the cause of the symptom, absence of histopathology-based esophageal motility disorders, and fulfillment of criteria for the last 3 months with symptom onset at least 6 months prior to diagnosis (Table 3.1). In these patients, it is reasonable to consider therapy with visceral analgesics, such as a tricyclic antidepressant, selective serotonin uptake inhibitor, or trazodone, as one theory for the cause of functional heartburn is esophageal hypersensitivity.

Surgical therapy is another treatment option for long-term therapy in patients with GERD. Before this is considered, objective documentation of gastroesophageal reflux via esophageal pH testing or endoscopy is mandatory as the highest surgical response is seen in those with typical symptoms who respond to a PPI or have abnormal pH testing with good symptom correlation. Response rates to surgical intervention are lower in those with atypical or extraesophageal symptoms.

According to the Society of American Gastrointestinal and Endoscopic Surgeons, once the diagnosis of GERD is objectively confirmed, surgical therapy should be considered in certain individuals. These include patients who have failed medical management (inadequate symptom control or medication side effects), patients who opt for surgery despite successful medical management (due to lifelong need for medications or expense of medications), patients who have complications of GERD (e.g., Barrett's esophagus or peptic stricture), and those patients who have extraesophageal manifestations (e.g., cough, aspiration, chest pain). A preoperative workup with the goal of selecting appropriate patients in order to optimize outcomes may include upper endoscopy, esophageal pH testing, esophageal manometry, barium swallow, and, in selected patients, a 4-h solid phase gastric emptying scan.

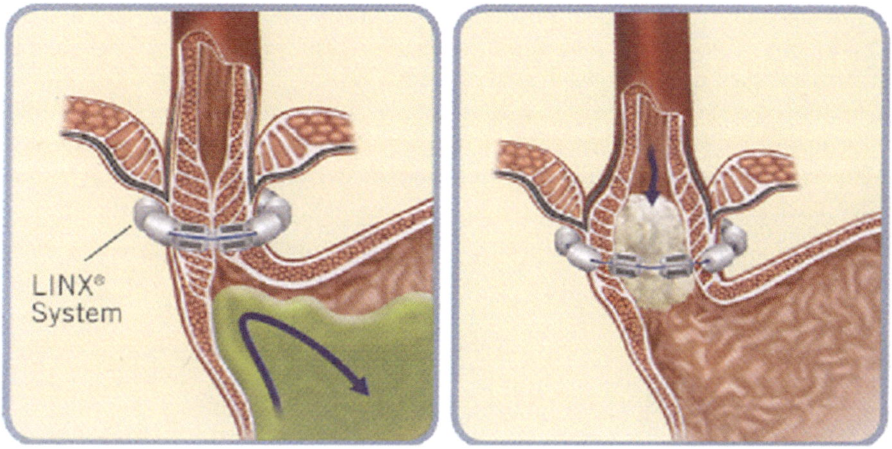

Fig. 4.3 Sphincter augmentation with the LINX system demonstrating both closed and open positions. Note how the system of magnetized titanium beads expands to accommodate a food bolus

The typical anti-reflux surgery is laparoscopic Nissen fundoplication; however, gastric bypass for the obese patient is the recommended treatment for GERD in the morbidly obese patient (body mass index [BMI] >35 kg/m^2) due to concerns over higher failure rates after Nissen fundoplication in this population. Finally, therapies such as sphincter augmentation with the LINX Reflux system, which entails laparoscopic placement of a bracelet of titanium beads with magnetic cores around the LES, are an option in some patients (see Fig. 4.3). This device is US Food and Drug Administration (FDA) approved and appears promising based on initial studies. Lastly, endoscopic therapies for GERD, including transoral incisionless fundoplication, have been developed but data on long-term efficacy is limited.

Case Resolution

Laparoscopic Roux-en-Y gastric bypass was performed. Twelve months following the surgery, he has lost substantial weight and no longer requires treatment for his sleep apnea, hypertension, or gastroesophageal reflux disease.

Key Clinical Teaching Points

- Empiric medical therapy is appropriate in those patients with typical GERD symptoms who have no alarm symptoms (e.g., dysphagia) and no symptoms suggestive of GERD-related complications.

- An ambulatory esophageal pH study (either catheter- or capsule-based) is the only way to objectively measure the degree of esophageal acid exposure and to correlate patient symptoms to acid reflux episodes.
- Before considering surgery, objective documentation of gastroesophageal reflux is mandatory as the highest surgical response is seen in those with typical symptoms who respond to PPI or have abnormal pH testing with good symptom correlation.

Teaching Questions

1. All of the following are associated with GERD, except:
   (A) Hiatal hernia
   (B) Scleroderma
   (C) Obesity
   (D) All are associated with GERD
2. The diagnosis of GERD can be made by clinical symptoms.
   (A) TRUE
   (B) FALSE
3. Which one of the following should be considered as the next step in a 59-year-old obese white male with a 15-year history of heartburn and intermittent solid dysphagia?
   (A) Lifestyle modification and H2R blocker
   (B) Upper endoscopy
   (C) Twice daily PPI
   (D) Esophageal manometry

Key References

1. Becher A, El-Serag H. Systematic review: The association between symptomatic response to proton pump inhibitors and health-related quality of life in patients with gastro-oesophageal reflux disease. Aliment Pharmacol Ther. 2011;34:618–27. A nice analysis of studies measuring improvement in quality of life for GERD patients treated with PPIs.
2. Dent J, El-Serag HB, Wallander MA, Johansson S. Epidemiology of gastro-oesophageal reflux disease: a systematic review. Gut. 2005;54:710–7. A summary of papers evaluating the incidence and prevalence of GERD in different populations.
3. Giannini EG, Zentilin P, Dulbecco P, Vigneri S, Scarlata P, Savarino V. Management strategy for patients with gastroesophageal reflux disease: A comparison between empirical treatment with esomeprazole and endoscopy-oriented treatment. Am J Gastroenterol. 2008;103:267–75. A well-written article comparing medical therapy to endoscopic therapy for the treatment of GERD.

4. Kaltenbach T, Crockett S, Gerson LB. Are lifestyle measures effective in patients with gastroesophageal reflux disease? An evidence-based approach. Arch Intern Med. 2006;166:965–71. This article reviews the evidence supporting lifestyle modification for treatment of GERD, a commonly discussed topic with patients.
5. Katz PO, Gerson LB, Vela MF. Guidelines for the diagnosis and management of gastroesophageal reflux disease. Am J Gastroenterol. 2013;108:308–28. These are the latest published guidelines for diagnosing and managing GERD.
6. Kahrilas PJ, Shaheen NJ, Vaezi MF, Hiltz SW, Black E, Modlin IM, et al. American Gastroenterological Association Medical Position Statement on the management of gastroesophageal reflux disease. Gastroenterology. 2008;135:1383–91. A state of the art review on the management of GERD by international experts in the field.
7. Vakil N, van Zanten SV, Kahrilas P, Dent J, Jones R, Global Consensus Group. The Montreal definition and classification of gastroesophageal reflux disease: A global evidence-based consensus. Am J Gastroenterol. 2006;101:1900–20. The consensus statement on defining GERD.

Part II
Gastroduodenal Disorders

Chapter 5
Aerophagia, Belching, and Rumination

Benjamin Stein and Brian E. Lacy

Case Study

A 62-year-old man is seen for evaluation of recurrent belching and burping. His symptoms started 1 year ago following an acute viral illness during which he experienced odynophagia, transient dysphagia, nausea, and vomiting. He was briefly hospitalized, supported with intravenous fluids, and treated empirically with antibiotics and an antiviral agent. Laboratory tests were normal, as were an abdominal X-ray and upper endoscopy. Viral cultures for Epstein–Barr virus, cytomegalovirus, and herpes simplex virus were also negative. All of his symptoms gradually resolved; however, when seen in follow-up, he reported a new symptom of frequent belching. He stated that some days he burped 75–100 times. Belching was typically absent in the morning upon awakening but progressed as the day went on. Physical examination was unremarkable. The patient was counseled to eat slower and to use over-the-counter simethicone as needed; however, he returned 4 weeks later with his wife who reported that he was constantly belching throughout the day. Interestingly, she also reported that he did not belch at night. No other gastrointestinal symptoms were present. The patient was treated empirically with a daily proton pump inhibitor. At follow-up 4 weeks later, his symptoms had not improved.

B. Stein, M.D., M.P.H. (✉)
Division of Gastroenterology and Hepatology, Dartmouth-Hitchcock Medical Center, Lebanon, NH, USA
e-mail: Benjamin.N.Stein@hitchcock.org

B.E. Lacy, M.D., Ph.D.
Division of Gastroenterology and Hepatology, Dartmouth-Hitchcock Medical Center, Lebanon, NH, USA

Geisel School of Medicine at Dartmouth, Lebanon, NH, USA

B.E. Lacy et al. (eds.), *Functional and Motility Disorders of the Gastrointestinal Tract*, DOI 10.1007/978-1-4939-1498-2_5

Introduction

The ingestion and expulsion of air are physiologically normal components of the digestive process. Belching or eructation is the process by which ingested air is expelled via the oropharynx. Aerophagia is a term derived from the Greek: *aer* meaning "air" and *phaegen* meaning "to swallow." In a clinical setting, aerophagia and excessive belching are only defined as pathologic if they have a significant negative impact on a patient's well-being. There is some discrepancy in the literature regarding the clinical "working" definition of aerophagia. Some authors define the term by symptoms related to excessive gastric and intestinal gas secondary to swallowed air. By Rome III criteria, both aerophagia and unspecified excessive belching are defined by the presence of excessive eructation with the distinction being that of objective air swallowing, which is present in aerophagia and not in unspecified belching. These disorders are typically diagnosed clinically and are treated with reassurance and behavioral modification.

Rumination is defined as recurrent effortless regurgitation of undigested food into the oropharynx. It is a normal part of digestion in animals with multi-compartment stomachs, a process commonly known as "chewing cud," but is considered abnormal in humans. Rumination was initially described in children and developmentally delayed adults, but it is now well recognized that this process may also occur in healthy adults. Similar to aerophobia and belching disorders, rumination is most often diagnosed clinically and treated with conservative measures.

Epidemiology

The incidence and prevalence of aerophagia, belching disorders, and rumination are not well defined. They are thought to be relatively rare, but it is likely that many patients do not seek medical attention and, when they do, may be misdiagnosed with other functional gastrointestinal disorders.

Pathophysiology

Belching or eructation is the audible, retrograde expulsion of air from the esophagus into the oropharynx. Normal physiological belching serves the function of preventing excessive accumulation of gas in the proximal gastrointestinal tract, which can result in bloating and excessive flatulence. Physiological belching typically occurs 25–30 times per day. The use of multichannel impedance monitoring has allowed for the classification of two distinct patterns of belching: gastric belching and supragastric belching.

Gastric belching is what we commonly think of as normal physiological eructation and involves the release of air from the stomach. Intragastric air accumulates following normal esophageal peristalsis and with the ingestion of air in food and drink, particularly carbonated beverages. The resultant proximal stomach distention activates a stretch-mediated vagal nerve reflex, leading to transient relaxation of the lower esophageal sphincter (TLESR) and reflux of gas in a mechanism similar to that seen in gastroesophageal reflux disease (GERD). This reflux leads to rapid distension in the lower esophagus triggering a reflex-mediated relaxation of the upper esophageal sphincter (UES), thereby allowing release of air into the oropharynx.

In contrast, supra-gastric belching occurs when air is ingested into the oropharynx and esophagus but does not enter the stomach and instead is rapidly expelled in a retrograde fashion. This pattern of belching is not thought to be a physiological reflex but rather a learned behavior whereby air influx occurs via a contraction of the diaphragm resulting in decreased intraesophageal pressure. The precipitant for the diaphragmatic contraction is not clear but may be related to visceral irritation such as that encountered during GERD. It should be noted that belching disorders are seen more commonly in patients with psychiatric comorbidities, and it has been demonstrated that distraction can reduce the frequency of belching; both of these observations support the hypothesis that this is primarily a behavioral disorder.

The pathophysiology of aerophagia appears to originate from excessive volitional air swallowing. Excessive bloating and distension are common symptoms of other gastrointestinal disorders such as irritable bowel syndrome, but excessive air swallowing can be demonstrated by impedance testing in patients with true aerophagia.

The physiological mechanism underlying rumination is not completely understood. The use of new technologies such as high-resolution manometry and intraluminal impedance has elucidated the process, however. During rumination events, there is a rise in intragastric pressure and a concomitant rise in pressure 2–3 cm above the gastroesophageal junction. This facilitates retrograde movement of food into the lower esophagus during what is coined a "common cavity phenomenon." Liquid and solid material then moves up the esophagus in a retrograde manner accompanied by UES relaxation, allowing movement of the food bolus into the oral cavity. This is followed by normal antegrade peristalsis when the food is re-swallowed. It is thought that the initial rise in intragastric pressure is dependent upon voluntary contraction of the abdominal wall musculature, thus forming some of the basis of treatment interventions described below.

Diagnosis and Evaluation

Clinically significant belching is almost always secondary to supra-gastric belching and can be diagnosed with a careful history and observation of the patient. Patients describe repetitive and bothersome eructation, typically without symptoms of pyrosis, nausea, or vomiting. Although belching is commonly seen in other conditions such as GERD and functional dyspepsia, the presence of symptoms associated with

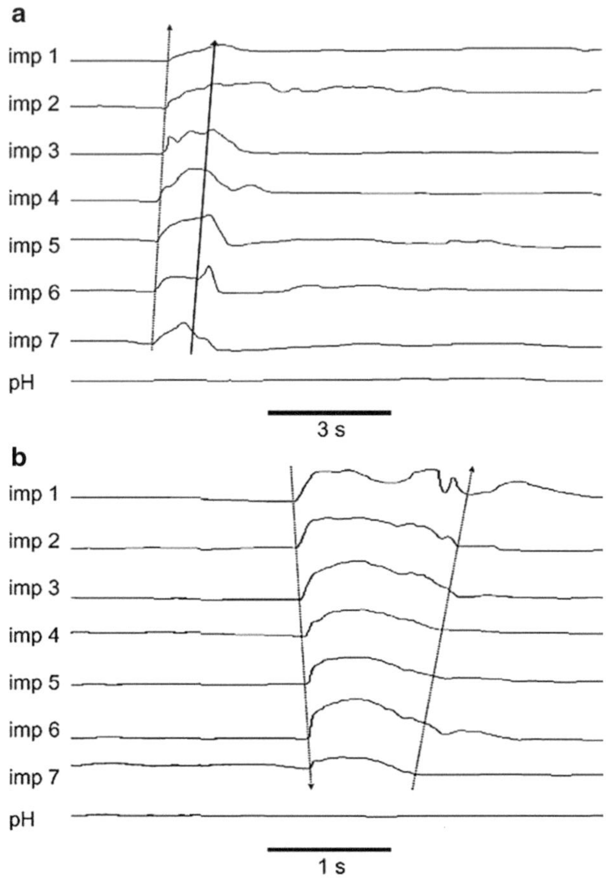

Fig. 5.1 Impedance monitoring tracing during a supra-gastric belch demonstrates a pattern of rapid increase from the proximal to the distal esophagus followed by a retrograde decline

these other disorders should prompt consideration of an alternative diagnosis. The clinician will typically observe frequent belching, sometimes more than 20 times per minute, during the patient encounter. The physical exam is essentially normal other than the observation of frequent diaphragmatic contractions. With typical symptoms, further diagnostic testing is unnecessary. When symptoms are atypical, esophageal manometry and/or combined impedance–pH testing may help distinguish between alternative diagnoses. Patients with excessive supra-gastric belching demonstrate a pattern of rapid increase in impedance from the proximal to the distal esophagus (representing "air sucking") followed by a retrograde decline in impedance (see Fig. 5.1).

In addition to belching, patients with aerophagia often complain of bloating and abdominal discomfort. They often describe excessive flatulence and constipation as well. Indeed, these symptoms may predominate, and belching may be a secondary complaint. Physical examination may reveal abdominal tympani with normal bowel sounds. Abdominal radiographs in patients with aerophagia may demonstrate intestinal air without air–fluid levels. The Rome III criteria for aerophagia and excessive belching are shown in Table 5.1.

Table 5.1 Rome III diagnostic criteria for Aerophagia and unspecified excessive belching[a]

Aerophagia (must include both of the following)	Unspecified excessive belching (must include both of the following)
1. Troublesome repetitive belching at least several times a week 2. Air swallowing that is objectively observed or measured	1. Troublesome repetitive belching at least several times a week 2. No evidence that excessive air swallowing underlies the symptom

[a]Criteria fulfilled for the last 3 months with symptom onset at least 6 months before diagnosis

Table 5.2 Rome III diagnostic criteria for rumination syndrome[a]

Rumination syndrome (must include both of the following)
1. Persistent or recurrent regurgitation of recently ingested food into the mouth with subsequent spitting or remastication and swallowing 2. Regurgitation is not preceded by retching
Supportive criteria 1. Regurgitation events are usually not preceded by nausea 2. Cessation of the process when the regurgitated material becomes acidic 3. Regurgitant contains recognizable food with a pleasant taste

[a]Criteria fulfilled for the last 3 months with symptom onset at least 6 months before diagnosis

Similar to belching disorders, rumination can usually be diagnosed by clinical history without the need for diagnostic tests. Rumination may be difficult to distinguish from other functional disorders such as GERD and gastroparesis. The regurgitation associated with rumination typically occurs during or shortly following a meal. Regurgitation is effortless; it is not preceded by retching as is seen with emesis, and nausea is uncommon. These features differentiate rumination from gastroparesis. The regurgitated food typically is recognizable and has a pleasant taste. The process generally ceases once the food becomes acidic differentiating it from GERD. Nevertheless, rumination may be accompanied by heartburn secondary to the caustic effects of gastric contents in the esophagus. The disorder is frequently accompanied by weight loss, particularly in adolescents. It may be difficult to distinguish rumination from bulimia and/or anorexic behavior, and a high index of suspicion should be present in patients, particularly younger women, with other risk factors for these eating disorders. On examination, patients may be noted to have voluntary contraction of the abdominal musculature. The Rome III criteria for rumination syndrome are shown in Table 5.2. When the diagnosis remains uncertain, esophageal manometry with intraluminal impedance can distinguish rumination from other disorders. Rumination is characterized by a rise in manometric intragastric pressure, followed by retrograde esophageal flow as measured by impedance (see Fig. 5.2). Much less commonly performed, and much less widely available, antroduodenal manometry can also be used to diagnose rumination syndrome. During this procedure, the classic "R" wave indicative of rumination can be demonstrated. The R wave indicates a Valsalva maneuver, where intra-abdominal pressure increases, intrathoracic pressure increases, and esophageal pH drops. The differential diagnoses to be considered in belching, aerophagia, and rumination are given in Table 5.3.

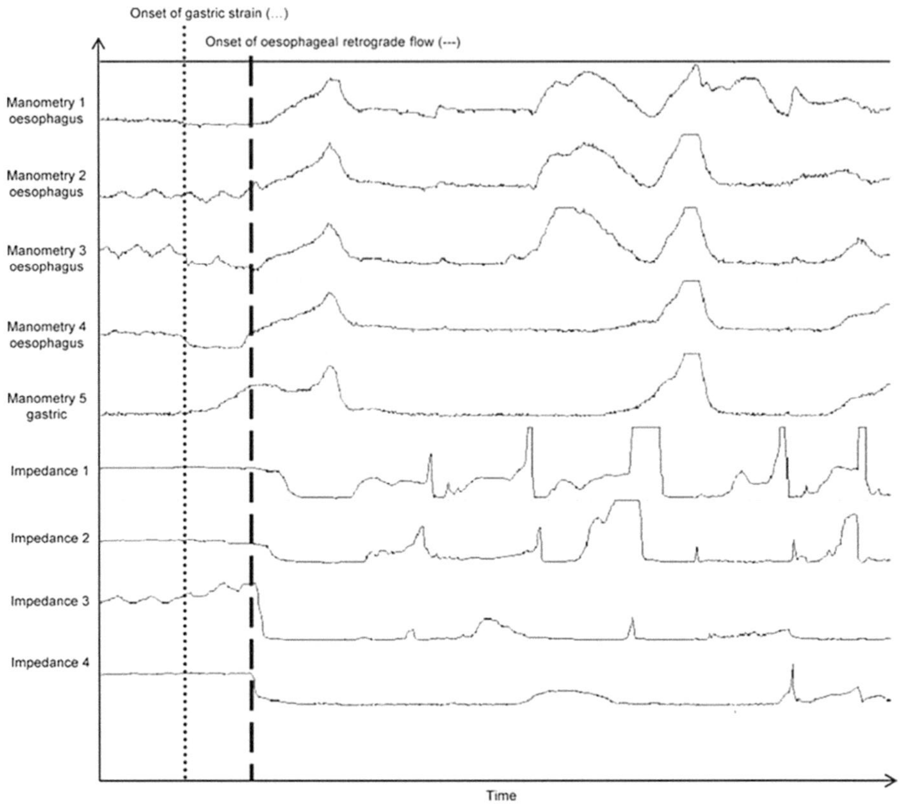

Fig. 5.2 Combined manometry and impedance monitoring from a patient with rumination demonstrates a rise in intragastric pressure, followed by retrograde esophageal flow

Table 5.3 Differential diagnosis for aerophobia, excessive belching, and rumination

Aerophagia	Excessive belching	Rumination
GERD	GERD	GERD
Functional dyspepsia	Functional dyspepsia	Nausea and vomiting disorders
IBS		Gastroparesis
Ileus		Bulimia nervosa
Functional constipation		

GERD gastroesophageal reflux disorder, *IBS* irritable bowel syndrome

Treatment

The mainstay of treatment of excessive belching and aerophagia is reassurance and explanation of the underlying disorder. In those with belching disorders, treatment is aimed at decreasing the voluntary but often unintentional diaphragmatic contraction that initiates the influx of esophageal air. Behavioral therapy may be useful;

patients can be taught to recognize and reduce the frequency of diaphragmatic contractions through biofeedback training. Referral to a speech therapist may occasionally be of benefit, particularly if the therapist has experience in teaching esophageal vocalization—a therapeutic option for post-laryngectomy patients. An empiric trial of gastric acid suppression to treat underlying GERD is also a reasonable consideration, although this approach has not been studied specifically.

In patients with aerophagia, several interventions may be of benefit, although none are well studied. Dietary modification with reduced intake of carbonated beverages and instructions to eat slowly and avoid talking while eating will reduce the amount of air reaching the stomach. The use of medications which reduce the surface tension of gas bubbles, such as simethicone, may be helpful. Referral to speech and or behavioral therapy is recommended if the abovementioned are unsuccessful or if symptoms are severe. A suggested algorithm for the work-up, diagnosis, and treatment of clinically significant belching is shown in Fig. 5.3.

Recommendations for the treatment of rumination syndrome are based mainly on reports from case series and expert opinion. The key aspect of treatment is explanation of the underlying mechanism of the disorder. Rumination starts with a voluntary, although unintentional, contraction of the abdominal musculature, and behavior

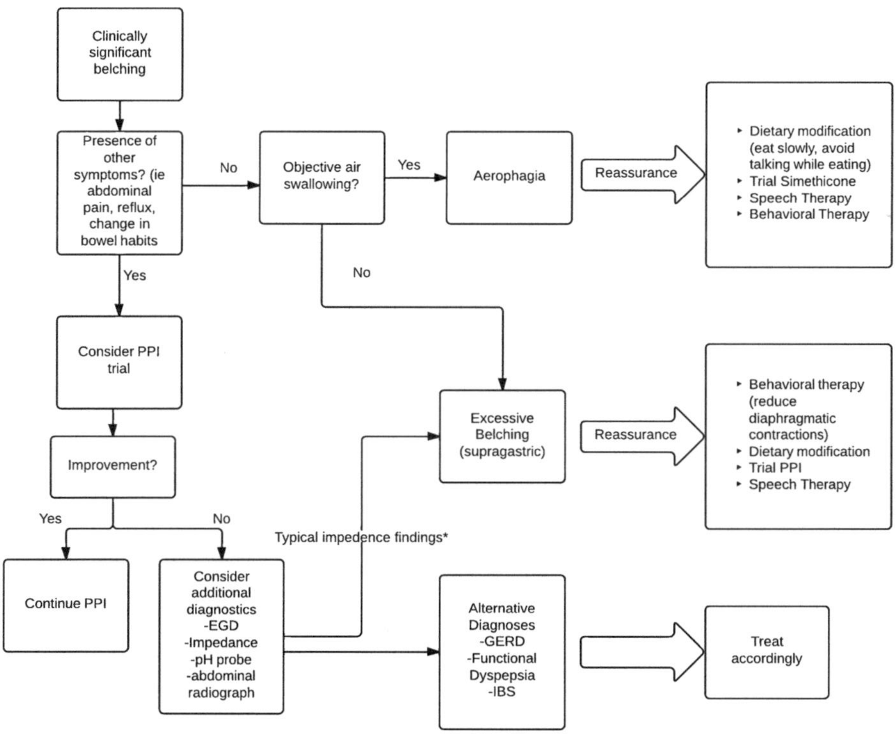

Fig. 5.3 Suggested algorithm for the approach to the patient with excessive belching. *Rapid increase in impedance from the proximal to the distal esophagus followed by a retrograde decline

modification aimed towards inhibiting this contraction is often helpful. Diaphragmatic breathing, which focuses on diaphragmatic and abdominal muscle relaxation, is one example and may be best taught to a patient by a behavioral psychologist.

The role of acid suppression using proton pump inhibitors is controversial. Rumination typically ceases once the regurgitated food becomes acidic tasting and, thus, proton pump inhibitor therapy may actually prolong the rumination cycle.

It has been suggested that improving LES tone, either surgically or pharmacologically, may be effective at treating rumination. There are limited data to support surgical fundoplication, however, and given the risks associated with surgical intervention, it is not a recommended treatment. Baclofen, which reduces the frequency of TLESRs, has been studied in a small series of patients with rumination and has been demonstrated to reduce the frequency of impedance-measured rumination episodes.

Case Resolution

At follow-up, the proton pump inhibitor was stopped as it provided no benefit, and the physiology of belching was explained at length. Given the absence of warning signs and symptoms suggestive of other disorders, no tests were ordered. The patient was counseled on ways to minimize gulping air including avoiding carbonated beverages and eating slowly and encouraged to use simethicone on an as-needed basis. He was also counseled to avoid initiating a belch and was taught diaphragmatic breathing in the office. Although skeptical, he promised to try these suggestions. Two weeks later, he reported that his symptoms were about 30 % better. He was then referred to speech therapy to help him minimize air swallowing and belching. His symptoms had nearly resolved when seen two months later.

Key Clinical Teaching Points

- Belching disorders, aerophagia, and rumination are relatively rare disorders. The key to an accurate diagnosis is a careful history and observation; specialized testing is rarely necessary.
- Following exclusion of other gastrointestinal disorders, the treatment of aerophagia, belching, and rumination should focus on explanation of the underlying mechanisms to the patient, combined with behavioral modification techniques.
- Pathological belching is more often a result of "supra-gastric" belching rather than "gastric" belching. This is significant in that treatment is aimed at behavioral modification of air sucking rather than reducing intragastric air.

Teaching Questions

1. Which one of the following is required to diagnose aerophagia?
   (A) Upper endoscopy
   (B) A good clinical history
   (C) A good clinical history and direct observation
   (D) High-resolution esophageal manometry
2. Which of the following treatment option(s) is appropriate for patients with aerophagia?
   (A) Education and reassurance
   (B) Dietary interventions
   (C) Empiric therapy with a proton pump inhibitor
   (D) Behavioral therapy
   (E) All of the above
3. Transient lower esophageal sphincter relaxations are the primary pathophysiologic event leading to rumination syndrome.
   (A) True
   (B) False
4. Which one of the following tests or procedure is best to diagnose rumination syndrome?
   (A) Upper endoscopy
   (B) Barium swallow
   (C) 48-h wireless pH study
   (D) Impedance–pH monitoring with esophageal manometry
   (E) 4-h solid-phase gastric emptying scan

Key References

1. Bredenoord AJ. Management of belching, hiccups, and aerophagia. Clin Gastroenterol Hepatol. 2013;11:6–12. Excellent review of the clinical features, pathophysiology and treatment of belching and aerophagia.
2. Bredenoord AJ, Weusten BL, Sifrim D, Timmer R, Smout AJ. Aerophagia, gastric, and supragastric belching: A study using intraluminal electrical impedance monitoring. Gut. 2004;53(11):1561–5. The first study to identify the distinction between gastric and supragastric belching using impedance monitoring.
3. Chitkara DK, Van Tilburg M, Whitehead WE, Talley NJ. Teaching diaphragmatic breathing for rumination syndrome. Am J Gastroenterol. 2006;101:2249–52. An excellent review of the diagnosis and treatment of rumination syndrome.

4. O'Brien MD, Bruce BK, Camilleri M. The rumination syndrome: Clinical features rather than manometric diagnosis. Gastroenterology. 1995;108:1024–9. Retrospective study that established the clinical features used to define the diagnosis of rumination.
5. Tack J, Talley NJ, Camilleri M, Holtmann G, Hu P, Malagelada JR, Stanghellini V. Functional gastroduodenal disorders. Gastroenterology. 2006;130:1466–79. Summarizes the Rome III consensus with regards to the definition, evaluation and treatment of gastroduodenal disorders including aerophagia, unspecified belching and rumination.

Chapter 6
Dyspepsia

Kelly Everhart and Brian E. Lacy

Case Study

A 49-year-old woman is referred for the evaluation of a 2-year history of upper gastrointestinal discomfort. She describes a daily, persistent ache or discomfort that waxes and wanes. She complains that eating tends to worsen her pain and that she feels very full, even after eating only a modest-sized meal. Her weight is unchanged, and her medical history is notable only for occasional migraine headaches. Her surgical history includes an appendectomy (age 7) and wisdom teeth extraction (age 16). She does not use tobacco products and rarely drinks alcohol. Her family history is noncontributory. She is an appropriate, interactive woman (body mass index [BMI] is 23.4 kg/m^2). Physical examination is notable only for mild epigastric tenderness to palpation. There is no evidence of ascites, organomegaly, a succussion splash, abdominal mass, or bruit. An upper gastrointestinal (UGI) series (2 years ago), abdominal ultrasound and hepatobiliary iminodiacetic (HIDA) scan (18 months ago), upper endoscopy (12 months ago), and 4-h solid-phase gastric emptying scan (4 months ago) were normal. She is *Helicobacter pylori*-negative. Extensive laboratory tests (complete blood count [CBC], erythrocyte sedimentation rate [ESR], liver function tests [LFTs], lipase, and electrolytes) have all been normal on at least two occasions. The patient asks you what her diagnosis is and how her symptoms can be treated.

K. Everhart, B.A., M.S. (✉)
Division of Gastroenterology and Hepatology, Dartmouth-Hitchcock Medical Center, 1 Medical Center Drive, Lebanon, NH 03756, USA
e-mail: Kelly.K.Everhart.MED@dartmouth.edu

B.E. Lacy, M.D., Ph.D.
Division of Gastroenterology and Hepatology, Dartmouth-Hitchcock Medical Center, 1 Medical Center Drive, Lebanon, NH 03756, USA

Geisel School of Medicine at Dartmouth, Lebanon, NH USA

B.E. Lacy et al. (eds.), *Functional and Motility Disorders of the Gastrointestinal Tract*, DOI 10.1007/978-1-4939-1498-2_6

Introduction

Dyspepsia is a common medical disorder that poses a diagnostic and therapeutic challenge to all healthcare providers. Clinically, patients often present with a variety of complaints including abdominal pain or discomfort, bloating, belching, early satiety, epigastric fullness, nausea, and "reflux." Healthcare providers must determine if these symptoms meet criteria for dyspepsia or if they point toward another diagnoses, such as chronic pancreatitis or choledocholithiasis. The investigation and treatment of dyspepsia is complicated by the fact that dyspeptic symptoms are nonspecific, such that they cannot be used to reliably distinguish organic disorders from functional gastrointestinal disorders. Further complicating matters is the fact that once a patient is identified as having functional dyspepsia (FD), the pathophysiology of FD is complex and incompletely understood, and symptom response to treatment is unpredictable. Indeed, healthcare providers are often uncomfortable making the diagnosis of dyspepsia and selecting empiric therapy. Finally, dyspepsia is frequently a chronic disorder that is frustrating for patients and physicians alike.

In the following sections, we'll review the diagnosis, evaluation, and treatment of dyspepsia, emphasizing the differences between uninvestigated dyspepsia, investigated dyspepsia, and functional dyspepsia. Given the variety of upper gastrointestinal symptoms classified as dyspepsia, an extensive differential diagnosis exists (see Table 6.1). Subsequent diagnostic evaluation, which often includes laboratory,

Table 6.1 Differential diagnosis of dyspepsia

Mucosal disorders
Esophagitis
Occult acid reflux disease
Gastritis
Duodenitis
Peptic ulcer disease
H. pylori infection
Gastric cancer
Neuromuscular dysfunction
Gastroparesis
Visceral hypersensitivity
Impaired fundic relaxation
Abnormalities in the brain-gut axis
Others
Psychological disorders
Medications
Abdominal wall pain
Hepatobiliary disorders
Pancreatic disorders
Vascular disorders (median arcuate ligament syndrome; SMA syndrome)
Ischemic heart disease

Table 6.2 Rome III criteria for functional dyspepsia (Modified from Tack et al 2006)

For the 2 categories noted below, criteria must be fulfilled for the last 3 months with symptom onset at least 6 months prior to diagnosis. Patients must have one or more of the following symptoms:
Postprandial fullness
Early satiety
Epigastric burning
In addition, patients cannot have any evidence of structural disease that is likely to explain symptoms (i.e., upper endoscopy is normal)
A. Postprandial distress syndrome
Diagnostic criteria must include **both** of the following:
Bothersome postprandial fullness, occurring after ordinary sized meals, at least several times per week
Early satiation that prevents finishing a regular meal, at least several times per week
Other supporting criteria:
Upper abdominal bloating or postprandial nausea or excessive belching can be present
Epigastric pain syndrome may coexist
B. Epigastric pain syndrome
Diagnostic criteria must include **all** of the following:
Pain or burning localized to the epigastrium, of at least moderate severity at least once per week
The pain is intermittent
Not generalized or localized to other abdominal or chest regions
Not relieved by defecation or passage of flatus
Not fulfilling criteria for biliary pain
Supportive criteria:
The pain may be of a burning quality, but without a retrosternal component
The pain is commonly induced or relieved by ingestion of a meal, but may occur while fasting
Postprandial distress syndrome may coexist

endoscopic, and radiologic studies, differentiates uninvestigated from investigated dyspepsia and further subdivides investigated dyspepsia into those patients with an organic etiology of their symptoms and those with functional dyspepsia (FD).

Functional dyspepsia accounts for the majority of patients with dyspeptic symptoms; approximately 70 % of dyspeptic patients have a normal initial diagnostic evaluation. The Rome III criteria (see Table 6.2) currently define FD as the presence of symptoms thought to originate in the gastroduodenal region in the absence of any organic, systemic, or metabolic disease likely to explain the symptoms. The Rome committee recently introduced two new subcategories for FD into their diagnostic criteria: postprandial distress syndrome (PDS) and epigastric pain syndrome (EPS). Importantly, while epigastric pain or discomfort is the hallmark symptom in patients with FD, many patients with FD will not complain of pain but will rather state that they have burning, pressure, or fullness in their epigastric area or that they cannot finish a normal-sized meal (early satiety). Postprandial nausea, belching, and abdominal bloating are also often present in FD. Patients with abdominal pain or discomfort relieved with defecation are currently excluded from the Rome III FD definition as these symptoms are most consistent with the diagnosis of irritable bowel syndrome (IBS; see Chap. 16). It is important to note that there is a large overlap between FD and IBS, and approximately 30–40 % of patients with FD have overlapping IBS, while approximately 40 % of patients with IBS have overlapping FD.

Epidemiology

Dyspepsia is one of the most commonly encountered problems in medical practice. Population studies from the United States and Europe demonstrate that 20–25 % of adults suffer from dyspepsia at any given time. Once investigated, most patients with dyspeptic symptoms are diagnosed with FD. In these populations, the prevalence of FD is approximately 12–15 %, while its incidence is 2–5 %. The natural history of FD is not well understood, likely because it is a disorder of multiple, potentially coincident pathophysiologies. Patient cohort analyses report a wide range of time to resolution, from 30 to 50 % resolution at 1–2 years post-diagnosis to 80 % with persistent symptoms at 18–24 months.

Pathophysiology

The underlying pathophysiology of FD includes heightened or otherwise abnormal visceral sensation (see Fig. 6.1) and abnormalities in gastric emptying and fundic accommodation. On gastric scintigraphy, 30–40 % of FD patients have a mild delay in gastric emptying, while 5–10 % demonstrate rapid gastric emptying. Impaired fundic accommodation, identified by a gastric barostat or single-photon emission computed tomography (SPECT) study (only performed at specialized centers), is present in 30–40 % of patients with FD. Some patients with FD are likely hypersensitive to normal amounts of gastric acid, which may explain the small but positive response of dyspeptic patients to treatment with histamine type 2 receptor antagonists (H2RA's) or proton pump inhibitors (PPIs). Others are hypersensitive to duodenal lipids or to the presence of duodenal eosinophilia.

Infection with *Helicobacter pylori* (*H. pylori*) has long been implicated in the pathogenesis of dyspepsia. The prevalence of *H. pylori* is, however, generally the same between subjects with and without dyspepsia, and several large, randomized, placebo-controlled trials have shown little or no long-term benefit in the resolution of FD symptoms after eradication of *H. pylori*. Finally, FD may share the postinfectious etiology that is well described in patients with IBS. Although neither anxiety nor depression directly causes FD, their coexistence may exacerbate the experience and increase the reporting of FD symptoms.

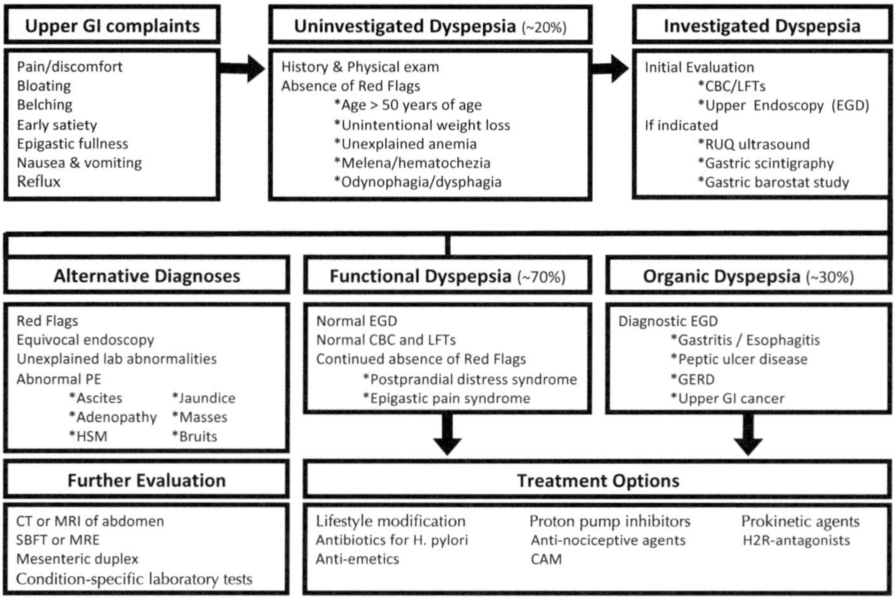

Fig. 6.1 The pathophysiology of FD

Diagnosis and Evaluation

Because the differential diagnosis of dyspepsia is broad (see Table 6.1 and Fig. 6.2), a careful history and thorough physical examination are important first steps to distinguish dyspepsia from other disorders and to help determine whether dyspeptic symptoms represent an underlying organic process or are functional in nature. A careful review of the patient's medication list should be performed as nonsteroidal anti-inflammatory agents (NSAIDs), aspirin products, antibiotics, alternative medications, and iron supplements can cause dyspeptic symptoms. The presence of classic symptoms of pyrosis and regurgitation makes gastroesophageal reflux disease the most likely diagnosis. Postprandial pain or discomfort raises the possibility of peptic ulcer disease and, when coupled with unintentional weight loss, raises the possibility of gastroparesis, gastric outlet obstruction, or even gastric cancer. Realizing that dyspeptic symptoms are nonspecific, clinicians should be particularly attentive to "red flags" in the history or on physical examination that may suggest the presence of underlying systemic or malignant disease (see Table 6.3). For example, findings of hepatosplenomegaly, ascites, adenopathy and masses, jaundice, an abdominal bruit, or a succussion splash should make the clinician consider alternative diagnoses and initiate an appropriate investigation.

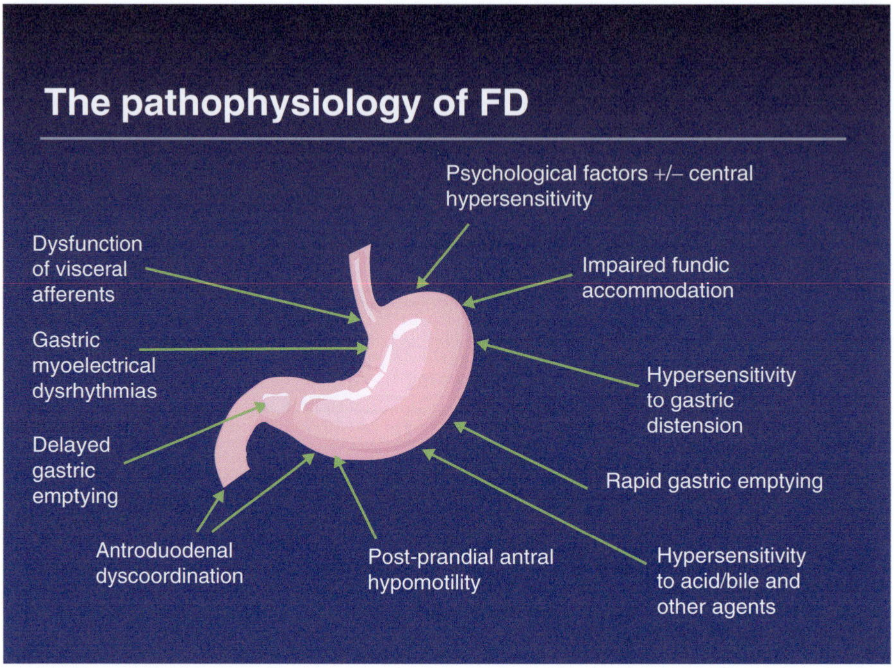

Fig. 6.2 Diagnostic algorithm

Table 6.3 Warning symptoms and signs in the evaluation of dyspepsia

Dysphagia
Odynophagia
Hematemesis
Intractable nausea and vomiting
NSAID use
Unintentional weight loss (>10 % of body weight)
History of ulcer disease or pancreatitis
Jaundice
Anemia
Hematochezia
Presence of an abdominal mass
Age >45

In the patient younger than 45 years old and without worrisome signs or symptoms, an assessment for *H. pylori* is recommended. When positive, multiple placebo-controlled trials have demonstrated that it is appropriate to initiate *H. pylori* eradication in hopes of relieving dyspeptic symptoms. A follow-up appointment should be scheduled 4 weeks after completion of antibiotic therapy, and if symptoms persist, then treatment with an antisecretory agent (e.g., a PPI) is a reasonable next step. Patients with symptoms refractory to *H. pylori* eradication and antisecretory therapy should be referred for upper endoscopy with biopsies to document *H. pylori* eradication and eliminate other upper gastrointestinal mucosal disorders, such as celiac disease. Should EGD be unrevealing, and symptoms persist, then a right upper quadrant ultrasound is reasonable, followed by the initiation of symptom-based therapy (e.g., an antiemetic or antinociceptive agent). A "test and treat" strategy such as the one described is considered safe because ulcer disease is uncommon in patients not taking anti-inflammatory agents. Furthermore, the risk of gastric cancer is low (<1:1,000) in patients with dyspeptic symptoms who do not have warning signs and are younger than 45 years of age.

In patients older than 45 years and in those with warning signs, EGD should be performed at the outset in order to exclude significant pathology (e.g., ulcer disease, gastric neoplasm). If endoscopy is normal, including biopsies to exclude *H. pylori*, and basic laboratory tests are normal, then a trial of an antisecretory agent should be initiated. If symptoms persist, then further diagnostic imaging with a right upper quadrant is reasonable (although data documenting the clinical utility of ultrasound is limited) and therapy based upon the predominant symptom (e.g., pain or nausea or bloating) should be initiated.

Treatment

In the absence of signs or symptoms indicative of an organic process, empiric treatment can be initiated in a young patient based upon the patient's predominant complaint. Alternatively, a wait-and-watch approach can be adopted as many cases of acute dyspepsia resolve spontaneously. Lifestyle modification and pharmacotherapy are also treatment options that may benefit some patients. In all cases, follow-up should be scheduled 3–4 weeks later to reassess symptoms, identify warning signs if present, and assess response to therapy (Table 6.4).

Table 6.4 Treatment options for functional dyspepsia

Proton pump inhibitors (PPIs)
Tricyclic antidepressants (TCAs)
Prokinetic agents (metoclopramide, domperidone)
Antinociceptive agents (tramadol, gabapentin, pregabalin)
Buspirone
CAM (Iberogast, capsaicin)

Watchful Waiting

Dyspepsia is a self-limited process in some patients that may occur as a consequence of an acute infectious process, a side effect of a medication, or a reaction to stress; these symptoms usually resolve spontaneously within days to weeks. In a young patient (<40 years) without warning signs on history or physical examination, it is reasonable to delay further diagnostic testing in favor of a period of observation. Sufficient education and reassurance about when further investigation is warranted, and the risks of delayed investigation, must be provided to patients. Unfortunately, although a trial of observation is safe, it is not effective for most patients as it is rare for symptoms to resolve completely over this timeframe.

Lifestyle Modifications

The success of lifestyle modifications in the treatment of dyspepsia is not well described. Prospective, randomized, studies comparing different interventions are not available to guide therapy in an evidence-based manner, although anecdotal evidence suggests that exercise and certain dietary guidelines may mitigate symptoms in some patients. Several small studies have noted that FD patients may be more sensitive to dietary fats than their unaffected peers. Minimizing dietary fat and eating smaller, more frequent meals may benefit some patients. A dietary history or patient-recorded diary might identify symptom triggers like caffeine, fats, spices or alcohol which can then be eliminated.

Coating Agents and Simethicone

Theoretically, coating agents such as bismuth and sucralfate are attractive treatment options for dyspeptic patients since they prevent injury to the stomach mucosa by acid or other caustic substances. Although they are commonly used, bismuth products and sucralfate have not yet been proven effective agents in the treatment of dyspeptic symptoms. Simethicone, however, was found to be more effective than either cisapride or placebo at relieving upper abdominal pain during an 8-week period in a single trial.

Antisecretory Therapy

Histamine type 2 receptor antagonists (H2RAs) are generally safe and inexpensive; however, their benefit to symptoms associated with FD is modest at best and otherwise absent when compared to placebo. Proton pump inhibitors (PPIs) are more effective than H2RAs in treating dyspepsia, especially if the predominant symptom is pyrosis. In the setting of FD, PPIs have consistently been shown to be more effective than placebo, although the benefit is modest (10–16 % improvement in symptom frequency and/or severity). Twice-daily PPIs have not been shown to be more effective than once-daily dosing for symptom resolution.

Helicobacter pylori *Eradication*

H. pylori is clearly associated with an increased risk for peptic ulcer disease and gastric adenocarcinoma. *H. pylori* eradication is, therefore, a required and effective component of therapy for dyspeptic patients with coexisting gastritis or peptic ulcer disease. Unfortunately, *H. pylori* eradication rarely leads to symptom improvement in patients with FD.

Prokinetic Agents

Prokinetic agents are most useful in the treatment of symptoms associated with gastroduodenal dysmotility such as early satiety, epigastric fullness, nausea, and vomiting. Since these are common complaints of patients with FD, prokinetic agents are reasonable options when H2RAs/PPIs fail, especially if nausea is the predominant symptom. Metoclopramide, a dopamine antagonist, is the most common prokinetic agent used to treat nausea in FD. Compared to placebo, metoclopramide has not been shown to improve global dyspeptic symptoms. It is also associated with a number of side effects including fatigue, somnolence, depression, anxiety, dystonia, and, rarely, the development of tardive dyskinesia. Domperidone, another dopamine antagonist but with a better adverse event profile, is commonly used to treat dyspeptic symptoms in countries outside of the Unites States since it is not Food and Drug Administration approved in the United States. Like metoclopramide, domperidone improves dyspeptic symptoms, especially nausea, in some patients; however, its benefit compared to placebo is equivocal.

Smooth Muscle Antispasmodic Agents

Smooth muscle antispasmodic agents such as hyoscyamine, dicyclomine, and glycopyrrolate are used to treat irritable bowel syndrome (IBS). Unlike the pathophysiology of IBS, the abdominal discomfort associated with FD does not appear to originate from smooth muscle spasm along the gastrointestinal tract. These agents are unlikely to benefit patients with dyspepsia, although their efficacy has not been evaluated in this patient population.

Antinociceptive Agents

Patients with dyspepsia often present to healthcare providers seeking relief from abdominal pain. By the time that they are formally evaluated, patients have often tried over-the-counter agents like acetaminophen, aspirin, and NSAIDs without success. Importantly, aspirin and NSAIDs have been associated with the development of dyspeptic symptoms. Tricyclic antidepressants (TCAs) such as amitriptyline and desipramine have been shown to alleviate dyspeptic symptoms in patients with functional gastrointestinal disorders including FD. Large, randomized trials comparing different TCAs are lacking. Gabapentin, carbamazepine, tramadol, and selective-serotonin reuptake inhibitors have been used in the treatment of difficult-to-treat dyspepsia; however, anecdotal reports regarding their clinical utility have been conflicting, and their efficacy has not been subjected to formal study in most circumstances. One prospective study evaluating venlafaxine showed no benefit compared to placebo.

Complementary and Alternative Medicines

Complementary and alternative medicine (CAM) is an expanding feature of many dyspeptic patients' treatment regimens. Ginger, peppermint oil, caraway oil, and pressure bands are notable CAM options; however, their efficacy and safety in FD have not been formally evaluated in randomized, placebo-controlled trials. One small randomized study found that red pepper (capsaicin) was more effective than placebo. A meta-analysis of randomized clinical trials found that Iberogast, a combination of nine different herbs, was more effective than placebo in treating some symptoms of FD.

Psychological Therapies

Hypnotherapy can effectively treat some patients with IBS when compared to supportive care or medical therapy over both short (16 weeks) and long (56 weeks) time intervals. Whorwell and colleagues compared hypnotherapy to supportive care or medical therapy in a randomized study of 126 patients with FD. Hypnotherapy was found to be significantly more effective than both medication and supportive care over both the short term and the long term. Similarly, cognitive behavioral therapy (CBT) was more effective than educational sessions with a therapist in managing the symptoms of patients with functional abdominal pain. See Chap. 20 for more information on CAM use and CBT in functional gastrointestinal disorders.

Novel Therapies

Buspirone, an anxiolytic, acts on gastric 5-hydroxytryptamine receptors, relaxing the fundus and improving gastric accommodation. It has been shown to improve dyspeptic symptoms more than placebo, likely by improving gastric accommodation in the postprandial period. Acotiamide, an acetylcholinesterase inhibitor and antimuscarinic agent, also improves symptoms of postprandial distress; however, it is not yet available for use in the United States.

Case Resolution

The patient was diagnosed with FD and reassured that the natural history of the disorder is benign. A once-daily PPI trial for 8 weeks was not helpful. She was subsequently started on a low-dose bedtime TCA and referred for cognitive behavioral therapy. She reported a 50 % reduction in her dyspeptic symptoms at a follow-up appointment 3 months later.

Key Clinical Teaching Points

- A careful history and physical examination is a critical component in the initial evaluation of patients with dyspeptic symptoms. "Red flags" indicate that the patient may be suffering from an organic disorder.
- An extensive battery of tests is neither required nor recommended for all patients with dyspeptic symptoms. Rather, diagnostic testing should be guided by the patient's predominant symptom or to rule out more serious disorders. CBC, LFTs, EGD, and abdominal ultrasonography are reasonable first-line studies when clinically indicated.
- Although some patients with dyspeptic symptoms may benefit from empiric therapy to eradicate *H. pylori*, this treatment option rarely eliminates symptoms in patients with FD.
- PPI therapy improves dyspeptic symptoms in patients with underlying esophagitis, reflux symptoms, and gastritis but is less effective in patients with a normal endoscopy and no pyrosis.
- TCAs may improve the symptoms of FD in those patients who are *H. pylori-negative* and who have failed PPI therapy.

Teaching Questions

1. In the evaluation of a patient with dyspepsia, upper endoscopy (EGD) helps distinguish between an organic process (e.g., gastritis) and functional dyspepsia (FD), in which the endoscopy is normal. What percentage of patients with dyspepsia have a normal endoscopy and thus are categorized as having FD?

   (A) 10 %
   (B) 30 %
   (C) 50 %
   (D) 70 %

2. The pathophysiology of functional dyspepsia (FD) is multifactorial. Which 2 categories are thought to account for the majority of cases?

   (A) *H. pylori* infection and bile gastritis
   (B) Impaired fundic accommodation and a mild delay in gastric emptying
   (C) Rapid gastric emptying and gastric acid hypersensitivity
   (D) Delayed gastric emptying and *H. pylori* infection

3. In a young patient (35 years or age or less) with symptoms of dyspepsia and no warning signs on exam or history, which tests are required before treatment can be initiated?

   (A) Upper endoscopy.
   (B) Laboratory tests including CBC and LFTs.
   (C) Right upper quadrant ultrasound.
   (D) No testing is required.
   (E) CT scan of abdomen.

4. True or False—Prokinetics are generally considered the best therapy for patients with FD since this generally reflects a motility disorder of the stomach.

   (A) True
   (B) False

Key References

1. Brook RA, Kleinman NL, Choung RS, et al. Functional dyspepsia impacts absenteeism and direct and indirect costs. Clin Gastroenterol Hepatol. 2010;8:498–503. One of 2 recent articles highlighting the costs associated with dyspepsia.
2. Calvert EL, Houghton LA, Cooper P, Morris J, Whorwell PJ. Long-term improvement in functional dyspepsia using hypnotherapy. Gastroenterology. 2002;123:1778–85. A nice article on the use of hypnotherapy in FD.
3. Castillo EJ, Camilleri M, Locke III GR, Burton DD, Stephens DA, Geno DM, Zinsmeister AR. A community-based, controlled study of the epidemiology and pathophysiology of dyspepsia. Clin Gastroenterol Hepatol. 2004;2:985–96. A nice epidemiologic study on the prevalence of dyspepsia.

4. El-Serag HB, Talley NJ. Health-related quality of life in functional dyspepsia. Aliment Pharmacol Ther. 2003;18:387–93. A nice article summarizing quality of life studies.
5. Lacy BE, Talley NJ, Locke GR, Bouras EP, DiBaise JK, El-Serag HB, Howden C, Moayyedi P, Prather C. Functional dyspepsia: A review of current treatment options and management. Aliment Pharmacol Ther. 2012;36:3–15. A comprehensive recent review on treatment options for FD.
6. Moayyedi P, Soo S, Deeks J, Delaney B, Harris A, Innes M, et al. Eradication of helicobacter pylori for non-ulcer dyspepsia. Cochrane Database Syst Rev. 2008 (CD002096). The recent Cochrane analysis summarizing articles on the low yield of improving dyspeptic symptoms after *H. pylori* eradication.
7. Tack J, Talley NJ, Camilleri M, Holtmann G, Hu P, Malagelada JR, Stanghellini V. Functional gastroduodenal disorders. Gastroenterology. 2006;130:1466–79. The Rome III criteria for FD.

Chapter 7
Chronic Nausea

Maria I. Vazquez-Roque and Ernest P. Bouras

Case Study

A previously healthy 34-year-old woman developed postprandial fullness, early satiety, and nausea about 6 months prior to her current evaluation. There was no history of an antecedent gastrointestinal illness. Examination at that time, including laboratories and upper gastrointestinal barium study, was unremarkable. She did not improve with an empiric course of acid suppression. Following a study showing poor gallbladder emptying, she underwent a cholecystectomy 4 months ago, but this did not lead to clinical improvement.

Currently, her most bothersome symptom of nausea is constant. There is no associated vomiting. She also feels bloated and has lost about 5 pounds since her symptoms began. Although she describes a vague mid-abdominal discomfort that developed after her cholecystectomy, she denies actual pain. Her history is otherwise remarkable only for the use of nonsteroidal anti-inflammatory agents and occasional narcotic pain medications for headaches and neck pain following an injury sustained at work two months prior to the current appointment. She notes that she will also occasionally use the pain medications for the abdominal discomfort. Lastly, she has developed constipation, which she attributes to decreased food intake. Physical examination reveals a non-distended abdomen with normal bowel sounds. Her mood and affect appear normal, and she has no neurological abnormalities. She is searching for relief from her nausea, which has limited her ability to work and is making it difficult for her to interact with friends and family.

M.I. Vazquez-Roque, M.D. • E.P. Bouras, M.D. (✉)
Division of Gastroenterology, Mayo Clinic Florida, 4500 San Pablo Road, Jacksonville, FL 32224, USA
e-mail: bouras.ernest@mayo.edu

B.E. Lacy et al. (eds.), *Functional and Motility Disorders of the Gastrointestinal Tract*, DOI 10.1007/978-1-4939-1498-2_7

Introduction

Nausea is a subjective symptom, best described as a queasiness or sick sensation with the feeling of the imminent need to vomit. Epigastric discomfort, systemic symptoms (e.g., sweating and light-headedness), and emotional symptoms (e.g., fatigue and depression) have been associated with nausea.

Nausea is a nonspecific symptom and is associated with numerous disorders and therapies. The differential diagnosis for nausea, either alone or accompanied by vomiting, is extensive (see Table 7.1). In the acute setting, it is often easier to identify the etiology for nausea. The diagnosis is more challenging, however, for those presenting with chronic nausea as it is often a pathologic response to a variety of

Table 7.1 Differential diagnosis of nausea and vomiting

Medications and toxic etiologies
Cancer chemotherapy
Aspirin
Nonsteroidal anti-inflammatory drugs
Auranofin
Antigout drugs
Digoxin
Antiarrhythmics
Antihypertensives
β-Blockers
Calcium channel antagonists
Diuretics
Oral antidiabetics
Oral contraceptives
Erythromycin
Tetracycline
Sulfonamides
Antituberculous drugs
Acyclovir
Sulfasalazine
Azathioprine
Nicotine
CNS-active drugs
Narcotics
Anti-Parkinsonian drugs
Anticonvulsants
Antiasthmatics
Theophylline
Radiation therapy
Ethanol abuse
Hypervitaminosis

(continued)

Table 7.1 (continued)

Infectious causes
Gastroenteritis (Viral or Bacterial)
Otitis media
Disorders of the gut and peritoneum
Gastric outlet obstruction
Small bowel obstruction
Gastroparesis
Chronic intestinal pseudo-obstruction
Nonulcer dyspepsia
Irritable bowel syndrome
Pancreatic adenocarcinoma
Inflammatory intraperitoneal disease
Peptic ulcer disease
Cholecystitis
Pancreatitis
Hepatitis
Crohn's disease
Mesenteric ischemia
Retroperitoneal fibrosis
Mucosal metastases
CNS causes
Migraine
Malignancy
Hemorrhage
Infarction
Abscess
Meningitis
Congenital malformation
Hydrocephalus
Pseudotumor cerebri
Seizure disorders
Demyelinating disorders
Emotional responses
Psychiatric disease
Psychogenic vomiting
Anxiety disorders
Depression
Pain
Anorexia nervosa
Bulimia nervosa
Labyrinthine disorders
Motion sickness

(continued)

Table 7.1 (continued)

Labyrinthitis
Tumors
Meniere's disease
Fluorescein angiography
Endocrinologic and metabolic causes
Pregnancy
Uremia
Diabetic ketoacidosis
Hyperparathyroidism
Hypoparathyroidism
Hyperthyroidism
Addison's disease
Acute intermittent porphyria
Postoperative nausea and vomiting
Cyclic vomiting syndrome
Miscellaneous causes
Myocardial infarction
Congestive heart failure
Radiofrequency ablation
Starvation

Adapted from Douglas A, Drossman M., Ed. (2006). Rome III: The functional gastrointestinal disorders. McLean, Virginia: Degnon Associates

Table 7.2 Diagnostic criteria for chronic idiopathic nausea (CIN)

Must include all of the following
Bothersome nausea occurring at least several times per week
Not usually associated with vomiting
Absence of abnormalities at upper endoscopy or metabolic disease that explains the nausea
Criteria need to be fulfilled for past 3 months, with symptom onset at least 6 months before diagnosis

Adapted from Douglas A. Drossman, M., Ed. (2006). Rome III: The functional gastrointestinal disorders. McLean, Virginia: Degnon Associates

disorders ranging from organic disease to psychological conditions. Moreover, adverse medication reactions are among the most common causes of nausea.

Nausea is considered chronic when it persists for >1 month. Chronic idiopathic nausea (CIN) has been recently defined as bothersome nausea occurring at least several times per week that is not associated with vomiting or an obvious metabolic or gastrointestinal disorder (see Table 7.2). For consistency purposes in this chapter, we will use the term CIN to refer to chronic nausea without an identifiable cause. When nausea is associated with vomiting, other diagnoses such as gastroparesis or cyclic vomiting syndrome need to be considered. It is not clear whether patients with CIN represent a distinct syndrome, a heterogeneous collection of different unidentified etiologies, or part of a spectrum of gastric sensorimotor dysfunction.

Epidemiology

Given the ubiquitous nature of chronic nausea, the exact incidence, prevalence, and natural history are unknown. In one study, 8 % of otherwise normal subjects reported nausea. Decreased awareness contributes to gaps in knowledge regarding demographics, age, and gender distribution of CIN. In a recent study, no differences in patient demographics, lifestyles, or anthropometric characteristics were appreciated in patients with chronic unexplained nausea and vomiting (CUNV) compared to their counterparts with gastroparesis. Similarities were also found for severity, pattern, and nature of symptoms. Forty-five percent of patients with CUNV (and 26 % of patients with gastroparesis) met Rome III criteria for the diagnosis of CIN. In addition, there appeared to be stability in the disorder, as little change in diagnosis was noted over the course of a year. At present, there are no published quality of life studies for CIN; however, studies of other disorders associated with nausea have demonstrated decreased activity, increased fatigue, sleep disturbance, and irritability. Furthermore, increased nursing care and health-care expenses and lost productivity have been demonstrated in patients with chronic nausea.

Pathophysiology

The exact mechanisms underlying CIN remain unclear but are likely to be multiple given the variety of its causes. Indeed, CIN may arise due to central or peripheral abnormalities or a combination of both. To better approach its evaluation and management, it is helpful to have a basic understanding of the functional anatomy and physiology involved in the pathogenesis of nausea and vomiting (see Fig. 7.1). Motor and sensory function of the gut is controlled by the interaction among the extrinsic nervous system (parasympathetic and sympathetic), central nervous system, and gut smooth muscle cells. The area postrema, located on the floor of the fourth ventricle, is sensitive to neurotransmitters, peptides, drugs, and toxins. The nucleus tractus solitarius (NTS) in the medulla serves a central role, receiving input from visceral afferents (via the vagus nerve) and humoral factors (via the area postrema). Neurons from the NTS project into paraventricular nuclei of the hypothalamus and limbic and cortical regions, impacting electromechanical events, sensation, and emotion. Afferent neural pathways also arise from non-digestive locations such as the pharynx, heart, bile ducts, and vestibular apparatus. Aberrant afferent signaling of vagal or splanchnic nerves, altered neuronal communication, environmental triggers, gut inflammation, alterations in the gut microbiome, visceral hypersensitivity, and numerous medications can impact this intricate network and lead to the generation of nausea and vomiting and the emotional experience of those symptoms.

The neural circuitry that mediates nausea and vomiting involves multiple receptors and neurotransmitters. Stimulation of the serotonin type 3 (5-HT_3) receptor provokes dopamine release which in turn stimulates the dopamine D2 receptor in

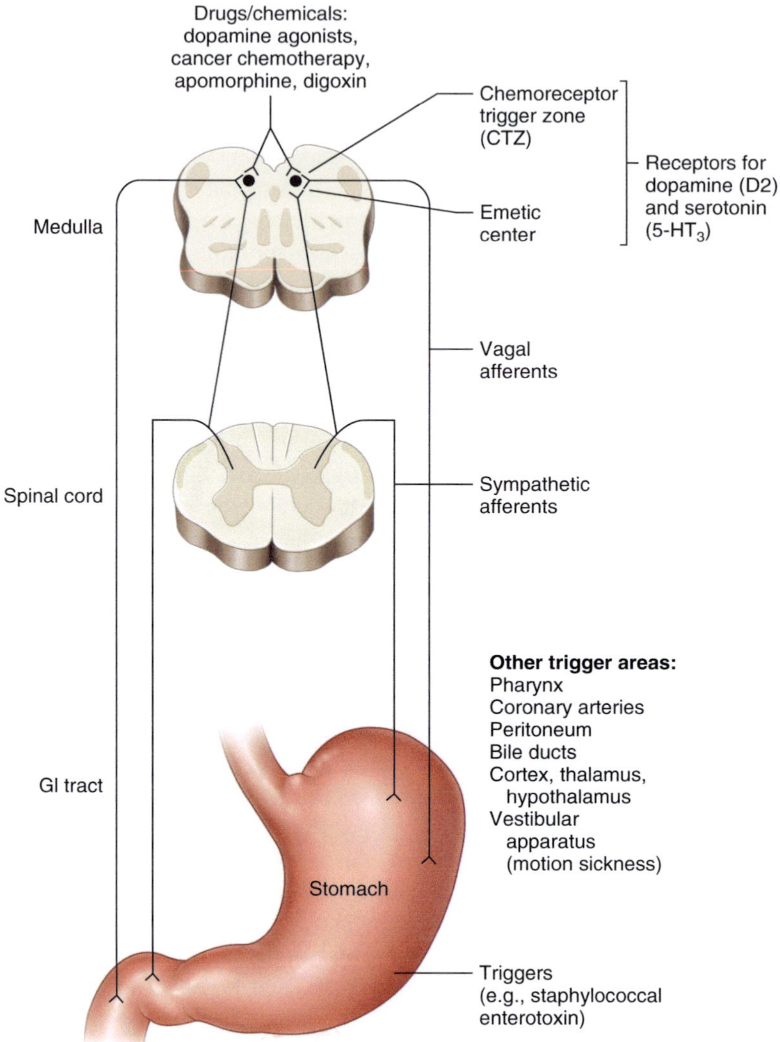

Fig. 7.1 Neural pathways that control nausea and vomiting

the emetic center, thereby activating the sequence that leads to the sensation of nausea. Activation of the histamine (H_1) and muscarinic (M_1) receptors, found in greater density in the vestibular center, triggers the sensation of nausea related to motion sickness and vestibular nausea. Cannabinoid receptors (CB1), mostly found in the dorsal vagal complex, inhibit the emetic reflex. The terminal emetic pathway involves the neurokinin-1 (NK-1) receptor that binds to substance P in the area postrema and NTS. Modification of these receptors and pathways form the basis of many therapeutic approaches for nausea described below. Table 7.3 highlights the anatomic localization and receptor mediation of various clinical emetic stimuli.

Table 7.3 Anatomic localization and receptor mediation of various clinical emetic stimuli

Anatomic site	Clinical stimuli	Receptors activated	Receptor-directed therapy
Area postrema	Medications (e.g., opiates, nicotine, cytotoxics), metabolic (e.g., uremia, hypercalcemia, hypoxemia), bacterial toxins, radiation therapy	Dopamine D2, Serotonin 5-HT_3, Histamine H1, Muscarinic M1	Antidopaminergics, 5-HT_3 antagonists
Labyrinths	Motion sickness, labyrinthine tumors or infections; Meniere's disease	Histamine H1, Muscarinic M1	Antihistamines, anticholinergics
Peripheral afferents	Gastric irritants (e.g., salicylate, antral distention); nongastric stimuli (i.e., colonic, biliary, intestinal distention); chemotherapy; pharyngeal stimulation	Serotonin 5-HT_3	5-HT_3 antagonists
Cerebral cortex Somatic pain	Noxious odors, visions, or tastes	Poorly characterized	

Adapted from Douglas A, Drossman M., Ed. (2006). Rome III: The functional gastrointestinal disorders. McLean, Virginia: Degnon Associates

Diagnosis and Evaluation

Given the complex biopsychosocial factors that are frequently present in patients presenting with chronic nausea, and the lack of controlled trials to guide a diagnostic approach, recommendations are based largely on expert opinion. A comprehensive history is the most critical aspect of the evaluation. The etiology of nausea can often be determined from a careful history and physical examination. Some historical features to consider include the presence and timing of nausea (e.g., constant or meal-related), associated vomiting, abdominal pain and distention, medication usage, heartburn, pregnancy, neurologic symptoms, vertigo, nystagmus, imbalance, eating disorders, sleep quality, and antecedent history of an infectious illness, among others. Psychological features should be explored, as elevated scores for hypochondriasis, depression, and hysteria have been reported on formal testing in patients with nausea of presumed psychogenic origin. Symptoms of functional dyspepsia, gastroparesis, and vomiting disorders need to be considered.

In addition to a thorough abdominal exam, the clinician should be mindful of the differential diagnosis, searching for signs of jaundice, lymphadenopathy, and metabolic, vestibular, and neurologic disorders. Importantly, a careful neurologic examination should include examination of the cranial nerves, a fundoscopic examination, and assessment of nystagmus and gait, and exclusion of focal deficits is essential. An attentive clinician may also recognize signs of anxiety or depression.

As a simple diagnostic marker for CIN does not exist, testing should be guided by the findings of the history and physical examination. Baseline biochemical testing should be performed to evaluate for the presence of anemia, renal dysfunction, hepatitis, and electrolyte abnormalities that may accompany nausea; serologic tests for hypercalcemia, hypothyroidism, and markers of inflammation should be checked. Cortisol levels, serum drug levels, and pregnancy tests should also be considered where appropriate. Empiric acid suppression may have both diagnostic and therapeutic utility in patients with heartburn or reflux symptoms, as gastroesophageal reflux disease can occasionally present with nausea. Mucosal disease of the upper gut is most accurately diagnosed with upper endoscopy. If no significant abnormalities are identified, additional testing should be guided by symptom duration, frequency, severity, and other relevant characteristics.

Abdominal imaging to assess patients with abdominal pain and alarm features (e.g., weight loss) should be pursued when clinically indicated. Studies of gastric function, such as gastric emptying, may be considered in patients with meal-related symptoms; however, these tests may be of low yield as symptoms in patients with dyspepsia do not appear to correlate with gastric emptying parameters. Nevertheless, identification of delayed gastric emptying might direct the clinician to other lines of therapy (see Chap. 20 on gastroparesis). Electrogastrography (EGG) can detect abnormalities of gastric myoelectric activity. However, this technique is not widely used and has not been shown to direct treatment in patients with nausea. Systemic illnesses, central nervous system lesions, and psychological factors should be considered when appropriate. Observation is indicated when no clear etiology for nausea is identified, as the cause may become more apparent over time. A suggested diagnostic algorithm for patients presenting with chronic nausea is provided in Fig. 7.2.

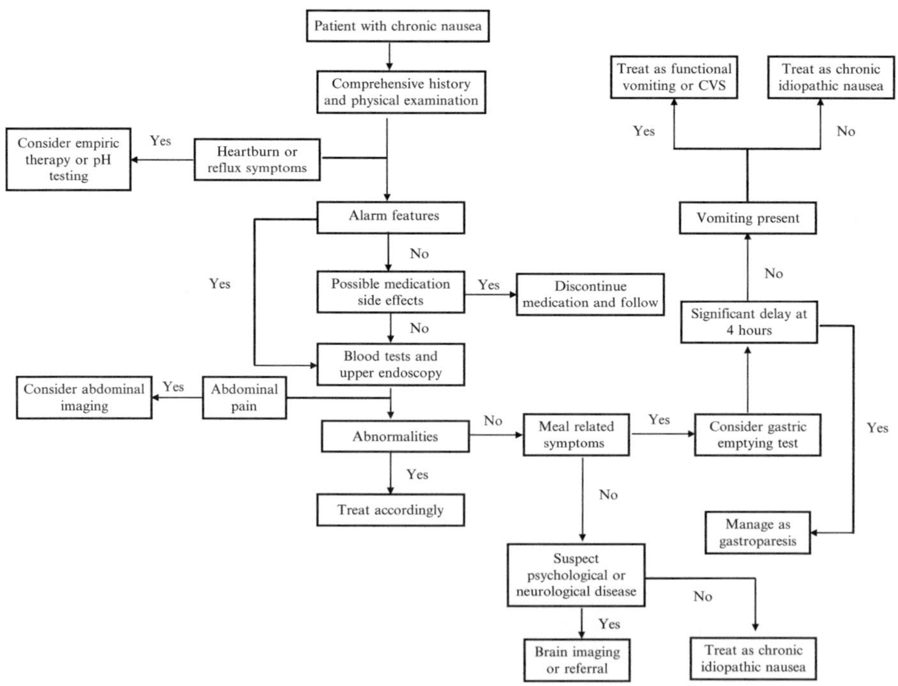

Fig. 7.2 Algorithm for diagnosis and evaluation for patients with chronic nausea

Treatment

Guiding management principles for CIN include focusing both on managing complications (e.g., weight loss, nutritional issues) and providing targeted therapy whenever possible. CIN is a challenge to treat, as patients are often resistant to both therapeutic and prophylactic pharmacologic interventions. Unlike acute nausea associated with certain conditions or therapies, there is limited data on the pharmacologic and non-pharmacologic treatments for CIN. Specific treatments and treatment duration are not defined. Empiric therapy to relieve symptoms is used if the diagnostic evaluation reveals no specific etiology. Antiemetics and prokinetics remain commonly used treatments; however, a variety of alternative therapies are also available (see Table 7.4). As a general rule, non-pharmacologic measures (e.g., behavioral therapy) are favored when available.

From a practical standpoint, it is often useful to determine if nausea is associated with meal ingestion and to differentiate these patients from those with more persistent or constant nausea. For patients with meal-generated symptoms, dietary modifications, acid suppressive therapy, and prokinetic agents may be reasonable options. As with a dyspeptic patient, dietary alterations may include small, frequent, low-fat, and low-fiber meals, while avoiding the ingestion of large amounts of liquid during meals. Antacids and acid suppression should be considered in patients with reflux symptoms and other acid-related issues.

Metoclopramide and domperidone are dopamine antagonists with central and peripheral actions. With both prokinetic and antiemetic properties, these agents are differentiated by the fact that domperidone does not cross the blood-brain barrier and is, therefore, free of the centrally mediated extrapyramidal side effects that are

Table 7.4 Therapeutic options for patients with chronic nausea

Therapy	Details	Comments/Examples
Dietary modification	Small, frequent meals Low fat and low residue Limit fluid intake with meals	May be most helpful for those with meal-related symptoms
Drugs	Acid suppression	Proton pump inhibitors, H_2 blockers, antacids
	Antiemetics	Phenothiazines, 5-HT_3 antagonists, histamine-1 antagonists, muscarinic antagonists, NK-1 antagonists, benzodiazepines, cannabinoids
	Prokinetics	Dopamine antagonists: metoclopramide, domperidone
	Antidepressants/viscerosensory modulators	Tricyclic antidepressants Other antidepressants
Behavioral	Diaphragmatic deep breathing, biofeedback, and relaxation techniques	Minimal risk Tailor to history
Alternative	Ginger, hypnosis, acupuncture/pressure	Efficacy in small trials

Table 7.5 Pharmacologic options for patients with chronic nausea

Drug class	Examples	Mechanism of action	Comments
Phenothiazines	Prochlorperazine, promethazine	Central and peripheral effects, D2 and 5-HT	Side effects may limit use
5-HT_3 antagonists	Ondansetron, granisetron	Central 5-HT_3 effects	Well tolerated Constipation
Histamine-1 antagonists	Diphenhydramine, meclizine, dimenhydrinate	Central vestibular H-1 effects	Motion sickness and vestibular nausea
Muscarinic-1 antagonists	Scopolamine	Peripheral and central effects	Motion sickness
Tricyclic antidepressants	Amitriptyline, nortriptyline	Serotonin and norepinephrine reuptake inhibitor	Low dose (10–50 mg daily)
Neurokinin-1 antagonists	Aprepitant	Peripheral and central effects	Chemotherapy-induced nausea and vomiting
Benzodiazepines	Lorazepam, diazepam	Central effects, $GABA_A$ receptor	Anxiolytic, chronic use not favored for nausea
Cannabinoids	Dronabinol, Cesamet	Central and peripheral effects in the CB receptor	Prominent side effects Chronic use not favored

associated with metoclopramide use. Although useful in some patients with nausea and vomiting in various clinical contexts (e.g., gastroparesis, chemotherapy), the side effect profile of metoclopramide and limited availability of domperidone in the United States often limit their usefulness. For patients without an obvious relationship to meals, consideration should be given to using medicines with purely antiemetic properties or those thought to impact visceral sensation.

Table 7.5 reviews various pharmacologic options for patients with chronic nausea. For all of these medications, their efficacy and safety in the therapy for chronic nausea is poorly described and their ultimate role in the management of chronic nausea remains to be defined. No single antiemetic drug or class of drugs has emerged as the best option. Ultimately, the decision regarding which medication to use should be based on mechanism of action, patient response, tolerance, and cost. Of note, some medications have different delivery routes that may be more advantageous in some situations (e.g., transdermal therapy). The clinician should try to avoid medications with strong adverse effect profiles that may complicate overall patient management. In particular, issues of sleep quality may impact drug choice, given the sedative effect of many of these drugs. Any drug choice should also follow a careful review of possible drug interactions.

Phenothiazine compounds mediate their actions primarily though a central anti-dopaminergic mechanism in the area postrema. They are available in various formulations and have been shown to be useful in a variety of clinical situations. 5-HT_3 antagonists, whose mechanism of action involves both central and peripheral components, are well tolerated and effective in many clinical situations (e.g., chemotherapy). Antihistamines and anticholinergics may be useful, especially when the nausea is associated with motion sickness or labyrinthitis. Associated drowsiness may limit their use, however.

Low-dose amitriptyline has been shown to decrease the sensation of nausea in healthy volunteers. Accordingly, tricyclic antidepressants (TCA) and other medications that may work on gastric sensation, via either central or peripheral mechanisms, could be considered for refractory nausea. Although open-label treatment trials using TCAs have reported improved symptom control in patients with idiopathic and diabetic gastroparesis, a recent double-blind, placebo-controlled trial did not demonstrate significant benefits of a TCA compared to placebo. Importantly, these medications are used at lower doses (e.g., 10–50 mg) compared with doses used in the management of anxiety and depression. Therefore, relevant psychological concerns should be addressed separately. A single case study reported mirtazapine, a 5-HT_2 receptor antagonist, to be efficacious in the symptoms of severe gastroparesis unresponsive to conventional prokinetic treatment.

Behavioral medicine approaches including biofeedback, relaxation techniques, and diaphragmatic deep breathing exercises should be considered in those patients with more persistent and difficult to treat nausea. Risks of therapy are minimal, and both published data and clinical experience suggest that this line of therapy can be helpful. Other treatment approaches to consider include ginger, acupuncture/acupressure, and hypnosis, each of which has shown efficacy in small trials involving patients with nausea and vomiting. Cannabinoids, which appear to work centrally in the region of the medulla oblongata, and benzodiazepines have also been shown to be of use in some patients with nausea and vomiting. Nevertheless, given prominent side effects and risk of dependency, chronic use is not recommended. Neurokinin-1 antagonists have shown efficacy in both acute and delayed nausea and vomiting associated with chemotherapy.

Case Resolution

Routine laboratory studies were normal, and there was no evidence of complications from her cholecystectomy. Upper endoscopy revealed no mucosal disease. Following a discussion regarding management of her chronic pain syndrome, she began a physical therapy program and was tapered off of her narcotic and nonsteroidal anti-inflammatory medications. Her nausea subsequently gradually resolved, and her bloating and constipation are no longer problematic. She was able to return to work with a greatly improved quality of life.

Key Clinical Teaching Points

- The differential diagnosis for patients presenting with chronic nausea is extensive, and adverse medication effects are among the most common etiologies.
- A careful history, including details about the nature and timing of nausea, is essential in the evaluation and treatment of the patient with chronic nausea.
- No one specific therapy has emerged as a single best option, and targeting therapy based on the findings and quality of symptom presentation should be a goal.
- Avoid pharmacologic therapies with strong side-effect profiles that may lead to additional symptoms that complicate patient management.

Teaching Questions

1. In a patient presenting with chronic nausea, a gastrointestinal etiology should be the main focus of the evaluation.

   (A) True
   (B) False

2. A 42-year-old female teacher presents with a 6-month history of nausea. Which one of the following is the most important component of her diagnostic evaluation?

   (A) History
   (B) Upper endoscopy
   (C) Gastric emptying test
   (D) Brain imaging

3. You are evaluating a 70-year-old man that has a 3-month history of nausea. On further history, he describes balance problems since the onset of the nausea. He denies vomiting, abdominal pain, or unintentional weight loss. He has been on a stable dose of an antihypertensive medication for 5 years. His evaluation reveals benign positional vertigo. Which of the following would be the best initial option to treat his nausea?

   (A) Ondansetron
   (B) Aprepitant
   (C) Meclizine
   (D) Omeprazole

Key References

1. Douglas A, Drossman M, editors. Rome III: The functional gastrointestinal disorders. McLean, Virginia: Degnon Associates; 2006. This book contains the guidelines and recommendations for all adult and pediatric functional gastrointestinal disorders.
2. Hasler WL, Chey WD. Nausea and vomiting. Gastroenterology. 2003;125(6):1860–7. A useful review on nausea and vomiting that remains applicable to clinical practice.
3. Pasricha PJ, Colvin R, Yates K, et al. Characteristics of patients with chronic unexplained nausea and vomiting and normal gastric emptying. Clin Gastroenterol Hepatol. 2011;9:567–76 e1–4. Recent article characterizing patients with CUNV, a new diagnostic category being proposed by some researchers.
4. Quigley EM, Hasler WL, Parkman HP. AGA technical review on nausea and vomiting. Gastroenterology. 2001;120:263–86. Comprehensive review covering the topic of nausea and vomiting.
5. Stapleton J, Wo JM. Current treatment of nausea and vomiting associated with gastroparesis: Antiemetics, prokinetics, tricyclics. Gastrointest Endosc Clin N Am. 2009;19(1):57–72. A recent review on medical therapy for nausea and vomiting associated with gastroparesis.

Chapter 8
Gastroparesis

Blake Scott and Kenneth L. Koch

Case Study

A 37-year-old Caucasian female is referred to gastroenterology for the evaluation of chronic nausea, vomiting, early satiety, and epigastric pain. Nausea is intermittent, located in the epigastric area, and often worse after ingestion of food. The patient describes forceful emesis after meals, and the vomitus consists of partially and/or undigested food. Her epigastric pain is sometimes worsened by eating without any particular food group implicated. Additionally, her abdominal pain is sometimes located in the right upper quadrant and exacerbated by twisting and/or bending movements. The patient's medical history is significant for cholecystectomy, gastroesophageal reflux disease, and major depressive disorder. She takes escitalopram for depression and ondansetron for relief of nausea. She denies alcohol, tobacco, and illicit substance use. Physical examination is remarkable for local RUQ tenderness at a port site (from her prior cholecystectomy); pain increases with palpation during head flexion, indicating a positive Carnett's sign. Routine hematologic and chemistry studies, TSH, and hemoglobin A1c testing are normal. An upper endoscopy is completely normal and the pylorus is patent. She undergoes further diagnostic testing with a 4 h solid phase gastric scintigraphy study which reveals 25 % meal retention at 4 h (normal 0–9 %). An electrogastrogram (EGG) with water load test reveals a normal 3 cpm electrical rhythm. Her diagnosis is idiopathic gastroparesis with a normal EGG rhythm.

B. Scott, M.D.
Wake Forest School of Medicine, Winston-Salem, NC, USA

K.L. Koch, M.D. (✉)
Section of Gastroenterology, Wake Forest Baptist Medical Center, Winston-Salem, NC, USA
e-mail: kkoch@wakehealth.edu

B.E. Lacy et al. (eds.), *Functional and Motility Disorders of the Gastrointestinal Tract*, DOI 10.1007/978-1-4939-1498-2_8

Introduction

Gastroparesis is now more widely recognized as a cause of chronic nausea and vomiting due to an increased physician awareness of the disease and the availability of standardized testing to objectively evaluate patients for delayed gastric emptying. For primary care physicians, endocrinologists, and gastroenterologists, the increasing incidence/prevalence of diabetes mellitus has resulted in an increase in the number of patients with gastroparesis. Recognizing symptoms of gastroparesis, having a basic knowledge of the underlying pathophysiology of gastroparesis, and establishing an accurate diagnosis enable providers to manage their patients effectively.

Epidemiology

The estimated incidence of gastroparesis in diabetic patients is approximately 2.4 new cases per 100,000 based on data collected in Olmsted County, MN, between years 1996 and 2006 in male patients. The incidence is estimated at 9.8 cases per 100,000 in women using the same data registry. The prevalence for both genders is 9.6 cases per 100,000 in men and 37.8 per 100,000 cases for women [1]. These estimates are based on definite cases of gastroparesis which means that these patients had both documented delayed gastric emptying on scintigraphic testing and typical symptoms associated with gastroparesis.

There are six general causes of gastroparesis (see Table 8.1). Diabetes mellitus and idiopathic gastroparesis are the two most widely reported gastroparesis subtypes. Diabetic gastroparesis is a widely recognized complication much like retinopathy, neuropathy, and nephropathy. The incidence of gastroparesis increases in patients who have had diabetes for over a decade. Idiopathic gastroparesis often develops after a febrile illness and may represent a post-infectious complication, similar to post-infectious IBS or functional dyspepsia. Other less common causes of gastroparesis include obstructive etiologies (e.g., pylorospasm or pyloric stenosis), chronic mesenteric ischemia, and complications of prior surgery (e.g., after fundoplication or vagotomy).

Table 8.1 Six categories of gastroparesis and underlying causes

Category	Causes
Obstructive	Pylorospasm; pyloric stenosis; post duodenal bulb tumors
Ischemic	Chronic mesenteric ischemia
Diabetic	Loss of ICCs and enteric neurons; pylorospasm
Idiopathic	Possibly post-viral; possibly degeneration of enteric neurons, loss of ICCs, smooth muscle
Postsurgical	Fundoplication; vagotomy; partial gastrectomy
Miscellaneous	Pseudo-obstruction secondary to scleroderma, SLE, Addison's disease, hypothyroidism

ICCs interstitial cells of Cajal, *SLE* systemic lupus erythematosus

Since obstructive and ischemic gastroparesis are potentially reversible, it is important to identify and treat these patients expeditiously. Miscellaneous and much less common causes of gastroparesis include scleroderma, systemic lupus erythematosus (SLE), Addison's disease, severe hypothyroidism, Parkinson's disease, amyloidosis, and a paraneoplastic process.

Pathophysiology

The neuromuscular basis for normal gastric emptying is complex and involves the coordinated interaction of the central nervous system, peripheral nervous system, enteric nervous system, pacemaker cells (called interstitial cells of Cajal (ICCs)), and gastric smooth muscle. The interactions of nerve and muscle allow the stomach to perform three major tasks in order to accomplish gastric emptying after the ingestion of food. First, the fundus relaxes in order to accommodate the food bolus presented from the esophagus. Second, the corpus and antrum mill the ingested food into chyme, 1–2 mm bits of food in suspension. Third, the nutrient suspension is emptied through the pylorus via corpus-antral peristaltic waves and antropyloroduodenal coordination.

Fundic accommodation is regulated by the vagus nerve in coordination with intramuscular ICCs located within the fundic wall. The fundus normally maintains a state of sustained contraction (high tone) via vagal efferents. This is in contrast to the antrum which has low tone. Ingested solids stimulate mechanoreceptors within the fundus, initiating a vagovagal reflex using nitric oxide, leading to smooth muscle relaxation within the fundus. In some gastroparesis patients a loss of neuronal nitric oxide synthetase impairs normal fundic relaxation. This same reflex arc may be injured in those patients who develop gastroparesis secondary to vagal nerve damage after fundoplication.

The second major function of the stomach is trituration, which refers to the mixing of ingested food to form chyme. This takes place in the corpus/antrum and is mediated primarily by the interaction between ICCs within the myenteric plexus (MY-ICCs), IM-ICC, enteric neurons, and circular smooth muscle cells. MY-ICCs located between the circular and longitudinal layers of smooth muscle are responsible for the generation of slow waves and act as pacemaker cells to coordinate circular muscle contraction. MY-ICCs establish a frequency of slow waves which occur normally at three cycles per minute. In the appropriate neurohumoral setting, gastric peristalsis occurs, which means that a wave of circular muscle contraction migrates from the proximal corpus to the pylorus at a rate of 3 contractions per minute. Thus, normal 3 cpm electrical pattern recorded in the EGG signal indicates normal integrated enteric neuron and ICC activity. The peristaltic contractions mix the ingested food with gastric acid, gastric lipase, and other various enzymes and break it down to form to chyme, the nutrient suspension that will empty into the duodenum. Loss of ICCs contributes to gastric dysrhythmias and uncoordinated and/or reduced gastric peristalsis which results in impaired emptying and the clinical diagnosis of gastroparesis.

The final step in emptying chyme from the gastric antrum into the duodenum is regulated by antral peristalsis coordinated with pyloric sphincter relaxation and reduced duodenal contractions, all of which is termed antropyloroduodenal coordination. Antral peristalsis and the emptying of chyme are affected by the size of food particles. Undigested solids require high-amplitude antral contractions to empty. Normally, pyloric tone increases to prevent large particles from emptying prematurely. Ordinarily, nitric oxide stimulates pyloric sphincter relaxation. Reduced nitric oxide has been implicated in the mechanism of pylorospasm or tonic contraction of the pylorus.

Gastric emptying is affected by many factors ranging from meal characteristics to pathologic changes in key gastric neuromuscular components. Neuromuscular disorders which tend to delay gastric emptying include gastric dysrhythmias, impaired fundic accommodation, antral hypomotility, and pylorospasm. Meal-related factors which tend to delay gastric emptying include increased acidity of ingested foods, fat content in foods, and indigestible fibers. Fats delay emptying more than carbohydrates or proteins. When high fat-containing meals are consumed, gastric lipases help break triglycerides into fatty acids and mono- and diglycerides which then enter the duodenum. Longer-chain fatty acids stimulate cholecystokinin (CCK) release which causes fundic relaxation, diminished antral contractions, and an increase in pyloric tone, the end result being a delay in gastric emptying. Monosaccharides stimulate the duodenum to release incretins (e.g., glucagonlike peptide (GLP-1)). These promote insulin secretion and induce antral hypomotility further delaying gastric emptying. Indigestible fibers delay gastric emptying due to their size, while hyperglycemia decreases antral contractions and induces gastric dysrhythmias leading to a delay in gastric emptying.

Diagnosis and Evaluation

Gastroparesis is a syndrome characterized by a documented delay in gastric emptying in the absence of mechanical obstruction. Symptoms associated with gastroparesis are nonspecific and include early satiety, postprandial fullness, nausea, vomiting, bloating, and upper abdominal pain. Note that there is significant symptom overlap with functional dyspepsia (see Chap. 5—this will be added at final edit).

The broad differential diagnosis of chronic nausea and vomiting, shown in Table 8.2, must be considered when evaluating patients who may have gastroparesis. For example, prominence of abdominal pain in conjunction with nausea and vomiting may herald the presence of peptic ulcer disease, biliary colic, mesenteric ischemia, pancreatitis, sphincter of Oddi dysfunction, or abdominal wall syndrome. The pain may be a trigger for nausea and vomiting, and if the underlying disease is addressed, the nausea and vomiting typically improves. Abdominal pain is the predominant symptom in approximately 20 % of patients with gastroparesis.

In patients with predominant nausea and vomiting, the differential diagnosis includes gastrointestinal entities such as GERD, cyclic vomiting syndrome, and rumination syndrome [2]. As noted in Table 8.2, non-gastrointestinal causes include

Table 8.2 Differential diagnosis of chronic nausea and vomiting

Gastrointestinal diseases
Bowel OBSTRUCTION due to mechanical causes
Peptic ulcer disease; mucosal inflammation (e.g., gastritis, esophagitis)
Gastroparesis
Gastric dysrhythmias
GERD
Rumination syndrome
Cyclic vomiting syndrome
Chronic mesenteric ischemia
Pancreatitis
Cholecystitis
Intestinal malignancies (e.g., gastric carcinoma, colonic carcinoma, etc.)
Non-gastrointestinal disease/causes
CNS disease (e.g., migraines, cerebrovascular disease, tumors, seizures)
Psychiatric disease (e.g., bulimia nervosa, anorexia nervosa)
Endocrinopathies (e.g., hyper/hypothyroidism, diabetes mellitus, adrenal insufficiency)
Hyperemesis gravidarum
Uremia
Medications (e.g., NSAIDs, chronic opiates, progesterone, lubiprostone, L-dopa, CCBs, digitalis, antiarrhythmics)
Extraintestinal malignancies (e.g., ovarian carcinoma, bronchogenic carcinoma, etc.)

entities such as medications (e.g., narcotics), Addison's disease, thyroid disease, uremia in the setting of chronic kidney disease, bulimia nervosa, and diseases originating from the central nervous system such as tumors and infections.

The history and physical examination are paramount to the initial evaluation of these patients. In patients with primary symptoms of pain, the presence of hematemesis, melena, and/or anemia should prompt evaluation for peptic ulcer disease. Postprandial pain associated with fatty food intake or abnormal liver function tests should prompt consideration for possible biliary colic. Sitophobia in a patient with risk factors for vascular disease such as dyslipidemia, smoking, diabetes mellitus, or other vascular disease should prompt consideration of mesenteric ischemia. Patients whose pain is localized to a highly specific location on the abdomen, often associated with a surgical scar, and related to position changes (e.g., twisting and/or bending) should be assessed for Carnett's sign. Carnett's sign is elicited by palpating the localized area of tenderness and then asking the patient to left their head off the pillow. With head flexion the abdominal wall contracts and the abdominal pain immediately worsens. This is considered a positive Carnett's sign and is suggestive of abdominal wall syndrome.

In patients with primary symptoms of nausea and vomiting, the history of forceful ejection of gastric contents is characteristic of vomiting, whereas the effortless return of undigested liquid or solids into the patient's mouth without burning or nausea is more characteristic of rumination. Regurgitation in the setting of GERD should be clearly differentiated from vomiting and rumination (and see Chap. 20).

Cyclic vomiting syndrome is characterized by intense episodes of nausea and vomiting which last for days with periods in between episodes where patients are totally symptom free. GERD is not always accompanied by characteristic heartburn. Nausea may be the atypical manifestation of GERD in the occasional patients. If asked to locate their nausea, these patients will indicate that they feel their nausea in the substernal area.

A careful history is important in elucidating the cause of gastroparesis. Patients with type 1 or 2 diabetes mellitus and non-gastric diabetic complications may have gastroparesis. Prior fundoplication, partial gastrectomies, vagotomy, and other intrathoracic or intra-abdominal procedures can all predispose to the development of gastroparesis. Symptoms that begin after a gastrointestinal febrile illness suggest post-infectious gastroparesis. Medications such as opioids, calcium channel blockers, GLP-1 agonists (exenatide in particular), cannabinoids, potent anticholinergic, and calcineurin inhibitors (e.g., cyclosporine) may all demonstrate delayed gastric emptying as a side effect.

Physical examination should include an assessment of volume status and nutrition. Careful inspection of the patient's dentition may reveal eroded enamel possibly implicating GERD or bulimia. Abdominal examination may reveal bruits suggestive of underlying vascular stenosis, tenderness suggestive of visceral inflammation, or a positive Carnett's sign implicating an abdominal wall syndrome.

The initial diagnostic testing performed once gastroparesis is suspected includes a complete blood count, metabolic profile, esophagogastroduodenoscopy (EGD), and gastric scintigraphy. Solid-phase gastric scintigraphy should be performed using a standardized solid meal and a 4 h exam [3]. Medications which could affect gastric emptying should be stopped 48–72 h prior to the exam. Typical offending agents include prokinetics, opioid analgesics, anticholinergics, and GLP-1 agonists. Patients must refrain from smoking the morning of the test and throughout the exam. For diabetic patients, the blood glucose should be less than 270 mg/dL [4]. Meal retention of >60 % at 2 h and >10 % retention at 4 h is considered diagnostic of delayed gastric emptying.

In evaluating patients with unexplained nausea and vomiting or gastroparesis, we find it helpful to obtain an electrogastrogram (EGG) with water load test to determine presence of gastric dysrhythmias or normal 3 cpm rhythm. The presence of a gastric dysrhythmia suggests depletion of ICCs and is congruent with delayed gastric emptying. On the other hand, the presence of normal 3 cpm activity after the water load is noncongruent and suggests the possibility of obstructive gastroparesis from mechanical pyloric obstruction (e.g., pyloric stenosis) or pylorospasm [4].

Treatment

The goals of gastroparesis therapy include maintaining hydration, electrolyte balance, ideal weight, and nutrition, improving patient symptoms, and preventing complications (e.g., bezoars, Mallory–Weiss tear). The armamentarium to achieve these goals is shown in Table 8.3 and includes the use of dietary modification,

Table 8.3 Drug and device treatments for symptoms of gastroparesis

Therapy	Mechanism	Adverse effects
Prokinetics		
Macrolide antibiotics Erythromycin 150–250 mg QID	Motilin receptor agonist	Nausea, diarrhea, abdominal cramping, antibiotic resistance, use limited by tachyphylaxis
Metoclopramide 5–20 mg AC and QHS	Dopamine$_2$ receptor antagonist, 5-HT3 receptor antagonist, 5-HT4 receptor agonist	Tardive dyskinesia, acute dystonias, extrapyramidal symptoms, depression, anxiety,
Domperidone 10–20 mg AC and QHS	Dopamine$_2$ receptor antagonist (peripheral acting)	galactorrhea, mastalgia, prolonged QT
Antispasmodics		
Dicyclomine 5–20 mg QAC & QHS	Muscarinic antagonist	Drowsiness and dry mouth
Antiemetics		
Ondansetron 4–8 mg QID PRN	5-HT$_3$ receptor antagonist	Headaches, increase LFTs
Granisetron 2 mg QD	5-HT$_3$ receptor antagonist	Hypotension, extrapyramidal symptoms
Prochlorperazine 5–10 mg TID PRN	Multiple CNS receptors	Drowsiness
Promethazine 25 mg TID PRN	H1 receptor antagonist	
<u>*Antiemetic/appetite stimulant*</u> Dronabinol 2.5–10 mg BID	Affects multiple CNS receptors; exact mechanism unclear	Palpitations, flushing, altered mentation/anxiety; can exacerbate nausea/vomiting, weakness
Antidepressants		
Amitriptyline 25–100 mg QHS Nortriptyline 10–75 mg QHS	Tricyclic antidepressant acting on multiple CNS receptors	constipation, sedation, arrhythmias
Benzodiazepines		
Alprazolam 0.25–0.5 mg TID Lorazepam 0.5–1 mg QID	GABA receptor antagonists	Sedation, dependence
<u>*Gastric electrical stimulation*</u>	Unclear	Complications of implanting the device, infection, lead migration, limited battery life
Endoscopic therapy		
Botulinum toxim A injection into pylorus	Relaxation of pylorus	None
Balloon dilation of pylorus	Stretch the pylorus	Bleeding, perforation
Dietary therapy		
Gastroparesis diet	Improve gastric empting based on physiology	None
High protein liquid supplements	Nutritional support, may reduce symptoms	
Surgical therapy		
Gastrostomy tube placement	Vent secretions to improve bloating, nausea, vomiting	Surgical complications, infection, tube dislodgement
Jejunostomy tube placement	Provides access to provide enteral nutrition	Same as gastrostomy
Gastrostomy tube with jejunal extension	Vent gastric secretions and provide enteral access for supplemental nutrition	Same as above; jejunal tubing can migrate retrograde causing gastric outlet obstruction
Pyloroplasty	Reduce gastric outflow resistance	Surgical complications

Table 8.4 Gastroparesis diet

Diet	Goal	Avoid
Step 1: in circumstances of severe nausea and vomiting Sports drinks, bouillon	Intake of salty liquids with caloric content to avoid dehydration Consume small volumes (120 mL/h) with overall goal to ingest 1000–1500 mL over 24 h	Highly sweetened drinks, citrus drinks
Step 2: begin once routinely tolerating step 1 Soup with noodles/rice, crackers with peanut butter/cheese, chewy confections (i.e., caramel) Consume in 6+ small volume meals/day	Consume 1,500 cal/day	Cream, milk-based liquids
Step 3: begin once routinely tolerating step 2 Starches, chicken, fish Starches include pastas, noodles, mashed/baked potatoes Chicken/fish (not fried) consume in 6 or more small volume meals/day	Consume solid foods which are palatable and easy to triturate yet do not provoke nausea/vomiting	High fat content, red meats and fresh vegetables, pulpy fibrous foods which are difficult to triturate

prokinetic agents, antiemetic agents, gastric electrical stimulators, and enteral nutritional support. In selected subpopulations botulinum A toxin injections and pyloroplasty may be considered.

Dietary modifications are safe and can be effective in patients who are counseled to adhere to the general principles. The typical dietary suggestions are shown in Table 8.4. The basic principles involve consumption of foods that are easy to triturate and empty. Foods high in fat content and fiber and large-volume meals delay gastric emptying and should be avoided. Patients are encouraged to eat smaller meals more frequently, e.g., six small meals per day [5]. The stepwise dietary program outlined in Table 8.4 focuses on the principles of rehydration and electrolyte restoration during acute flares of nausea and vomiting. As symptoms improve the diet is advanced by the patient to involve soups/smoothies and then more solid foods that are easily triturated.

The goal of drug therapy is to improve symptoms and improve the rate of gastric emptying. Prokinetic therapies are prescribed to improve gastric emptying [6]. Unfortunately improvement in gastric emptying does not reproducibly correlate with symptoms associated with gastroparesis. Metoclopramide is the only FDA-approved medication for the treatment of gastroparesis. Metoclopramide and domperidone are dopamine receptor antagonists which tend to promote gastric emptying. Dopamine inhibits release of acetylcholine which subsequently reduces gastric emptying as well as small bowel motility. Metoclopramide traverses the blood–brain barrier, and thus its use is often limited by side effects (anxiety, depression, insomnia, jitteriness, gynecomastia, change in libido, and rarely tardive dyskinesia).

Metoclopramide now has a black box warning due to the rare but well-documented side effect of tardive dyskinesia. Generally the smallest effective dose is preferentially used, and oral disintegrating tablets as well as liquid formulations are available to promote improved absorption. Domperidone affects peripheral dopamine receptors and has less CNS penetration than metoclopramide which gives domperidone a more favorable side effect profile. Domperidone is not approved in the United States, but is available via an investigational new drug (IND) application through the FDA.

Macrolide antibiotics stimulate motilin receptors within the stomach and promote gastric emptying. Erythromycin is the prototype for this class of medication, but the chronic use of these agents is limited by tachyphylaxis.

Antiemetic agents such as the phenothiazines (prochlorperazine), antihistamine agents (promethazine), as well as 5-HT_3 receptor antagonists (ondansetron) are all commonly used for symptomatic management of patients with gastroparesis, but there is a paucity of data to suggest any particular drug class is superior to another.

Patients with a pain component attributable to their gastroparesis are often times empirically treated with tricyclic antidepressants (TCAs) given their pain modification properties. Nortriptyline is typically the agent of choice given a lower incidence of observed anticholinergic activity as compared with amitriptyline, although a recent double-blind, placebo-controlled study did not show any significant benefit of TCAs compared with placebo.

Pylorospasm may produce functional gastric outlet obstruction. Injection of botulinum toxin A into the pyloric sphincter in patients with diabetic gastroparesis and idiopathic gastroparesis improved gastric emptying, but not symptoms, in some patients although it is not recommended for routine use. Patient selection is likely a key factor in treatment outcomes. In patients with gastroparesis and normal 3 cycle per minute EGG recordings, injection of botulinum toxin A into the pylorus reduced gastroparesis symptoms. In several patients, pyloroplasty resulted in sustained improvement in symptoms and improved gastric emptying.

Patients with refractory gastroparesis symptoms despite dietary modification and pharmacotherapy agents are challenging. Gastric electrical stimulation (GES) may be considered in these patients [7]. In gastric electrical stimulation, two leads are implanted into the antrum, and the generator device positioned in a subcutaneous pocket delivers high-frequency (12 cpm), low-energy (330 mv) electrical stimulation to the stomach. The device (Enterra, Medtronic Inc.) is allowed by the FDA for compassionate therapy in drug-refractory gastroparesis as a humanitarian device exemption. The mechanism of action of GES is unknown at this time. Complications of GES include lead migration, gastric perforation and pocket infection, and the risks of surgical implantation of the device. Patients with drug-refractory diabetic gastroparesis appear to respond better with GES compared with idiopathic gastroparesis.

In patients who are unable to maintain adequate nutritional status, surgical treatments may be necessary to ameliorate symptoms and provide access for enteral feedings. Venting gastrostomy and feeding jejunostomy tubes are used to manage vomiting and to provide enteral feedings for nutrition support in patients with refractory gastroparesis.

Case Resolution

The patient was diagnosed with idiopathic gastroparesis. However, the possibility of functional gastric outlet obstruction secondary to pylorospasm was considered because the EGG recording showed a normal 3 cpm rhythm. Prokinetic therapy with metoclopramide and gastroparesis dietary counseling resulted in minimal relief of symptoms. The patient underwent endoscopy with intrapyloric injection of botulinum toxin A and pyloric balloon dilation. Three weeks later she returned to clinic endorsing an improvement in nausea, vomiting, and early satiety. Symptoms recurred months later, and repeat endoscopy with botulinum A toxin injection resulted in similar improvement in her symptoms. Ultimately the patient had pyloromyotomy and subsequently gained weight, had normal gastric emptying, and reported sustained improvement in symptoms.

Key Clinical Teaching Points

- Gastroparesis is defined as the presence of typical symptoms (early satiates, prolonged fullren, nausea, vomiting) in the setting of a documented delay in gastric emptying in the absence of mechanical obstruction.
- Symptoms associated with idiopathic gastroparesis overlap with functional dyspepsia symptoms.
- The initial goals of therapy are to maintain hydration, correct electrolyte imbalances, maintain an adequate weight, and improve symptoms of nausea and vomiting.
- Prokinetic agents improve gastric emptying in some patients, but this does not always translate into an improvement in symptoms.
- Well-designed, prospective, placebo-controlled trials to evaluate the safety and efficacy of antiemetic agents are lacking.

Teaching Questions

1. A 55-year-old woman with a known history of type I diabetes mellitus presents for evaluation of recent onset of nausea, postprandial non-bloody emesis, and occasional abdominal pain which is epigastric and non-radiating. She has chronic loose stools, but does not endorse melena. Lab work is obtained, and she is not anemic. What diagnostic test would you perform next?

   (A) Right upper quadrant ultrasound
   (B) 4 h gastric scintigraphy
   (C) Esophagogastroduodenoscopy (EGD)
   (D) CT scan of the abdomen

2. A 48-year-old obese female is evaluated by her primary care provider for chronic nausea and vomiting. She has a 15-year history of progressively difficult to manage type II diabetes mellitus which is presently controlled with metformin, glipizide, and exenatide. She takes Vicodin for chronic back pain. She is referred for consultation. EGD is normal. A 4 h gastric scintigraphy is ordered. Which of the following instructions should be stressed to the patient prior to performing the gastric emptying test?

   (A) She should be instructed to stop using her Vicodin at least 48 h prior to the test.
   (B) She should be instructed to stop using her exenatide at least 48 h prior to the test.
   (C) She should stop using all of her diabetic medications prior to the test.
   (D) Both A and B are correct.
   (E) All of the above are correct.

3. A 55-year-old woman with idiopathic gastroparesis possibly secondary to a viral infection presents for evaluation and management of nausea and vomiting. She has 20 % retention of solid food at 4 h as assessed by a 4 h gastric emptying test. Her EGD is normal. She has been symptomatic for 4 months since a viral-type illness. She is currently taking ondansetron for nausea management with some improvement in symptoms. She eats three meals a day and tells you that she has two young children, and both she and her children are terribly busy and frequently eat on the go at local fast food restaurants. She has not lost any significant amount of weight since her diagnosis. What therapeutic recommendations would you make at this time?

   (A) Review the gastroparesis diet (eat smaller, more frequent meals, and avoid eating at fast food restaurants) and refer to a dietician.
   (B) Refer her to a general surgeon for gastric electrical stimulation therapy.
   (C) Refer her to a general surgeon for gastrostomy tube for venting.
   (D) Refer her to gastroenterology for pyloric botulinum toxin A injections.

4. A 44-year-old male with diabetic gastroparesis is referred to your clinic for management of chronic nausea and vomiting. His past medical history is significant for diabetes mellitus complicated by diabetic retinopathy and nephropathy manifested by microalbuminuria with normal estimated glomerular filtration rate. Review of systems reveals that he is generally constipated and strains to have a bowel movement every 3–4 days. He denies abdominal pain. His workup reveals a hemoglobin A1c of 9 %, a normal EGD, and 30 % meal retention on a 4 h solid-phase gastric emptying test. His endocrinologist intensifies his insulin regimen to improve his blood glucose levels. He is referred to a dietician for counseling regarding a gastroparesis diet. At a 3-month follow-up visit, his hemoglobin A1c is 7.2 %, and he reports strict compliance with the gastroparesis diet. He continues to experience nausea. Which treatment would be a reasonable addition for treatment of his ongoing nausea?

(A) Metoclopramide 5 mg AC and QHS
(B) Dicyclomine 20 mg AC and QHS
(C) Amitriptyline 100 mg QHS
(D) All of the above

Key References

1. Camilleri M, Bharucha A, Farrugia G. Epidemiology, mechanisms and management of diabetic gastroparesis. Clin Gastroenterol Hepatol. 2011;9(1):5–e7. A nice study describing the epidemiology of gastroparesis.
2. Camilleri M, Parkman H, Shafi M, Abell TL, Gerson L, American College of Gastroenterology. Clinical guideline: Management of gastroparesis. Am J Gastroenterol. 2013;108:18–37. A very thorough review of treatment options for gastroparesis.
3. Abell T, Camilleri M, Donohoe K, Hasler WL, Lin HC, Maurer AH, et al. Consensus recommendations for gastric emptying scintigraphy: A joint report of the American Neurogastroenterology and Motility Society and the Society of Nuclear Medicine. J Nucl Med Technol. 2008;36:44–54. A consensus document highlighting the need to perform gastric emptying scans in a standardized manner.
4. Brzana RJ, Koch KL, Bingaman S. Gastric myoelectrical activity in patients with gastric outlet obstruction and idiopathic gastroparesis. Am J Gastroenterol. 1998;93(10):1803–09. An interesting article on the electrophysiology of the stomach in the subset of patients with gastroparesis due to outlet obstruction.
5. Koch K. Gastric neuromuscular function and neuromuscular disorders. Sleisenger and Fordtran's gastrointestinal and liver disease 9th Ed 2010; 789–815. A nice review of the abnormal physiology that underlies gastroparesis.
6. Hejazi R, McCallum R, Sarosiek I. Prokinetics in diabetic gastroparesis. Curr Gastroenterol Rep. 2012;14:297–305. A recent review article on the use of prokinetics in patients with diabetic gastroparesis.
7. McCallum RW, Snape W, Brody F, Wo J, Parkman HP, Nowak T. Gastric electrical stimulation with Enterra therapy improves symptoms from diabetic gastroparesis in a prospective study. Clin Gastroenterol Hepatol. 2010;11:947–54. A recent prospective study demonstrating the efficacy of gastric electrical stimulation for the treatment of diabetic gastroparesis.

Chapter 9
Cyclical Vomiting Syndrome

Nicholas J. Talley and Kate E. Napthali

Case Study

A 45-year-old woman was referred with symptoms of recurrent vomiting and diarrhea. Her background medical history was significant for abnormal liver function tests, an elevated BMI, and a liver biopsy which showed hyperglycogenosis and mild predominantly portal inflammation. Her past medical history was significant for recurrent severe migraine headaches. She was on thyroxine replacement therapy for hypothyroidism, was a nonsmoker, and did not consume alcohol. Her symptoms started a year ago after an episode of acute gastroenteritis; only *Blastocystis hominis* was found in her stools. She was treated with metronidazole; however her symptoms of recurrent vomiting and diarrhea persisted despite convalescent stool specimens which showed that the *Blastocystis* had resolved. The vomiting pattern was intermittent occurring fortnightly. Each episode began usually in the morning with intense nausea and headache. She was perfectly well in between vomiting attacks except for loose stools and mild abdominal pain relieved by defecation. She denied cannabis use or compulsive bathing. Investigations including a complete blood count, electrolyte panel, esophagogastroduodenoscopy (EGD) and colonoscopy including biopsies, and a hormonal screen, including vasoactive intestinal peptide and chromogranin A, were all normal. The patient was diagnosed as having cyclic vomiting syndrome (with associated migraine) and post-infectious irritable bowel syndrome (IBS).

N.J. Talley, M.D., Ph.D. (✉)
Faculty of Health and Medicine, University of Newcastle,
New Lambton, NSW, Australia
e-mail: nicholas.talley@newcastle.edu.au

K.E. Napthali, FRACP
John Hunter Hospital, University of Newcastle, Newcastle, NSW, Australia

B.E. Lacy et al. (eds.), *Functional and Motility Disorders of the Gastrointestinal Tract*, DOI 10.1007/978-1-4939-1498-2_9

Introduction

Cyclical vomiting syndrome (CVS) is a highly characteristic disorder, and the diagnosis can readily be made if an accurate history is obtained. CVS is characterized by episodic vomiting and associated intense nausea which resolves spontaneously. The episodes can last from 24 h to up to 2 weeks. Characteristically patients have no nausea or vomiting between episodes, but they may report abdominal pain. First described by French physicians in the mid-nineteenth century in children, CVS is now increasingly recognized in adults. Despite the episodic nature of CVS, it results in significant morbidity with up to 50 % of patients requiring admission and intravenous hydration during each attack and a mean of 20 days' school missed per academic year.

Epidemiology

There are limited data available to accurately assess the prevalence of CVS. Although generally considered to be rare, CVS is diagnosed more frequently in children than in adults and, as such, a larger number of cross-sectional studies are available to assess prevalence of the condition in the pediatric population.

A cross-sectional study from Aberdeen found that of 2,165 children 1.9 % fulfilled the diagnostic criteria for CVS, with an average age of onset of 5.3 years. In this population, the coexistent diagnosis of migraine headache was twice as likely as in the normal population, reinforcing a long held belief that the two entities are linked. A second, cross-sectional study undertaken in Sri Lanka assessed the prevalence of all functional gut disorders in 427 adolescents aged between 12 and 16. Of the patients included in the study, 0.5 % fulfilled criteria for the diagnosis for CVS. Similarly, in a Turkish study of 1,263 children aged 7–14 years of age, 1.9 % of children fulfilled the criteria for CVS and, of these, 29 % had a family or personal history of migraine. The epidemiology in adults is less well defined, but the median age of onset of CVS in adults was 34 years.

Pathophysiology

The pathogenesis of CVS is incompletely understood, but associations with migraine, metabolic syndromes, hypothalamic–pituitary axis dysfunction, chronic cannabis use, and autonomic dysregulation have been reported. Precipitants for CVS include episodes of heightened emotional response such as birthdays, outings, or emotional stress. Also reported to be a trigger for episodes of vomiting are periods of heightened metabolic demand such as intercurrent illness, fever, or exercise.

Migraine

Based on the cross-sectional studies described above, there is broad consensus that a relationship exists between pediatric CVS and pediatric migraine. Furthermore, an association has been established between those pediatric patients with CVS and those with a genetic polymorphism in mitochondrial DNA (mtDNA) usually observed in adults with migraine. Subsequent studies found that the mtDNA polymorphisms 16519T and 3010A were not associated with adult-onset CVS; however the association with pediatric migraine was again observed.

Metabolic Syndromes

The relationship between episodes of CVS and heightened metabolic demand led to the identification of an association between CVS and mitochondriopathies including mitochondrial encephalomyopathy, lactic acidosis, and stroke-like episodes (MELAS) and medium chain acyl-CoA dehydrogenase deficiency (MCAD). The association between mtDNA and CVS has been supported by the observation that elevated levels of Krebs cycle intermediates are found in the peripheral circulation of children during acute attacks of CVS, and this profile is similar to that of people with known mitochondrial disorders. As the association between mtDNA polymorphism and CVS in children has been established, a similar association between CVS and other disorders of mitochondrial inheritance has been suggested, but these are all rare. These syndromes can be identified through mtDNA analysis and identification of a point mutation.

Hypothalamic–Pituitary–Adrenal Axis Dysfunction

Elevated corticotrophin-releasing factor (CRF) is known to impair gastric emptying, and elevations in serum CRF are observed during periods of emotional or physical stress. CVS is precipitated by stimuli or states associated with stimulation of CRF release, and the resulting endocrine, autonomic, and visceral changes are suggestive of central CRF activation. Although further studies are needed to establish the role of elevated CRF as a pathogenic mediator of CVS, the hypothesis is supported by observations that children have elevated levels of CRF in the peripheral circulation. Furthermore, tricyclic antidepressants (TCAs), frequently used to treat CVS, are also known to inhibit the promoter activity of the CRF gene. The relevance of central CRF activation in the pathophysiology of CVS deserves further consideration.

Chronic Cannabis Use (Cannabinoid Hyperemesis)

Cannabis is a very widely taken drug in many countries with a lifetime prevalence of over 40 % in the USA. Often used for its antiemetic properties, chronic cannabis use has also been associated with a specific syndrome of cyclic vomiting, abdominal pain, and compulsive bathing. In a case series published in 2004, of 9 patients with cannabis hyperemesis, 7 patients had their symptoms resolve completely with cessation of cannabis use. Similarly, in 98 patients presenting to hospital with a history of daily to weekly cannabis use, they all experienced protracted nausea and vomiting, comorbid abdominal pain, and compulsive bathing. It should be noted that the patterns of vomiting in cannabinoid hyperemesis (CH) do not necessarily fulfill the Rome III criteria for CVS, and it should probably be considered a distinct entity.

Diagnosis and Evaluation

A positive diagnosis should be made on the history (Tables 9.1 and 9.2). There are no specific investigations available to diagnose CVS, but essential to the diagnosis is the exclusion of serious surgical or medical causes of nausea and vomiting. Warning signs for an alternative cause of recurrent vomiting include localized severe abdominal pain, hematemesis, fever, or central nervous system signs (e.g., meningism or visual disturbance). It is important to note that fever can occur in CVS from associated autonomic dysfunction, while hematemesis may develop from a Mallory–Weiss tear. Always ask about any history of cannabis use to exclude cannabis hyperemesis. On physical examination look for any evidence of other rare causes of vomiting such as Addison's disease (pigmentation). A brainstem tumor causing vomiting, also very rare, almost always also causes neurological symptoms or signs.

The initial testing approach that we recommend is a baseline blood panel which would include electrolytes, liver and pancreatic enzyme screening, and a urinalysis, and in children, an evaluation for metabolic disorders (which would include lactate, ammonia, and amino acids). Judicious use of imaging, limiting radiation exposure, and EGD should be considered. If there are no red flags and if the attacks follow a relatively predictable temporal pattern with identifiable triggers, then the diagnosis of CVS is established.

Table 9.1 The Rome III criteria for the diagnosis of CVS in adults

1. Stereotypical episodes of vomiting regarding onset (acute) and duration (less than 1 week)
2. Three or more discrete episodes in the prior year
3. Absence of nausea and vomiting between episodes
Supportive (minor) criteria for the diagnosis would be a personal or family history of migraine headache

Table 9.2 Clinical features of cyclic vomiting in children and adults

		Children	Adults
Female: Male		Slight female preponderance	Similar
Mean age of onset		4.8 years	35 years
Symptoms	Vomiting	6 times/h at peak, bilious (81 %), bloody (34 %)	Episodic stereotypical attacks
	Systemic	Lethargy (93 %), pallor (91 %), fever (30 %)	
	GI	Salivation (27 %), nausea (82 %), abdominal pain (81 %), anorexia (81 %), retching (79 %), diarrhea (30 %)	Abdominal pain (71 %), diarrhea (19 %)
	Neurological	Headache (42 %), photophobia (38 %), phonophobia (38 %), vertigo 26 %	None
Temporal pattern	Duration	24 h	3 days
	Prodrome, recovery	1.5 h, 6 h	Nausea, epigastric pain
	Periodic	49 % have regular intervals, usually 2–4 weeks	3 months
	Circadian	Early morning onset (42 %)	Not applicable
	Stereotypical	Usually	Usually
Precipitating events		Psychological stress (47 %), infection (31 %), exhaustion (24 %), dietary (23 %), menses (22 %)—1, or more triggers identified (76 %)	Menses (57 %)
Natural history		3.6+ years, 28 % progress to migraine	Unknown
Complications		Secondary esophagitis	Secondary to recurrent vomiting
Family history of migraine		82 %	24 %

Adapted from *Cyclic vomiting syndrome: a brain–gut disorder* B U.K. Li, Misiewicz, L Gastroenterol Clin N Am 2003; 32: 997–1019—permission granted 04/07/2013

Treatment

Once diagnosed, the treatment approach to CVS should address both the emetic and the non-emetic phases of the cycle.

Emetic Phase

Limited evidence is available to guide the management of the acute emetic phase of CVS. The evidence—such as it is—is limited to small case series and anecdotal reports which advocate symptomatic relief, intravenous fluid, and sedation to control symptoms.

Supportive Therapy

Intravenous dextrose is the fluid of choice in CVS. Given the postulated role of mitochondrial dysfunction, it is thought that the administration of dextrose solution intravenously may buffer the energy cycle malfunction in a subset of pediatric patients with CVS. As psychological and physical stimuli can exacerbate the vomiting and nausea during this phase of CVS, benzodiazepine sedation and use of a low stimuli environment such as a single darkened room should be considered.

Antiemetic Therapy

$5HT_3$ antagonists such as ondansetron or granisetron are generally more effective than dopamine antagonists such as prochlorperazine.

Antimigraine Therapy

Antimigraine medications can be used to terminate the acute emetic phase of the cycle. Triptans such as sumatriptan and zolmitriptan can be used at this time. If the acute migraine treatment does not settle the episode within a reasonable period of time (2–3 h), further supportive therapy should be considered.

Non-emetic Phase

In those patients—both pediatric and adult—who have a clear trigger, efforts should be made to remove these precipitants, but triggers are less common in adults. Cannabis must be stopped even if the patient believes its use is helping any nausea (they are often mistaken!). Ask about the role of sleep deprivation, over excitability, ingestion of certain foods such as cheese or chocolate, or menses.

In those patients who have a prior personal or family history of migraine headache, trialing antimigraine medications can be considered. Antimigraine medications are also sometimes considered in those patients with no specific personal or family history of headache. A systematic review of the management of CVS published in 2012 reviewed the management of 1,093 cases in 25 papers and found that TCAs and antimigraine therapies appeared to be helpful (Table 9.3).

As can be observed in Table 9.3, TCAs remain the medication of choice in both adult and pediatric CVS with the largest numbers studied and the most consistent effect. It is known that TCAs have some effect on migraine, and other antimigraine

Table 9.3 Response of pediatric cyclic vomiting syndrome to medications (uncontrolled studies)

Drug	No of patients	Response (%)
Tricyclic antidepressants	244	67.6
Propranolol	91	86.8
L-Carnitine and amitriptyline	30	76.7
Erythromycin	20	65
Coenzyme Q	18	66.7
Phenobarbital	14	78.6
Valproate	13	100
Pizotifen	8	50
Cyproheptadine	6	83.3
L-Carnitine	6	100
Response of adult cyclic vomiting syndrome to medication		
Tricyclic antidepressants	237	75.5
Sumatriptan	37	56.8
Zonisamide/levetiracetam	20	75
Coenzyme Q	7	71.4

Adapted from Lee L, Abbott L, Mahlangu B *et al* The management of cyclic vomiting syndrome: a systematic review. *European Journal of Gastroenterology and Hepatology*, 2012, Vol 24 No 9 p1004 (permission received 4/7/13 online)

medications such as propranolol and sumatriptan were found to also have some efficacy, albeit in smaller numbers. Case series' using coenzyme Q10, L-carnitine, clonidine, and cyproheptadine have been reported; however the numbers are small in these case series.

Consider first line a trial of amitriptyline if the attacks of CVS occur more than one to two times a month or if the attacks, when they occur, have a significant impact on the patients' day-to-day activities, manifest by prolonged hospital stays or time off work/school. Start at a dosage of 10 mg at night and then 25 mg 2 weeks later and increase if tolerated every few weeks by 25 mg up to 75 mg at night (higher doses may sometimes be needed). Consider switching to imipramine or another secondary tricyclic if amitriptyline is not tolerated. Similar to depression, it may take up to several weeks of therapy to see maximal benefit. Given the limitations of use of amitriptyline in the infant and pediatric population under 5 years of age, propranolol is an alternative agent.

In the pediatric population, an antimigraine (low amine) diet (LAD) has been put forward as an alternative approach. In one study of 21 children with CVS, 13 responded to the LAD with complete resolution of symptoms at 8 weeks, while 5 showed partial resolution, 2 had no response, and one was lost to follow-up. These results reflect a similar small single-center uncontrolled study in Italy which also showed an excellent response to an exclusion diet in children with CVS. The role of diet in adults is unknown.

Case Resolution

The patient was started on 10 mg per day of amitriptyline, which was slowly increased up to 75 mg and administered at night. She was reviewed several months later, and her symptoms had resolved. The plan is to wean her off the tricyclic in another 3 months. She also reported that her migraine headache had improved significantly after commencement of therapy.

Key Clinical Teaching Points

- Many clinicians mistakenly believe that CVS is a disorder only of children; although less well characterized, CVS can develop in adults.
- The clinical history of recurrent episodic nausea and vomiting with symptom-free intervals in-between acute episodes is nearly diagnostic of CVS. A thorough history should include questions about cannabis use, as cannabinoid hyperemesis can mimic CVS.
- An exhaustive, and costly, battery of tests need not be performed in every patient in order to accurately diagnose CVS. A careful history and examination to exclude an organic process and a review of the Rome III criteria, coupled with a limited number of diagnostic studies, are generally sufficient.
- CVS can be effectively treated; the art of effective medical management is finding the appropriate medication regimen for each patient. Many patients require multiple therapeutic interventions until the right medication is identified, and some patients will require combination therapy (e.g., a TCA and a triptan).

Teaching Questions

1. CVS is synonymous with cannabis hyperemesis.

   (A) True
   (B) False

2. The etiology of CVS in children is:

   (A) Secondary to a deficiency in amines
   (B) Due to an overproduction of serotonin
   (C) Multifactorial in nature
   (D) Predominantly psychogenic

3. True or false: CVS develops only in children, although it can extend in to adulthood.

   (A) True
   (B) False

4. Therapeutic options for CVS include:

   (A) Diet
   (B) Tricyclic antidepressants
   (C) Triptans
   (D) Beta-blockers
   (E) All of the above

Key References

1. Abell T, Adams K, et al. Cyclic vomiting syndrome in adults. Neurogastroenterol Motil. 2008;20:269–84.
2. Abraham M, Porter P. Clonidine in cyclic vomiting. JPGN. 2011;53:219–21.
3. Abu-Arafeh I, Russell G. Cyclical vomiting syndrome in children: A population based study. J Paediatr Gastroenterol Nutr. 1995;21:454–8.
4. Allen JH, deMoore GM, et al. Cannabinoid hyperemesis: Cyclical hyperemesis in association with chronic cannabis abuse. Gut. 2004;53:1566–70.
5. Andersen JM, Sugerman KS, Lockhart JR, Weinberg WA. Effective prophylactic therapy for cyclic vomiting syndrome in children using amitriptyline or cyproheptadine. Pediatrics. 1997;100:977–81.
6. Boles R. High degree of efficacy in the treatment of cyclic vomiting syndrome with combined coenzyme Q10, L carnitine and amitriptyline, a case series. BMC Neurol. 2011;11:102.
7. Boles RG, Zaki EA, Lavenbarg T, et al. Are paediatric and adult onset cyclic vomiting syndrome (CVS) biologically different conditions? Relationship of adult-onset CVS with the migraine and pediatric CVS-associated common mtDNA polymorphisms 16519 T and 3010A. Neurogastroenterol Motil. 2009;21:936–e72.
8. Chang Y, Windish D. Cannabinoid hyperemesis relieved by compulsive bathing. Mayo Clin Proc. 2009;84:76–8.
9. Degenhardt L, Chiu W, Sampson N, et al. Toward a global view of alcohol, tobacco, cannabis, and cocaine use: Findings from the WHO World Mental Health Surveys. PLoS Med. 2008;5(7):e141.
10. Devanarayana N, Adhikari C, Pannala W, Rajindrajith S. Prevalence of functional gastrointestinal diseases in a cohort of Sri Lankan adolescents: comparison between Rome II and Rome III criteria. J Trop Pediatr. 2011;57:34–9.
11. Ertekin V, Selimoglu MA, Altnkaynak S. Prevalence of cyclic vomiting syndrome in a sample of Turkish school children in an urban area. J Clin Gastroenterol. 2006;40:896–8.
12. Hejazi R, McCallum R. Cyclic vomiting syndrome in adults—rediscovering and redefining an old entity. Aliment Pharmacol Ther. 2011;34:263–73.
13. Lee L, Abbott L, Mahlangu B, et al. The management of cyclic vomiting syndrome: A systematic review. Eur J Gastroenterol Hepatol. 2012;24:1001–6.
14. Li BU, Lefevre F, Chelimsky GG. North American Society for Paediatric Gastroenterology, Hepatology, and Nutrition Consensus Statement on the Diagnosis and Management of Cyclic Vomiting Syndrome. J Paediatr Gastroenterol Nutr. 2008;47:379–93.
15. Lombard HC. Evrose de la digestion, caracteriseo par des crises periodiques de vomissements et une profonde modification de l'assimilation. Gazette Medicale de Paris 1861:312
16. Lucarelli S, Corrado G, et al. Cyclic vomiting syndrome and food allergy/intolerance in seven children: A possible association. Eur J Paediatr. 2000;159:360–3.
17. Olson AD, Li BU. The diagnostic evaluation of children with cyclic vomiting: A cost-effectiveness assessment. J Pediatr. 2002;141:724–8.

18. Paul S, Barnard P, Soondrum K. Antimigraine (low amine) diet may be helpful in children with cyclic vomiting syndrome. JPGN. 2012;54:698–9.
19. Rome III Diagnostic Criteria for Functional Gastrointestinal Disorders. Available at http://www.romecriteria.org/assets/pdf/19_RomeIII_apA_885-898.pdf. Accessed May 19, 2014.
20. Simonetto D, Oxentenko A, Herman M, et al. Cannabinoid hyperemesis: A case series of 98 patients. Mayo Clinic Proc. 2012;87:114–9.
21. Taché Y. Cyclic vomiting syndrome: The corticotropin-releasing-factor hypothesis. Dig Dis Sci. 1999;44(Suppl):79S–86S.
22. Van Calcar SC, Harding CO, Wolff JA. L-Carnitine administration reduces number on cyclic vomiting syndrome. Clin Paediatr. 2002;41:171–4.
23. Wang Q, Ito M, Adams K, et al. Mitochondrial DNA control region sequence variation in migraine headache and cyclic vomiting syndrome. Am J Med Genet. 2004;131:50–8.

Part III
Small Intestine Disorders

Chapter 10
Gas and Bloating

Cristina Almansa, Kenneth DeVault, and Lesley A. Houghton

Case Study

A 47-year-old female presents with bloating and distension. She has been suffering from this for the past 10 years, but it has been much worse over the past 18 months. She wakes up with minimal symptoms, eats a small breakfast, and then leaves for work. She is an administrative assistant and sits at a computer for most of the day. As the morning progresses, she begins to feel bloated and often does not eat lunch because of the discomfort. By the afternoon she is distended, feels her clothes are too tight, and occasionally will leave work early due to the discomfort. She states that she often feels *6 months pregnant* by the end of the day. She will burp at home, but not at work, in an attempt to obtain some relief from the bloating. She has no symptoms of dysphagia but describes mild heartburn that is relieved partially with antacids or proton pump inhibitors (PPIs). She feels nauseated at times but has not vomited. She reports infrequent bowel movements (two times each week) and rarely takes a laxative. She has recently gained 10 kg of weight despite what she feels to be a limited diet. Previous evaluation included upper endoscopy including small bowel biopsy, colonoscopy, upper abdominal ultrasound, and gastric emptying test, all of which were normal. Failed treatment trials include PPIs, lactose avoidance, and probiotics. She has recently changed jobs and was divorced 2 years ago after 20 years of marriage. Physical exam finds her to be pleasant and overweight

---

C. Almansa, M.D., Ph.D. • K. DeVault, M.D. • L.A. Houghton, Ph.D. (✉)
Division of Gastroenterology and Hepatology, Mayo Clinic,
Davis Building, 4500 San Pablo Road, Jacksonville, FL 32225, USA
e-mail: Houghton.Lesley@mayo.edu; Lesley.Houghton@manchester.ac.uk

B.E. Lacy et al. (eds.), *Functional and Motility Disorders of the Gastrointestinal Tract*, DOI 10.1007/978-1-4939-1498-2_10

(BMI: 29 kg/m^2). Her abdomen is slightly obese and nontender, and no masses or other abnormalities are noted. She asks you whether any tests are required to diagnose her problem and wonders what treatments are available.

Introduction

Bloating is commonly reported by patients with functional gastrointestinal disorders (FGIDs) such as irritable bowel syndrome, functional constipation, and dyspepsia. The term *bloating* refers to a subjective *sensation* of excessive gas/flatulence, fullness, abdominal hardness or tightness, or the feeling of abdominal inflation or swelling. This needs to be differentiated from *distension* which is reserved for an *actual* increase in abdominal girth. Not all patients with bloating exhibit a change in abdominal girth (i.e., distension; see Table 10.1). Both bloating and distension most frequently associate with irritable bowel syndrome (IBS), and thus, IBS has been the focus of bloating research with little knowledge of how this may translate to other conditions.

Epidemiology

Abdominal bloating is a common and bothersome symptom and is often ranked more troublesome than abdominal pain. It typically worsens as the day progresses, especially after meals, and improves overnight. Defecation and passage of gas can also afford some relief. Bloating affects between 24 and 97 % of patients with FGIDs and also commonly occurs in patients with gastroesophageal reflux disease, premenstrual syndrome, and intestinal dysmotility. It is considered a diagnosis per se (i.e., functional bloating) in patients who do not fulfill Rome criteria for other FGIDs (Table 10.1), with a prevalence ranging from 3 to 30 %. A significant but variable proportion (8–36 %) of subjects in the general community experience abdominal bloating. These wide variations in prevalence rates are undoubtedly

Table 10.1 Definitions

Abdominal bloating
Subjective *sensation* of excessive gas/flatulence, fullness, abdominal hardness or tightness or the feeling of abdominal inflation or swelling
Abdominal distension
Actual increase in abdominal girth
Functional abdominal bloating
Recurrent complaints of bloating with or without associated abdominal distension and absence of criteria for a diagnosis dyspepsia, IBS, or other functional gastrointestinal disorder

Rome III requires that symptoms are present at least 3 days/month in the last 3 months with symptom onset at least 6 months prior to the diagnosis

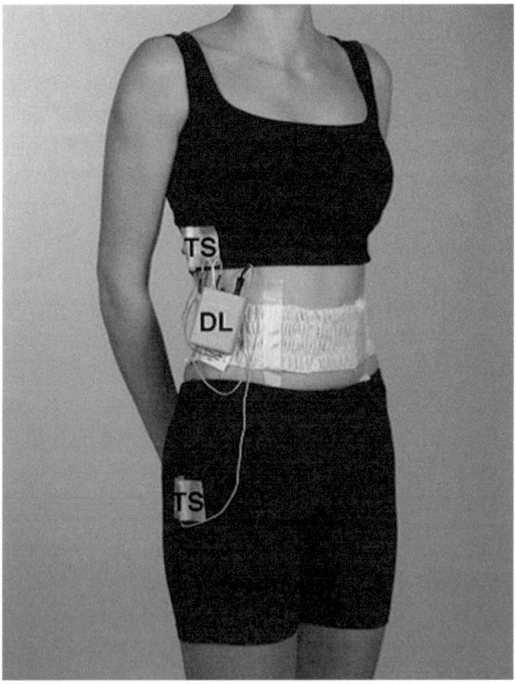

Fig. 10.1 Photograph of a subject wearing the ambulatory abdominal inductance plethysmography (AIP) equipment incorporating a belt into which is sewn a wire in zigzag fashion to allow for expansion and connected to an oscillator secured under the belt, data logger (DL), and tilt switches (TS) to record posture. It works on the principle that a loop of wire forms an inductor, the inductance of which is dependent on the cross-sectional area of the loop, from which circumference can be calculated. Reproduced with kind permission from Neurogastroenterol Motil 2005; 17: 500–511

influenced by the definition of bloating used as it is ambiguous and can mean different things to both patients and doctors. IBS patients with bloating consult more and have worse quality of life than those IBS patients without bloating. Despite this, bloating alone is seldom a reason for patients to seek health care and, compared with other functional and organic gastrointestinal disorders, presents only a moderate impact on the subject's quality of life and productivity.

The terms bloating and distension have often been considered synonymous; however, this is to be discouraged. Multiple surveys and studies objectively measuring abdominal girth (i.e., distension) over 24 h have shown that the symptom of bloating is often not accompanied by an objective increase in abdominal girth. Studies using the technique of abdominal inductance plethysmography (see Fig. 10.1) have shown that significantly more constipation-predominant IBS (IBS-C) patients (60 %) exhibit diurnal changes in girth beyond the normal reference range seen in healthy volunteers than diarrhea-predominant IBS (IBS-D) patients (40 %) with the average increase being about 3–4 cm but in some patients up to 10–12 cm (see Fig. 10.2). For reasons that remain unclear, the severity of the symptom of bloating only correlates with objective distension in IBS-C and not IBS-D patients. Interestingly, bloating alone has been reported to be more prevalent than distension in patients with functional constipation. Both women in health and with FGIDs are more likely to report distension and/or bloating than men. Other factors associated with an increased risk for distension over bloating alone include young age, presence of somatic symptoms, and multiple overlapping GI diagnoses.

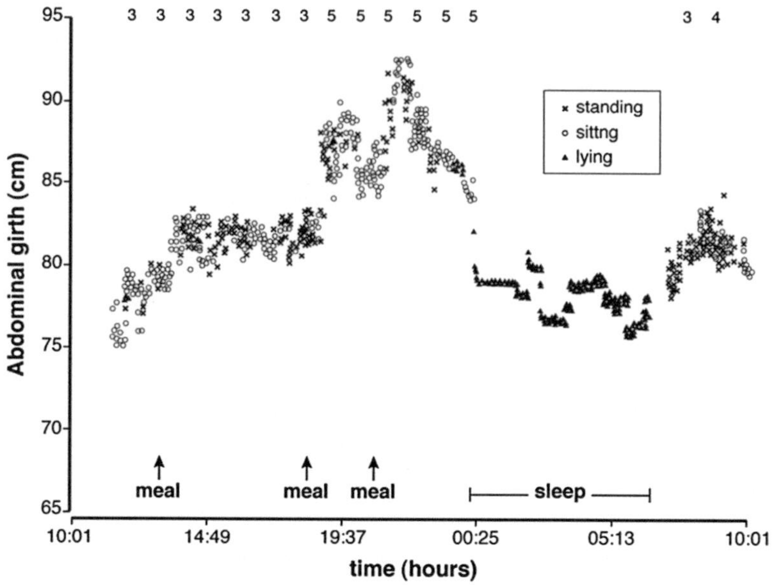

Fig. 10.2 Typical recording of abdominal girth over 24 h in a patient with IBS-C. Numbers across the *top* of the girth recording are the bloating scores (scale 0–5) obtained from a diary. Note how in this IBS-C patient girth changes tend to relate to the sensation of bloating, the increase in girth with meal ingestion, and the reduction in girth during sleep. Reproduced with kind permission from Gastroenterology 2006; 131:1003–1010

Pathophysiology

Distension

An understanding of the mechanisms associated with abdominal distension has greatly advanced in recent years. Using abdominal inductance plethysmography, it has been shown that IBS-C patients who have a diurnal change in girth beyond the 95th percentile limit for healthy volunteers (i.e., distenders) have slower gastrointestinal transit, particularly of the colon, compared with those who have changes in girth within the normal range (i.e., non-distenders). Moreover, abdominal distension directly correlated with orocecal and colonic transit times and with the hardness of stool. Accelerating transit with the probiotic *Bifidobacterium lactis* DC-173 010 has been shown to correlate with an improvement in abdominal girth, suggesting that gastrointestinal transit plays a role in abdominal distension.

The mechanism whereby intestinal content (e.g., solid, liquid, gas) leads to distension, however, appears to vary depending on the patient group assessed. In healthy volunteers, increased intra-abdominal content is associated with (1) relaxation and ascent of the diaphragm to enlarge the abdominal cavity and thus to accommodate the abdominal load, (2) contraction of the anterior abdominal muscles (upper and rectus, external oblique with the exception of the internal oblique which

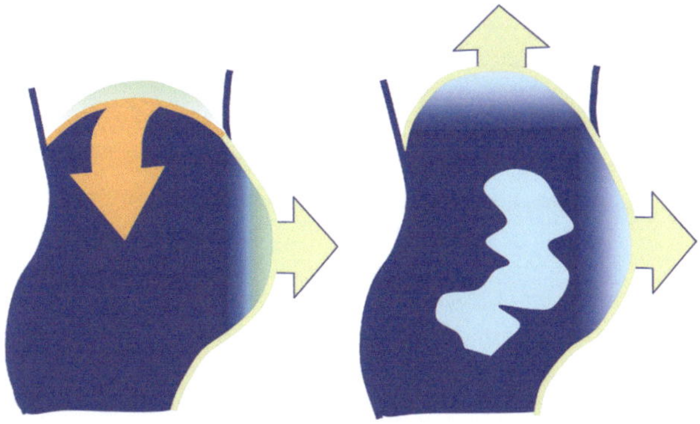

Fig. 10.3 Mechanisms of distension. In FGID patients, abdominal distension is related to abdomino-phrenic displacement and ventro-caudal distribution of contents, whereas in intestinal dysmotility patients, distension involves a true increment in intestinal content and abdominal expansion. Note the descent (contraction) of the diaphragm in the FGID patient but ascent (relaxation) of the diaphragm in the dysmotility patient. The latter is accompanied by expansion of the chest wall to compensate for the reduction in lung height preserving its air volume. Reproduced with kind permission from Gastroenterology 2009; 136:1544–1551

in an upright position is already contracted to counteract gravitational forces and support abdominal contents) to prevent excessive abdominal distension, and (3) expansion of the chest wall to compensate for the reduction in lung height caused by diaphragmatic ascent preserving air volume. This integrated *abdominothoracic response* appears to be related to volume rather than rate of expansion. In patients with intestinal dysmotility, a similar process takes place with the volume of pooled intestinal contents (particularly in the small bowel) directly correlating with ascent of the diaphragm and the degree of anterior protrusion of the abdominal wall. Thus, in patients with intestinal dysmotility, distension appears to be the result of a *true* increase in abdominal contents (see Fig. 10.3). These observations, however, contrast with those seen in patients with FGIDs. In patients with IBS and functional bloating, the degree of abdominal distension to a given intestinal load is significantly greater than that seen in patients with intestinal dysmotility or healthy controls. This appears to be related to impaired contraction of the lower rectus and external oblique abdominal muscles, and paradoxical *relaxation* of the internal oblique muscle and descent due to contraction of the diaphragm (see Fig. 10.3). Similar observations have been made in patients with functional dyspepsia with the exception that only the upper anterior wall (upper rectus and external oblique) and not the lower muscles (lower rectus and internal oblique) relax to a given gastric load. The cause of this *abdomino-phrenic dyssynergia* in FGIDs remains unknown, but IBS patients with the greatest diurnal changes in abdominal girth often exhibit rectal in- or hyposensitivity.

Lastly, patients with non-diarrhea IBS and functional constipation who report abdominal distension (not objectively measured) have prolonged rectal balloon expulsion times, higher resting anal sphincter pressures, higher maximum anal sphincter squeeze pressures, and longer times to onset of anal sphincter inhibition during rapid inflation of rectal balloon, suggesting a potential role for abnormal anorectal function in the pathophysiology of abdominal distension.

Bloating and Gas (Without Distension)

Unlike patients with intestinal dysmotility who have significant pooling of gut contents, particularly gas in the small bowel, patients with FGIDs have no more gas in their intestines than healthy controls or patients with organic gastrointestinal disease (e.g., Crohn's disease, colonic diverticulosis, peptic ulcer disease, GERD). Moreover, over ten times the normal amount of gas present in the gut, approximately 200 mL, can be infused into the intestine of healthy volunteers with less than a 2 cm change in girth, which is significantly less than the average 4 cm, and up to 10–12 cm seen in some IBS patients, suggesting that gas retention is not the cause of abdominal distension in these patients. Despite this, gas infused into the intestine of patients with IBS and functional bloating has been shown to be retained longer in the intestine and is not as well tolerated compared with similar gas loads infused in healthy volunteers. Patients with IBS-C retain gas longer than IBS-D patients, although the perception of the presence of the gas is greater in IBS-D. This may be related to the reduced transit and motility seen in IBS-C but increased prevalence of visceral hypersensitivity seen in IBS-D. Indeed, it has been shown that the sensation of bloating in the absence of abdominal distension is associated with increased visceral sensitivity compared with those who bloat and distend, with over 80 % of IBS patients who bloat alone exhibiting rectal hypersensitivity. Thus, ineffective gas propulsion and retention in patients with functional bowel disorders, particularly in a sensitized gut, may be responsible for the sensation of bloating and gas without visible distension.

Evidence supporting a role for small intestinal bacterial overgrowth (SIBO) and excess gas production in IBS is lacking. Studies assessing the presence of SIBO by culturing jejunal aspirate, the current gold standard, have shown that only 4 % of IBS patients are positive for SIBO, which is the same as controls. Qualitative differences in small bowel microbes, however, could lead to different symptom patterns. For example, IBS patients who are predominant methane producers report harder and more lumpy stools and have higher rectal sensory thresholds and baseline colonic phasic, nonpropulsive contractility than both healthy volunteers and those who predominantly produce hydrogen.

Diagnosis and Evaluation

A carefully performed history and physical examination may help clarify these symptoms. Classic bloating is not present in the morning and gets worse as the day goes on. An attempt should be made to determine if the patient actually has distension (an increase in girth) or rather a sensation of bloating without visible distension. It is often helpful to see the patient twice, once early in the day and then later in the day when they are bloated to see if there is a change on physical examination. Some patients provide *before and after* pictures which can be illustrative. The presence of FGIDs including dyspepsia, GERD, and IBS should be determined given the common presence of bloating in these disorders. Weight loss is unusual. A food history may help guide both testing and dietary advice. The abdominal exam should concentrate on percussion, palpation, and auscultation.

Testing in patients with bloating is challenging. The diagnostic yield of most tests is quite low, yet patients often get extensive testing that is frequently repeated. Furthermore, although a subset of patients will have abnormalities in one or more of these tests, whether they can be used to guide therapy is not clear. Some commonly obtained tests and their limitations include:

1. Abdominal X-rays: These rarely show a specific abnormality but may be useful during a distension episode to document intra-abdominal air content.
2. Endoscopy: These are often performed, but an organic process is rarely identified as the cause of symptoms. Small bowel biopsy and aspirate, although frequently performed, have a very low yield at identifying an etiology.
3. Ultrasound and CT: These are also frequently performed and may demonstrate increased abdominal fat, which can be reviewed with patients as a cause for their *distension*.
4. Transit tests: Nuclear medicine gastric emptying tests may show a delay in gastric emptying or, at times, rapid gastric emptying. Tests of small bowel and colon transit are available in some centers using scintigraphy, radiopaque markers, or capsule-based ambulatory pH/pressure-based technologies and may help guide therapy in the occasional patient.
5. Gastric accommodation studies: These include balloon distension studies (barostat) and nuclear medicine studies that label the gastric wall and drink-based satiety testing. These tests are not widely available, and their clinical role remains uncertain.
6. Breath testing: Hydrogen breath test are available for carbohydrate intolerance (e.g., lactose, fructose) and bacterial overgrowth (e.g., glucose, lactulose). Similarly, methane-based breath testing might identify constipation patients who might respond to attempts at changing the gut microbiota.

Treatment

Proven efficacious treatments for bloating and distension are limited, if nonexistent, making management of these symptoms difficult (see Table 10.2). This is partly due to treatment trials generally targeting pain and/or disordered bowel habit rather than bloating and distension, but also because patient, physician, and investigator alike often do not differentiate between bloating and distension or appreciate that the mechanisms responsible for them may be different. A number of medications have been

Table 10.2 Treatment options

Dietary changes (low FODMAP diet)
Mild exercise
Probiotics (*Bifidobacterium* and *Lactobacillus* species)
Prokinetics[a]
Antidepressants
Nonabsorbable antibiotics (rifaximin)

[a]Prokinetics are not widely available in the US market

evaluated in clinical trials and have evaluated changes in bloating but have rarely assessed changes in abdominal girth.

It might be expected that treatment with prokinetics to accelerate transit would alleviate distension. This treatment approach is supported by the experimental observations that use of an acetylcholinesterase inhibitor decreased both bloating and distension in FGID patients with increased gas retention. Prokinetics may also improve the symptom of bloating by aiding intestinal gas transit and expulsion and, in the case of postprandial bloating, by accelerating gastric emptying. Similarly, lubiprostone and linaclotide, which enhance luminal fluid secretion and intestinal transit, have been reported to improve bloating in patients with functional constipation and IBS-C. Laxatives and bulking agents, although commonly recommended, have failed to show a therapeutic benefit over placebo. Antidepressants, which have been shown to modulate visceral sensitivity, are also often prescribed in patients with FGIDs; however, clinical trials to date have offered mixed results. The probiotic *Bifidobacterium lactis* DN-173 010, which in addition to an effect on the gut microbiota accelerates transit, has also been suggested to improve objective abdominal distension in patients with IBS-C.

Increasing evidence that the gut microbiota is altered in IBS has resulted in many clinical trials of antibiotics, probiotics, and prebiotics. Many of these trials, however, have been poorly designed using small numbers of patients with no supporting physiological data to support a mode of action. Two probiotics that have been shown in animal models to reduce visceral sensitivity, *Bifidobacterium infantis* and *Lactobacillus acidophilus*, do appear to improve bloating in IBS. Seven to fourteen days of treatment with the nonabsorbable antibiotic, rifaximin, has also been shown to reduce the symptoms of gaseousness and bloating for up to 3 months in patients with IBS. Prolonged use of antibiotics for a condition like IBS cannot be advocated, especially after a recent meta-analysis showed that, although better than placebo, the therapeutic gain offered by rifaximin was modest, with a number needed to treat of 10.

Lastly, dietary changes such as the avoidance of carbonated drinks and foods that produce gas may help the symptom of bloating. The low fermentable, poorly absorbed, short-chain carbohydrate (fermentable; oligo-, di-, and monosaccharides; and polyols [FODMAP]) diet, in which highly fermentable substances such as wheat products, fruits rich in fructose (e.g., apples and pears), vegetables containing fructans (e.g., onions and asparagus), foods containing raffinose (e.g., legumes, cabbage), and products containing sorbitol (e.g., sugar-free gum) are avoided, appears to improve bloating. Moreover, mild exercise may also be of benefit by increasing intestinal gas clearance.

In summary, the treatment of bloating and distension remains challenging. Once obstruction and other structural lesions have been excluded, the focus should be on the *functional* nature of this condition and in improvement or relief of symptoms in contrast to *cure*. Initially focusing on diet and perhaps alterations in gut microbiota seems reasonable. Using transit tests to guide prokinetic therapy also seems a reasonable approach, as does trying agents that lower visceral sensitivity in the patient who has failed other trials. It needs to be born in mind, however, that accelerating transit may not improve the patient's perception of their bloating, if they are viscerally sensitive.

Case Resolution

The patient was provided reassurance and counseled that additional testing was not necessary. Several treatment approaches were discussed. She preferred a trial of the low FODMAP diet. In consultation with a dietitian, this diet was initiated, and upon return to clinic 3 months later, she reported a 50 % improvement in her symptoms and much less missed work. She elected to continue the diet on a long-term basis and was satisfied with her degree of improvement.

Key Clinical Teaching Points

- Bloating and distension are distinct entities.
- Mechanisms responsible for bloating and distension differ.
- Mechanisms for distension differ depending upon the associated disease (FGIDs versus intestinal dysmotility).
- Potential treatments include dietary changes, prokinetics, antimicrobial approaches, and agents that lower visceral sensitivity.

Teaching Questions

1. Which one of these statements about bloating and distension is true?

   (A) Bloating is always accompanied by an increase in abdominal girth (i.e., distension).
   (B) Females more frequently report abdominal distension than males.
   (C) Distension is frequently reported by patients with IBS-D.
   (D) Bloating per se is a frequent reason to seek health care.

2. Which one of these statements about the pathophysiology of bloating and/or distension is true?
   (A) Distension in patients with FGIDs is associated with increased abdominal gas.
   (B) The mechanism of distension is similar in patients with FGIDs and patients with intestinal dysmotility disorders.
   (C) Distension is associated with increased visceral sensitivity.
   (D) Distension is associated with increased colonic transit time.
3. Which one of these therapeutics options should <u>not</u> be initially recommended as a first line of treatment of patients with bloating?
   (A) Dietary changes
   (B) Mild exercise
   (C) Probiotics
   (D) Rifaximin

Key References

1. Accarino A, Perez F, Azpiriz F, Quiroga S, Malafelada JR. Abdominal distension results from caudo-ventral distribution of contents. Gastroenterology. 2009;136:1544–51. Key study showing anterior abdominal wall protrusion and diaphragmatic descent (contraction) during distension in patients with FGIDs.
2. Agrawal A, Houghton LA, Lea R, Morris J, Reilly B, Whorwell PJ. Bloating and distension in irritable bowel syndrome: The role of visceral sensation. Gastroenterology. 2008;134:1882–9. Found that bloating alone is associated with visceral hyper-sensitivity, whilst excessive distension appears to be associated with hypo- or in-sensitivity.
3. Agrawal A, Houghton LA, Reilly B, Morris J, Whorwell PJ. Bloating and distension in irritable bowel syndrome: The role of gastrointestinal transit. Am J Gastroenterol. 2009;104:1998–2004. Key study showing delayed colonic transit associates with distension in patients with irritable bowel syndrome.
4. Barba E, Quiroga S, Accarino A, Lahoya EM, Malagelada C, Burri E, Navazo I, Malagelada J-R, Azpiroz F. Mechanisms of abdominal distension in severe intestinal dysmotility: Abdomino-thoracic response to gut retention. Neurogastroenterol Motil. 2013;25:e389–94. Important study showing that pooling of gut contents, particularly the small bowel in patients with intestinal dysmotility, is associated with a coordinated abdomino-phreno-thoracic response, involving an accommodative ascent (relaxation) of the diaphragm and a compensatory expansion of the chest wall.
5. Caldarella M, Serra J, Azpiroz F, et al. Prokinetic effects in patients with intestinal gas retention. Gastroenterology. 2002;122:1748–55. Interventional study showing that neostigmine, a cholinesterase inhibitor with prokinetic effects, improves the symptoms of bloating and distension in FGID (IBS and functional constipation) patients with gas retention.
6. Houghton LA, Lea R, Agrawal A, Reilly B, Whorwell PJ. Relationship of abdominal bloating to distension in irritable bowel syndrome and the effect of bowel habit. Gastroenterology. 2006;131:1003–10. The first study showing the relationship between bloating and objectively measured abdominal girth (i.e., distension) in IBS-C and IBS-D patients.
7. Posserud I, Stotzer PO, Bjornsson ES, Abrahamsson H, Simren M. Small intestinal bacterial overgrowth in patients with IBS. Gut. 2007;56:802–8. Found that only 4 % of IBS patients have SIBO as detected using gold standard cultural techniques of jejunal aspirate.

8. Villoria A, Azpiroz F, Burri E, Cisternas D, Soldevilla A, Malagelada J-R. Abdomino-phrenic dyssynergia in patients with abdominal bloating and distensión. Am J Gastroenterol. 2011;106:815–9. Showed that distension in patients with FGIDs is associated with impaired contraction of the lower rectus and external oblique abdominal muscles, and paradoxical 'relaxation' of the internal oblique muscle and 'contraction (descent)' of the diaphragm.

Chapter 11
Small Intestinal Bacterial Overgrowth

Konstantinos Triantafyllou and Mark Pimentel

Case Study

A 78-year-old man with a 20-year history of type II diabetes mellitus is referred for the evaluation of postprandial fullness, bloating, and diarrhea (4–5 daily movements) of 1 year's duration. His body weight has not changed during this time. He has had no previous abdominal surgery and is well nourished, and a complete multisystem review and physical examination are unremarkable. Laboratory studies reveal a normal complete blood count and chemistry panel. Stool tests for pathogens and qualitative fecal fat are negative. The patient failed to improve following a 10-day course of loperamide, and he subsequently underwent both upper endoscopy and colonoscopy including small bowel and colon biopsies with unremarkable results. An abdominal CT scan was also completed and revealed fatty infiltration of the liver. The patient asks what his diagnosis is, whether any other tests are required, and if other treatments are available.

Introduction

Soon after birth, the previously sterile infant gastrointestinal tract becomes colonized by microbes. Because of the bactericidal action of gastric acid and the sweeping of the intestinal lumen by peristalsis, the proximal small intestine is normally colonized by

K. Triantafyllou, M.D., Ph.D.
Hepatogastroenterology Unit, Second Department of Internal Medicine and Research Institute, Attikon University General Hospital, Haidari, Greece

M. Pimentel, M.D., FRCP (C) (✉)
GI Motility Program, Division of Gastroenterology, Cedars-Sinai Medical Center, 8730 Alden Drive, Suite 201E, Los Angeles, CA 90048, USA
e-mail: pimentelm@cshs.org

B.E. Lacy et al. (eds.), *Functional and Motility Disorders of the Gastrointestinal Tract*, DOI 10.1007/978-1-4939-1498-2_11

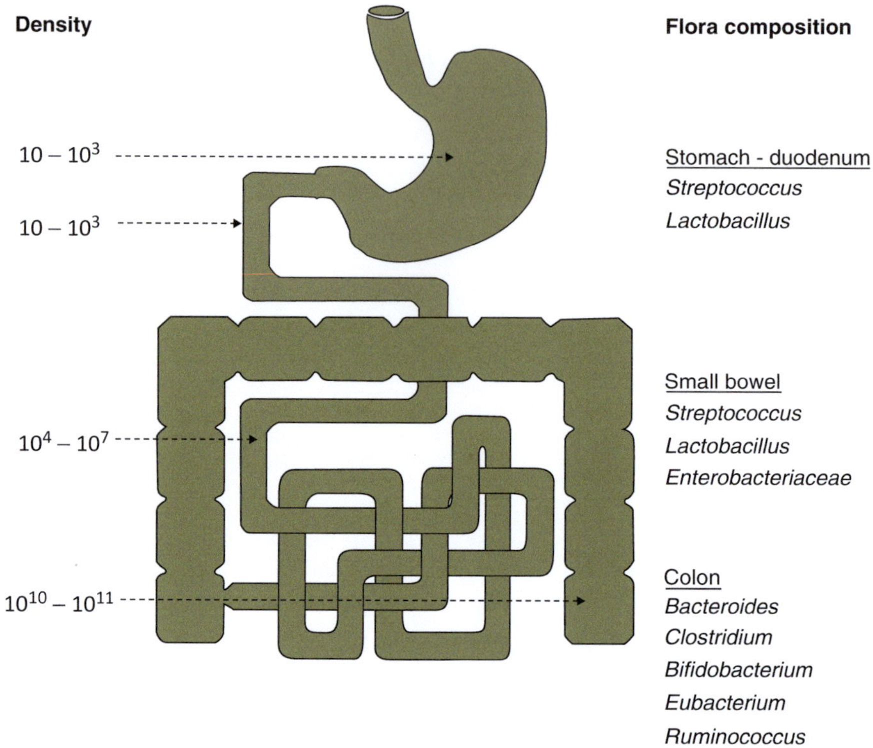

Fig. 11.1 Normal microbial distribution along the length of the gastrointestinal tract

a relatively small number of bacteria, consisting mainly of Gram-positive microbes and anaerobes from the oral cavity. In the ileum, an increase in microbial colonization of up to 10^9 colony-forming units (CFU)/mL occurs, due mainly to Gram-negative microbes and anaerobes. Finally, the colon contains an abundance of mostly anaerobic microbes at a concentration of up to 10^{12} CFU/mL (Fig. 11.1).

Small intestinal bacterial overgrowth (SIBO) is characterized by the presence of increased numbers of colonic-type bacteria in the small bowel. Traditionally, SIBO is defined by the detection of more than 10^5 CFU/ml of bacteria from an aspirate taken from the proximal small bowel. A revised definition lowering the concentration to 10^3–10^4 CFU/mL of colonic-type bacteria in association with characteristic symptoms has recently been proposed. SIBO is an increasingly recognized cause of malabsorption and is likely an under-recognized cause of a variety of nonspecific gastrointestinal symptoms.

Epidemiology

The prevalence of SIBO and its relationship to several clinical conditions are unclear because of controversies related to both its detection and definition. Moreover, the clinical manifestations of SIBO overlap with those of many other gastrointestinal disorders.

High clinical suspicion should be given to individuals with underlying disorders known to disrupt the protective elements that exist to prevent SIBO. The prevalence of SIBO varies depending on the population studied and the diagnostic methods used. In healthy individuals, SIBO has been described in 0–12 % using the glucose breath test and 20–22 % using the lactulose breath test. SIBO appears to be more prevalent in the elderly. In neonates and the elderly, SIBO may lead to significant morbidity or even death; however, exact mortality rates directly linked to SIBO are not available.

Pathogenesis

The most important factors contributing to the pathogenesis of SIBO are intestinal dysmotility, anatomical alterations of the gastrointestinal tract that predispose to stagnation of intestinal contents (e.g., large duodenal diverticula, prior gastric bypass surgery, resection of the ileocecal valve), low gastric acid production, and advanced age. To a lesser extent, bile, proteolytic pancreatic enzymes, and the innate immune system also protect against SIBO. Based on these factors, Table 11.1 presents the most common conditions associated with SIBO. It is not always easy, however, to detect a specific predisposing factor. SIBO may develop either in the presence of a specific pathogenetic mechanism (e.g., diabetes, blind loop syndrome, total gastrectomy, immunodeficiency states) or due to a combination of the aforementioned mechanisms. For example, chronic pancreatitis is associated with decreased intestinal motility and decreased production of pancreatic enzymes; advanced age is associated with gastric atrophy and intestinal dysmotility; obesity is related to altered gut flora and small bowel motility; and cirrhosis and nonalcoholic steatohepatitis are related to hypomotility and increased intestinal permeability.

Clinical Presentation

Originally, SIBO was a condition thought to be associated with diarrhea, malnutrition, vitamin deficiencies, and weight loss in the presence of conditions that induce stagnation in the intestinal lumen; however, this "classic" presentation is now uncommon. Indeed, the majority of SIBO patients present with nonspecific symptoms such as abdominal pain or discomfort, flatulence, bloating, and a change in bowel habits in the absence of an obvious risk factor. Children with SIBO may present with diarrhea and abdominal pain, while malnutrition and vitamin deficiencies are usually absent. In contrast, elderly SIBO patients may be asymptomatic, or they may present with unexplained weight loss and malnutrition. SIBO symptoms may develop through different mechanisms that include gas production, induction of diarrhea, and malabsorption, as shown in Table 11.2.

While SIBO has traditionally been linked to diarrhea and malabsorption, there is evidence that SIBO is implicated in the development of disorders with no

Table 11.1 Conditions associated with small intestinal bacterial overgrowth

Pathophysiologic mechanism	Condition
Anatomical	Blind loop Small intestinal diverticulosis Small intestinal strictures (Crohn's disease, radiation enteritis, chronic ischemic enteritis) Enteroenteric fistulae Short bowel syndrome Resection of the ileocecal valve
Hypomotility	Diabetes mellitus Scleroderma Amyloidosis Paraneoplastic syndrome Visceral myopathy (or neuropathy) Idiopathic intestinal pseudo-obstruction Hypomotility due to medication use Chagas disease
Reduced acid secretion	Atrophic gastritis Vagotomy Subtotal or total gastrectomy Gastric bypass Chronic proton pump inhibitor use[a]
Various	Irritable bowel syndrome Advanced age Chronic pancreatitis Cirrhosis with portal hypertension End-stage renal disease Nonalcoholic steatohepatitis Obesity Immunodeficiency states Celiac disease Rheumatoid arthritis Cystic fibrosis

[a]Questionable association

Table 11.2 Pathogenesis of symptoms in patients with small intestinal bacterial overgrowth

1. The fermentation of carbohydrates by enteric bacteria leads to the production of carbon dioxide, hydrogen, and methane which may induce, bloating, abdominal distension, abdominal pain, and flatulence
2. Short-chain fatty acids produced during fermentation stimulate the secretion of water and electrolytes leading to diarrhea
3. Deconjugation of bile salts may lead to fat malabsorption, steatorrhea, weight loss, and deficiencies of fat-soluble vitamins A, D, E, and K
4. Consumption of vitamin B12 by the intestinal microbes may result in macrocytic anemia and neurologic disturbances
5. Destruction of the brush border surface of the enterocytes may lead to carbohydrate and protein malabsorption, although these are very rare in SIBO

Table 11.3 Evidence supporting an association between small intestinal bacterial overgrowth (SIBO) and irritable bowel syndrome (IBS)

1.	Excessive fermentation and increased small bowel gas in IBS patients compared to controls
2.	Excessive colonic-type bacteria in the proximal small bowel of IBS patients
3.	Abnormal breath tests in IBS patients compared to controls
4.	Hydrogen production is associated with diarrhea in IBS; methane production is associated with constipation in IBS
5.	Antibiotic treatment results in an improvement of IBS symptoms that correlates with normalization of breath test
6.	At least 12-week response after antibiotic therapy in one controlled trial
7.	Animal model that unifies the SIBO hypothesis and post-infectious IBS. Rodents develop stool alterations together with SIBO and depletion of deep muscular plexus interstitial cells of Cajal long after acute *C. jejuni* infection

pathognomonic biochemical, immunological, and/or histological findings. Indeed, during the last decade, evidence has accumulated to support a role of SIBO for the development of irritable bowel syndrome (IBS). Table 11.3 summarizes the epidemiological, clinical, and translational evidence for this association. The controversy regarding the role of SIBO in IBS primarily originates from the accuracy of breath testing as the method to diagnose SIBO. As discussed in the SIBO diagnosis section below, hydrogen breath tests have lower accuracy for the detection of SIBO compared to the culture of proximal small intestinal contents, considered the diagnostic "gold standard." A recent systematic literature review, however, showed that no test is appropriately validated for the diagnosis of SIBO.

Diagnosis

Symptoms of diarrhea, weight loss, bloating, and flatulence in patients with a coexisting predisposition to SIBO, regardless of whether malabsorption has been demonstrated, should prompt the clinician to consider testing for bacterial overgrowth, especially if the patients have failed to respond to other empiric treatments. It is likely that SIBO is commonly overlooked in patients without known predisposing factors and in patients who have nonspecific symptoms. Table 11.4 shows the armamentarium of tests used to diagnose SIBO. In the absence of a "gold standard," the most practical method of evaluating SIBO has been suggested to be a "test, treat, and assess outcome" approach with breath testing being used to help discriminate patients that may benefit from antibiotics by the normalization of the breath test after treatment.

Culture of Aspirate from the Proximal Small Intestine

The "gold standard" for the diagnosis of SIBO has been considered the quantitative culture of fluid from the proximal small intestine with the presence of $>10^5$ CFU/mL considered abnormal. Recently, a lower threshold at $>10^3$ CFU/mL

Table 11.4 Diagnostic tests for small intestinal bacterial overgrowth (SIBO)

Diagnostic test	Criterion	PROS	CONS
Laboratory tests	Macrocytic anemia with low vitamin B12 levels and increased levels of folate Positive qualitative fresh stool examination for fat Positive three-day quantitative fecal fat collection	Easy to perform	Non-specific Absence of abnormality does not rule out SIBO Stool tests are not favorable in the lab
Culture and bacterial counts of proximal small intestinal aspirate	$>10^5$ CFU/ml of colonic type bacteria $>10^4$ CFU/ml of colonic type bacteria[a] $>10^3$ CFU/ml of colonic type bacteria[a]	The traditional gold standard	"Arbitrary" definition Invasive, costly procedure Does not detect SIBO in the distal small bowel or patchy SIBO Culture underestimates the actual bacterial numbers Anaerobic bacteria are not cultured
Breath tests			
Lactulose breath test	H_2 or CH_4 >10 ppm at baseline or Sustained rise of H_2 or CH_4 >20 ppm compared with baseline before 90 min	Easy to perform, non-invasive	Variable sensitivity and specificity False negative and false positive results Patient and procedure related limitation
Glucose breath test	H_2 or CH_4 >10 ppm at baseline or Sustained rise of H_2 or CH_4 >20 ppm compared with baseline		Variable sensitivity and specificity False negative results Patient and procedure related limitation
Culture independent techniques (16S rRNA)	Not specified	Accurate mapping of the microbiota	Only for investigational use
Antibiotic treatment	Resolution of symptoms and/or normalization of breath test	Easy to perform	Might not be appropriate to give antibiotics without prior diagnosis

CFU, colony-forming units; H_2, hydrogen; CH_4, methane; *ppm*, parts per million
[a]Alternative definition

of colonic-type microbes in the proper clinical context has been proposed. The culture of proximal small bowel aspirate, however, has many limitations that raise concerns regarding this test's sensitivity. This diagnostic approach is an invasive and costly procedure requiring endoscopy that exposes the aspirate to the risk of contamination from the oral cavity. Endoscopy also generally provides access only to the duodenum, and duodenal cultures may underestimate the prevalence of bacterial overgrowth in the more distal small bowel. Additionally, SIBO may not be a continuous process throughout the small intestine but rather may occur in discrete areas (i.e., be patchy), thus further limiting the role of aspirates. Moreover, anaerobic culture of samples is difficult and may be falsely negative when the aspirate is exposed to an aerobic environment prior to processing. Finally, using molecular techniques, it is estimated that only 40 % of the total gut flora can be identified using conventional culture methods.

Breath Testing

Breath testing is based on the principle that fermentation of a carbohydrate substrate by the luminal bacteria leads to the production of gas (hydrogen or methane) that is absorbed and ultimately excreted in the breath. Breath tests are safe, noninvasive, and easy to perform. Among them, hydrogen breath testing after ingestion of glucose or lactulose has been widely applied (Table 11.4). Other SIBO breath tests like the bile acid breath test and ^{14}C-xylose breath test are not widely available and have no established place in the diagnosis of SIBO.

There are several limitations to breath testing. To ensure accuracy of the hydrogen breath test, carbohydrate-containing food should be avoided for 12 h prior to testing. Cigarette smoking and vigorous physical exercise should also be avoided 2 h prior and during the testing. Pretest mouth washing with an antiseptic should be performed, and concurrent testing of breath methane levels should be performed to avoid false-negative results due to the presence of methanogenic bacteria that convert hydrogen into methane.

During the breath test, after an overnight fast, a baseline breath sample for hydrogen and methane measurement is obtained. Thereafter, the sugar substrate (10 g of lactulose or 50 g of glucose) is ingested, and additional breath samples are collected every 10–20 min for up to 3 h. Several criteria have been suggested to be consistent with SIBO using the lactulose breath test; however, it appears that an early rise (before 90 min) in breath hydrogen or methane after lactulose ingestion is the most reliable (Fig. 11.2). However, this criterion is not able to discriminate between SIBO and rapid transit. Normalization of the breath test after antibiotic treatment provides stronger evidence of SIBO. The sensitivity and specificity of breath testing vary from 17 to 90 % and 44 to 100 %, respectively.

When glucose is used as the substrate for hydrogen breath testing, a rise >20 ppm is generally considered to be consistent with SIBO. This test will only detect SIBO in the proximal small bowel since glucose is rapidly and completely absorbed there. The glucose will not be present in the distal small bowel unless rapid transit or a shortened small bowel is present. Thus, this test will be falsely negative if SIBO is limited to only the distal small intestine. The clinical relevance of the differentiation between proximal or distal SIBO, however, has not been validated and requires further study. The ranges for the test sensitivity and specificity have been reported from 27 to 93 % and 36 to 86 %, respectively.

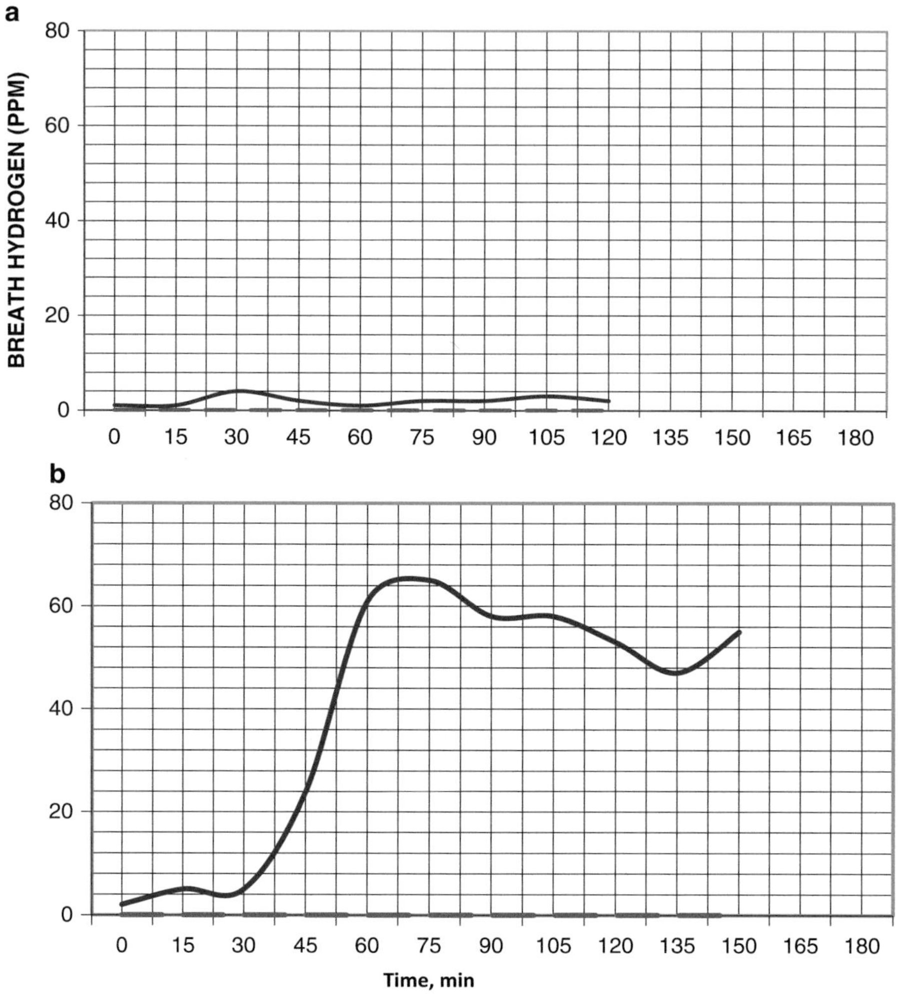

Fig. 11.2 Examples of lactulose hydrogen breath test results. (**a**) Negative test indicated by absence of rise in breath hydrogen; (**b**) positive test indicated by a rise >20 ppm in breath H_2 before 90 min

The Therapeutic Trial

In the absence of a true gold standard diagnostic test, an antibiotic treatment trial represents a reasonable diagnostic option especially in patients with typical symptoms and an underlying predisposing condition for SIBO. Symptom resolution after treatment is suggestive of SIBO. Of course, this can also be done in someone without an obvious increased risk of SIBO; however, the interpretation of the response and subsequent management plan may be more difficult. Another type of therapeutic trial may also be used to supplement an abnormal breath test in patients with atypical symptoms and without a known predisposing factor. Symptom resolution accompanied by breath test normalization is suggestive of SIBO.

Other Tests

Laboratory test abnormalities in SIBO are nonspecific, typically revealing a macrocytic anemia with low levels of vitamin B12. Levels of folate and vitamin K may be high since they are produced by the microbes. Steatorrhea may be present and can be confirmed by quantitative fecal fat collection or by qualitative microscopic examination of fresh stool for fat. If an anatomic defect is suspected as the cause of SIBO, appropriate imaging studies including barium contrast follow through, enteroclysis, and/or CT/MRI enterography may be used. Endoscopy and small bowel histology are usually normal in patients of SIBO; however, they are of value in order to exclude other diagnoses such as celiac disease and Crohn's disease that may also present as a malabsorptive syndrome. Stool testing can exclude infectious disorders, while motility/transit testing may reveal evidence of GI tract dysmotility.

Differential Diagnosis

Because many disorders that predispose to SIBO may present with symptoms identical to SIBO, the differential diagnosis is very broad. For example, gastroparesis, chronic pancreatitis, inflammatory bowel disease, celiac disease, and chronic mesenteric ischemia are known to have an increased prevalence of SIBO, and, at the same time, they may manifest clinically in a similar manner in the absence of SIBO.

Treatment

SIBO treatment requires attention to any predisposing conditions, nutritional support, antibiotic therapy, and prevention of SIBO recurrence. The main objective is to reverse the underlying small intestinal abnormality whenever possible. While infrequently the case, this can be done surgically when anatomic abnormalities or postsurgical complications exist. Treatment of motility disorders is also a challenge as there are few effective and well-tolerated prokinetic medications available. The successful use of low-dose subcutaneous octreotide for the treatment of scleroderma-associated SIBO has been described.

Nutritional support is usually complementary to the antibiotic treatment when SIBO presents with nutritional deficiencies. Usual measures include avoidance of lactose and reduction of nonabsorbed carbohydrates. Although without evidence to

Table 11.5 Antibiotics for the treatment of small intestinal bacterial overgrowth

Antibiotic	Oral dosage
Rifaximin	550 mg bid or tid
Metronidazole	250–500 mg bid to tid
Tetracycline	250–500 mg qid
Amoxicillin-clavulanate	500 mg/125 mg tid
Doxycycline	100 mg bid
Ciprofloxacin	250–500 mg bid
Norfloxacin	400 mg bid
Cephalexin	250 mg qid
Neomycin	500 mg bid

support its implementation, it has been suggested that a high-fat, low-carbohydrate, low-fiber diet supplies sufficient calories in those requiring supplemental nutrition, and this approach provides fewer fermentable substrates for the microbes. When a micronutrient deficiency exists, proper supplementation is recommended.

Antibiotic treatment is the cornerstone of SIBO treatment in order to reduce microbial load and to induce symptomatic improvement. The antibiotic regimen should target the broad spectrum of microbes associated with SIBO and should be effective against both aerobic and anaerobic enteric bacteria. There is no need for sensitivity testing when an aspirate is obtained since multiple microbes and microbial strains with different sensitivities are detected in patients with SIBO. Therefore, empiric treatment with one of the antibiotics listed in Table 11.5 for 7–10 days is recommended. When successful, antibiotic treatment usually leads to an improvement in symptoms that may last for months; however, some patients require prolonged therapy before evidence of response, and some, depending upon their predisposing condition, may require a course of therapy on a monthly basis (e.g., 7–10 days out of every month). In such a case, rotating three or four different antibiotics on a cyclical basis is recommended to prevent the development of resistance, although randomized, controlled trials to support this common practice are lacking.

Case Resolution

SIBO was considered as a cause of the patient's symptoms on the basis of older age and the potential effects of diabetes on gut motility. The diagnosis was confirmed by lactulose hydrogen breath testing that revealed an early hydrogen peak of 90 ppm at 60 min. The patient was treated with metronidazole 250 mg orally three times daily for 10 days with complete resolution of his symptoms. The symptoms recurred 4 months later, but the patient responded well to the same treatment.

Key Clinical Teaching Points

- SIBO is an increasingly recognized cause of malabsorption and is likely an under-recognized cause of a variety of nonspecific gastrointestinal symptoms.
- The prevalence of SIBO and its relationship to several clinical conditions are unclear because of controversies related to its detection and definition and the overlap of its clinical manifestations with those of many other gastrointestinal disorders.
- The most important factors contributing to the pathogenesis of SIBO are intestinal dysmotility, anatomical alterations of the gastrointestinal tract that predispose to stagnation of intestinal contents, and low gastric acid production.
- The "classic" presentation of SIBO as malabsorption is now uncommon with the majority of SIBO patients presenting with nonspecific symptoms such as abdominal pain or discomfort, flatulence, bloating, and a change in bowel habits in the absence of an obvious risk factor.
- The preferred diagnostic approach in SIBO remains controversial given limitations in available tests and the lack of true "gold standard."
- SIBO treatment requires attention to any predisposing conditions, nutritional support, antibiotic therapy, and prevention of SIBO recurrence.

Teaching Questions

1. Small intestinal overgrowth most commonly manifests clinically as which one of the following?

   (A) Florid malabsorption in the presence of a predisposing condition
   (B) Florid malabsorption without a predisposing condition
   (C) Asymptomatically
   (D) Nonspecific symptoms in the presence of a predisposing factor
   (E) Nonspecific symptoms without a predisposing factor

2. Which of the following is the most commonly used test for the detection of SIBO?

   (A) Culture of small bowel aspirate
   (B) Hydrogen breath test
   (C) Endoscopy with small bowel biopsy
   (D) Magnetic resonance enterography
   (E) Stool fat and vitamin B12 measurements

3. Which one is the corner stone of SIBO treatment?

   (A) Treatment of the underlying condition
   (B) Nutritional support
   (C) Probiotics
   (D) Antibiotics
   (E) Prokinetics

Key References

1. DiBaise JK. Nutritional consequences of small intestinal bacterial overgrowth. Pract Gastroenterol. 2008;69:15–29. Review of the nutritional aspects of SIBO including treatment recommendations.
2. Khoshini R, Dai S-C, Lezcano S, Pimentel M. A systematic review of diagnostic tests for small intestinal bacterial overgrowth. Dig Dis Sci. 2008;53:1443–54. Systematic review that questions the validity of available tests used to diagnose SIBO.
3. Pyleris M, Giamarellos-Bourboulis EJ, Tsivras D, Koussoulas V, Barbatzas C, Pimentel M. The prevalence of overgrowth by aerobic bacteria in the small intestine by small bowel culture: relationship with irritable bowel syndrome. Dig Dis Sci. 2012;57:1321–9. The strongest evidence to date linking SIBO with IBS using aspirate.
4. Quigley EMM, Abu-Shanab A. Small intestinal bacterial overgrowth. Infect Dis Clin N Am. 2010;24:943–59. Review of the clinical, diagnostic and treatment aspects of small bowel bacterial overgrowth.
5. Simren M, Barbara G, Flint HJ, Spiegel BMR, Spiller RC, Vanner S, Verdu EF, Whorwell PJ, Zoetendal EG. Intestinal microbiota in functional bowel disorders: A Rome foundation report. Gut. 2013;62:159–76. Extensive discussion of the association of gut microbiota and functional bowel diseases.
6. Yamini D, Pimentel M. Irritable bowel syndrome and small intestinal bacterial overgrowth. J Clin Gastroenterol. 2010;44:672–5. Comprehensive summary of the available evidence that links SIBO to IBS.

Chapter 12
Chronic Intestinal Pseudo-obstruction

Scott Gabbard and John K. DiBaise

Case Study

An 18-year-old woman was referred by her internist for a 3-year history of constipation and lower abdominal pain. A complete blood count (CBC) and thyroid-stimulating hormone level (TSH) were both normal. Based on her symptoms and a normal physical examination, she was diagnosed with IBS and treated with psyllium. She then noted occasional episodes of solid food dysphagia and upper abdominal bloating and distension. Upper endoscopy including biopsies of the duodenum, stomach, and esophagus was all normal. Six months later, her distension worsened, and she noted difficulty eating due to symptoms of early satiety and postprandial nausea. An abdominal X-ray revealed dilated loops of small intestine. A CT scan of the abdomen and pelvis with oral and intravenous contrast demonstrated diffusely dilated loops of small intestine without evidence of a transition point and no other abnormalities (Fig. 12.1). Over the next year, her symptoms progressed leading to a weight loss of 15 % of body weight.

Introduction

Intestinal pseudo-obstruction can be categorized as either acute or chronic. Chronic intestinal pseudo-obstruction (CIP) differs clinically from acute intestinal pseudo-obstruction by the presence of obstructive symptoms for at least 6 months (Table 12.1).

S. Gabbard, M.D. (✉)
Division of Gastroenterology and Hepatology, Cleveland Clinic,
9500 Euclid Avenue/A31, Cleveland, OH 44195, USA
e-mail: gabbars@ccf.org

J.K. DiBaise, M.D.
Division of Gastroenterology and Hepatology, Mayo Clinic, Scottsdale, AZ, USA

B.E. Lacy et al. (eds.), *Functional and Motility Disorders of the Gastrointestinal Tract*, DOI 10.1007/978-1-4939-1498-2_12

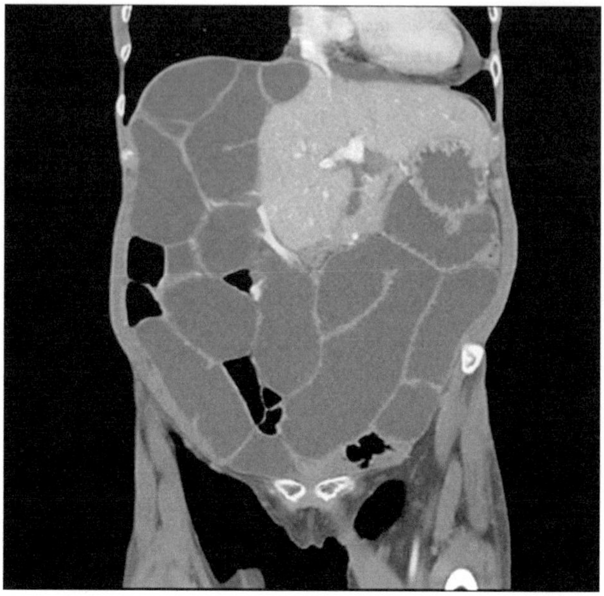

Fig. 12.1 Representative CT image demonstrating marked diffuse dilation of the small bowel without transition point

Table 12.1 Definition of chronic intestinal pseudo-obstruction

The following must be present	Dilation of small intestine on radiography
	Symptoms of obstruction for longer than 6 months
The following must be absent	Mechanical obstruction
Supporting studies	Delayed scintigraphy (i.e., gastric emptying scan)
	Abnormal esophageal or antroduodenal manometry
	Connective tissue disease serologies (i.e., anti-scl-70)
	Abnormal full-thickness biopsy of the small bowel

CIP is a rare yet debilitating neuromuscular disorder of the gastrointestinal tract characterized by impaired peristalsis with symptoms and imaging that may mimic mechanical bowel obstruction. Because the symptoms of CIP including abdominal pain, nausea, vomiting, bloating, and abdominal distension are nonspecific, CIP often goes undiagnosed for many years despite multiple potentially dangerous diagnostic tests and treatments. Thus, a high degree of clinical suspicion in conjunction with a careful history and physical examination remains paramount to establishing the diagnosis. Importantly, CIP is not a single disorder; rather, it refers to a heterogeneous group of disorders characterized by disordered intestinal peristalsis. Once mechanical obstruction is ruled out, dedicated imaging and motility testing can be utilized to help confirm the diagnosis. Unfortunately, a cure does not exist for CIP, and supportive care remains the cornerstone of disease management. Many patients with CIP have difficulty maintaining their normal weight and achieving adequate nutrition; a large percentage of CIP patients will eventually require nutritional support. For patients who fail symptomatic treatment or develop severe side effects from parenteral nutrition, small intestinal transplant has become a realistic treatment option.

Epidemiology and Natural History

CIP is a rare disorder. One estimate from a pediatric tertiary care center suggests that approximately 100 infants are born with CIP each year in the United States. The natural history for most CIP patients is that of a progressive worsening of their condition. In a recent report, the diagnosis of CIP was made a median of 8 years after symptoms first developed, and, during this time, each patient underwent an average of three surgeries related to their yet to be diagnosed CIP symptoms.

The long-term prognosis of CIP patients is poor. It is estimated that up to two-thirds of CIP patients develop a nutritional deficiency and that 30–50 % of adult CIP patients will require parenteral nutrition or small bowel transplantation. Many patients become opioid dependent due to chronic abdominal pain. CIP in the pediatric population has a similarly poor prognosis with a 10–25 % mortality rate before reaching adulthood.

Pathophysiology

The etiology of primary CIP is varied but may be characterized as a neuropathy, myopathy, or mesenchymopathy (i.e., affecting the interstitial cells of Cajal) depending upon the gut wall structure most affected. On the basis of these pathogenic abnormalities, a variety of both primary and secondary causes of CIP have been described. Secondary causes of CIP include but are not limited to collagen vascular disorders, endocrine disorders, neurologic disorders, and medications (Table 12.2). One of the more common secondary causes of CIP is primary systemic sclerosis. Importantly, certain malignancies (e.g., small cell carcinoma of the lung) may cause a paraneoplastic form of CIP. Irrespective of the etiology, the end result is that of impaired peristalsis and a poorly or nonfunctioning GI tract.

Diagnosis

The diagnosis of CIP may be elusive for a number of reasons. First, the symptoms do not typically develop at once but rather slowly evolve over a number of years. Second, CIP may affect all segments of the GI tract resulting in a variety of symptoms.

Table 12.2 Secondary causes of chronic intestinal pseudo-obstruction

Collagen vascular diseases
Primary systemic sclerosis
Systemic lupus erythematosus
Dermatomyositis/polymyositis
Periarteritis nodosa
Rheumatoid arthritis
Mixed connective tissue disease
Endocrine disorders
Diabetes
Hypothyroidism
Parathyroidism
Neurologic disorders
Parkinson's disease
Alzheimer's disease
Shy-Drager
Chagas' disease
Intestinal hypoganglionosis
Dysautonomia (familial or sporadic)
Medication associated
Tricyclic antidepressants
Anticholinergic agents
Ganglionic blockers
Antiparkinsonian agents
Clonidine
Phenothiazines
Miscellaneous
Celiac disease
Paraneoplastic syndromes (small cell lung carcinoma, carcinoid, thymoma)
Infiltrative disorders (amyloidosis, lymphoma)
Alcohol abuse
Post-infectious processes (viral, bacterial, parasitic)
Radiation
Vascular insufficiency
Metabolic (hypokalemia, hypomagnesemia)
Postsurgical
Post-organ transplant
Mitochondrial disorders

Adapted from: Gabbard SL, Lacy BE. Chronic intestinal pseudo-obstruction. Nutr Clin Pract. 2013;28:307–16. Permission for use granted

Third, these symptoms which include abdominal pain, bloating, distension, nausea, vomiting, constipation, and weight loss are nonspecific. Fourth, initial diagnostic tests (see below) are usually normal. Fifth, there are no biologic markers for CIP. Finally, there is a generalized lack of awareness of this disorder.

Thus, the diagnosis of CIP requires an awareness of the disorder combined with a carefully performed history and physical examination in addition to tests to exclude mechanical obstruction and, frequently, tests to assess gastrointestinal transit and the neuromuscular function.

Symptoms

The most common symptoms occurring in CIP are abdominal pain (80 %), nausea and vomiting (75 %), constipation (40 %), and diarrhea (20 %). The clinical picture tends to be dominated by abdominal pain and distension which are particularly severe during episodes of exacerbation. In CIP, symptoms should be present for a minimum of 6 months.

Imaging

Given the nonspecific nature of the symptoms of CIP, the initial evaluation centers on excluding mechanical obstruction. Evidence of obstruction essentially excludes the diagnosis of CIP. Although a plain X-ray of the abdomen may have findings suggestive of obstruction, cross-sectional abdominal imaging such as CT or MR is necessary to more thoroughly evaluate for mechanical obstruction. The use of barium contrast small bowel studies has largely been superseded by the development of CT and MR enterography protocols.

Endoscopy

Upper endoscopy, colonoscopy, and, occasionally, enteroscopy are useful in suspected CIP to identify intraluminal lesions, collect biopsy and fluid samples (e.g., to identify small bowel bacterial overgrowth), and, on occasion, provide treatment (e.g., placement of decompression tubes).

Motility Testing

For patients with persistent unexplained symptoms or to confirm the diagnosis of CIP, specialized tests to assess gastrointestinal motility and transit may prove useful. If symptoms of early satiety, nausea, and vomiting are predominant, a 4-h solid-phase gastric emptying scan should be performed to document the extent of delayed emptying. Similarly, colon transit testing, using either radio-opaque markers or scintigraphy, may provide useful information. The utility of small bowel transit testing remains poorly understood, and, when determined by lactulose hydrogen breath testing, accurate interpretation may be limited by the presence of small bowel bacterial overgrowth.

Further support for the diagnosis of CIP, and clues to the possible underlying etiology, may be obtained using intraluminal GI pressure recordings (i.e., manometry). Although esophageal manometry may demonstrate findings characteristic of scleroderma-related CIP, it mostly reveals nonspecific abnormalities. Indeed, nonspecific findings in esophageal motility have been found in more than 70 % of patients with CIP. Esophageal manometry may prove useful in predicting who will need parenteral nutrition as one study has shown that patients with ineffective esophageal motility were more likely to require parenteral nutrition than those with normal motility. Although not widely available, antroduodenal manometry (and small bowel manometry) may reveal characteristic neuropathic and myopathic abnormalities of the migrating motor complex (MMC) during the fasting and fed periods and may help to differentiate mechanical obstruction from CIP. Myopathic (smooth muscle) disorders are characterized by abnormally low-amplitude, coordinated contractions, whereas neuropathic processes are characterized by uncoordinated contractions and the absence of an MMC (Fig. 12.2). The presence of an MMC on antroduodenal manometry has been suggested to be predictive of successful tolerance to jejunal feeding in patients who have previously failed gastrostomy feeding. During antroduodenal manometry, patients with suspected CIP may be challenged with erythromycin (to stimulate gastric contractions) and octreotide (to stimulate small bowel motility); however, the clinical utility of these drug challenges remains to be demonstrated. Wireless motility capsule testing, the most recent addition to the motility testing armamentarium, transmits intraluminal pH, temperature, and pressure data allowing a determination of gastric, small bowel, and colon transit times. The role of this test in the evaluation of CIP, however, has not yet been established.

Pathology

The clinical utility of full-thickness intestinal biopsy has not been evaluated in a prospective manner, and its role in the diagnosis and management of CIP remains unclear. Nevertheless, obtaining a full-thickness biopsy of the intestinal wall should be considered if intra-abdominal surgery is being considered (e.g., to exclude obstruction or to place a tube for decompression). Biopsies may show smooth muscle atrophy in the primary myopathic processes, neuropathic degeneration in the primary neuropathic disorders, and various findings for the secondary causes of CIP including fibrosis in primary systemic sclerosis or evidence of amyloid or lymphoma. Importantly, although new information may be obtained, it may not change clinical management.

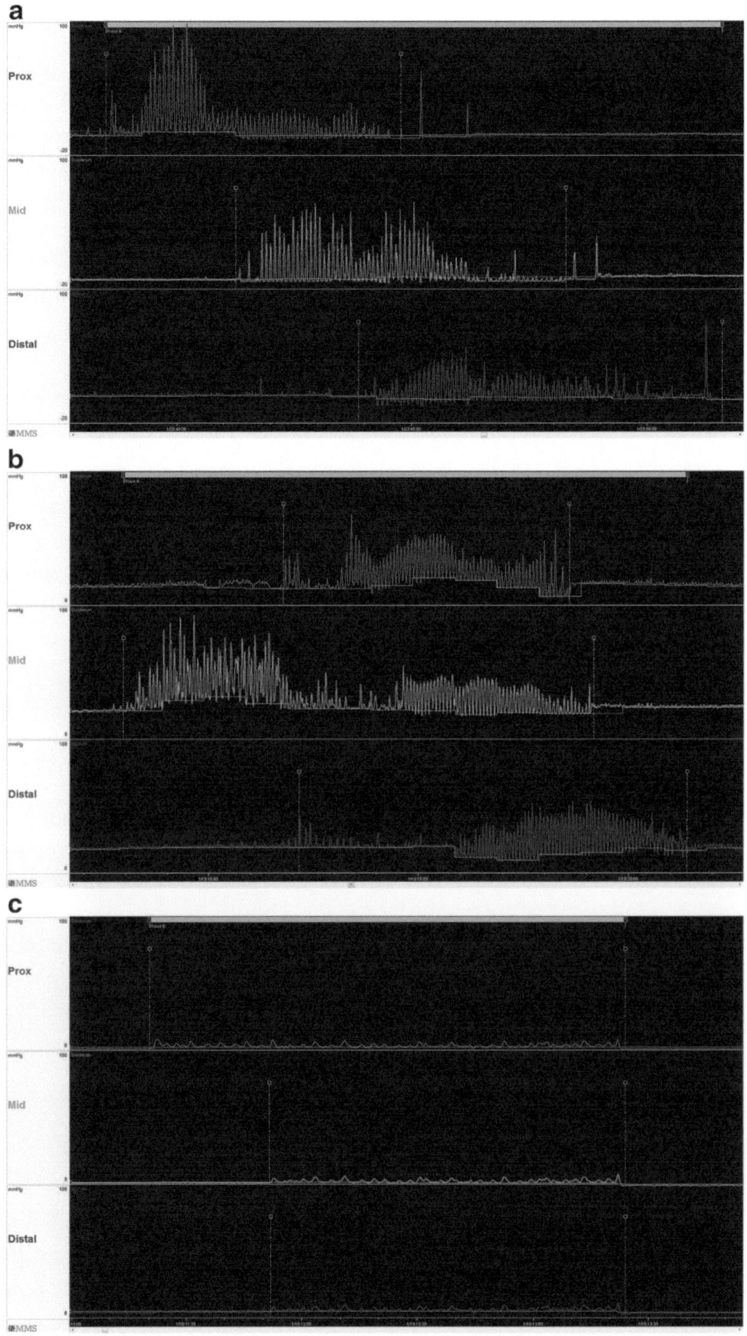

Fig. 12.2 Characteristic small bowel manometry findings showing (**a**) normal antegrade propagation and contraction wave amplitude and frequency of the phase III complex, (**b**) discoordinated phase III complex suggestive of intestinal neuropathy, and (**c**) marked reduction in the amplitude of the contractions including the phase III complex suggestive of intestinal myopathy. Note that the 3 sensors are each positioned 10 cm apart within the small intestine

Laboratory Testing

All patients diagnosed with CIP should have blood work performed to evaluate for evidence of secondary causes including autoimmune disorders, connective tissue disorders, and paraneoplastic process (e.g., anti-neuronal nuclear antibodies) and to assess nutritional status (i.e., micronutrient levels). Testing should include a complete blood count; erythrocyte sedimentation rate or C-reactive protein; serum electrolytes including calcium, magnesium, and phosphorous; glucose; albumin; thyroid-stimulating hormone; cortisol; and specialized testing for celiac disease, connective tissue disorders, and paraneoplastic process.

Treatment

CIP is often a challenge to treat as there is no curative medication or surgery available. Once the diagnosis of CIP is made, therapy should focus on maintaining fluid and electrolyte balance, improving nutritional status, relieving gastrointestinal symptoms (i.e., pain, nausea, vomiting, constipation, and bloating), and avoiding unnecessary surgery (Table 12.3).

Nutritional Assessment

The nutrition evaluation should begin with anthropometric measures such as weight and body mass index (BMI), details regarding weight loss, and a thorough dietary history including oral intake and diet restrictions. Because of poor intake or absorption, periodic assessment of micronutrient levels should be considered. The use of albumin and prealbumin to assess nutritional status, although commonly done, is unreliable and not recommended. Patients with CIP should undergo formal nutrition assessment by a registered dietitian with experience in treating patients with complex GI motility disorders.

Diet

Dietary treatment should begin with the correction of any nutritional deficiencies. A daily multivitamin is recommended, and additional supplemental micronutrients should be administered if depleted. Oral intake is preferred whenever possible. The ingestion of frequent meals (5–6 per day) of small portion size with an emphasis on liquid calories and protein, while avoiding foods high in fat and fiber, is recommended. High-fat foods (>30 % total calories) may delay gastric emptying and result in postprandial fullness and nausea, while high-fiber products are

Table 12.3 Treatment options for CIP

Diet	Low fiber, low fat, low osmolality
Access	G-tube, G-J tube, J-tube, central venous access
Diet supplementation	Tube feeding or parenteral feeding based on adequacy of oral intake
Decompression	Nasogastric/nasoenteric tube, rectal tube
	Percutaneous, gastrostomy, enterostomy, or cecostomy tube
Antiemetics	Antihistamines (diphenhydramine, meclizine)
	Phenothiazines (prochlorperazine, chlorpromazine promethazine)
	Anticholinergics (scopolamine)
	Serotonin receptor antagonists (ondansetron, granisetron, dolasetron)
	Trimethobenzamide
	Dronabinol
Prokinetics	Octreotide
	Erythromycin
	Metoclopramide
	Domperidone (not FDA approved)
	Prucalopride (not FDA approved)
	Tegaserod (not currently available)
	Cisapride (investigational use)
Antibiotics	Rifaximin
	Amoxicillin-clavulanate
	Fluoroquinolones
	Cephalosporins
	Metronidazole
Pain control	Tramadol
	Tricyclic antidepressants
	Serotonin-norepinephrine reuptake inhibitors
	GABA analogues
	Buprenorphine
Surgery	Intestinal resection, intestinal transplantation

associated with abdominal bloating, bezoar formation, and abdominal discomfort. Lactose and fructose consumption may worsen abdominal bloating and discomfort. A variety of oral nutritional supplements are available for use in malnourished patients and those unable to ingest sufficient calories with a regular diet. These supplements are high in calories and low in residue; however, the fat concentration varies among supplements.

Enteral Nutrition

If dietary intake remains inadequate to meet nutritional requirements, consideration of enteral feeding should be given. Before placement of a permanent feeding tube, however, a trial of nasogastric (if normal gastric emptying is present) or nasojejunal feeding should be considered. If tolerated without significant discomfort, nausea, or bloating, percutaneous enteral access may be obtained. An enteral feeding regimen infused continuously over the entire day or a cyclical regimen infused overnight is generally tolerated better than bolus administration and is required in those receiving post-pyloric feeding.

Parenteral Nutrition

Parenteral nutrition (PN) becomes necessary in those CIP patients with intestinal failure (i.e., intolerance to oral or enteral feedings due to a poorly or nonfunctioning gut). PN should otherwise be avoided as it is associated with a variety of complications, is expensive, and is complicated to manage both for the patient and their healthcare provider. Unfortunately, many CIP patients will eventually require PN given the lack of effective treatments and the progressive nature of the disease. A recent retrospective analysis of 51 CIP patients on PN for an average of 8.3 years found 180 episodes of catheter-related sepsis, nine episodes of acute pancreatitis (2/3 due to metabolic condition, 1/3 due to gallstones), five cases of D-lactic acidosis with encephalopathy, and 4 patients with progression to cirrhosis; there was one death directly related to a PN complication (catheter-related sepsis) in this population. Oral intake was a major independent factor associated with better survival. Thus, CIP patients on PN should be encouraged to continue some oral intake as tolerated.

Gastrointestinal Decompression

Decompression of distended intestinal segments is helpful for many CIP patients both to reduce symptom severity and to prevent hospitalizations and emergency department visits. There are no firm guidelines on when such intervention should be undertaken in the course of the disease and clinical judgment is necessary.

Antiemetics

Patients with CIP often suffer from recurrent bouts of nausea and vomiting during an episode of pseudo-obstruction and may complain of frequent or even constant bothersome nausea. There is no single agent that is universally effective and well tolerated for the treatment of nausea and vomiting in CIP. Therefore, each patient needs to be assessed individually, and trials of antiemetics while monitoring efficacy, adverse effects, and financial impact are needed.

Prokinetic Agents

CIP implies disordered gastrointestinal tract motility. Therefore, multiple prokinetic agents have been used in an attempt to improve gut motility. Nevertheless, mostly due to the rarity of CIP and the heterogeneous population affected, there have been few clinical trials conducted to determine the efficacy of any of these agents in CIP.

Erythromycin, a macrolide antibiotic that acts as a motilin receptor agonist, has been shown to be effective in accelerating gastric emptying and improving symptoms of CIP in case reports. Metoclopramide and domperidone, dopamine antagonists that exert prokinetic effects by increasing acetylcholine release, have also been used in clinical practice; however, clinical data for their use in CIP is lacking. Additionally, metoclopramide has a black box warning from the FDA due to the risk of tardive dyskinesia, although this has been estimated to be <1 % with chronic use. Domperidone is not FDA approved for use in the United States; however, it is available in the United States through an Investigational New Drug Application pathway. Recently, the 5-hydoxytryptamine 4 receptor agonist prucalopride, also not FDA approved for use in the United States, was shown in a small controlled trial to provide symptom relief in selected patients with CIP.

Somatostatin has well-described effects on motor activity on the small intestine. The long-acting somatostatin analogue, octreotide, has been used in patients with CIP secondary to both scleroderma and idiopathic causes. At a dose of 50 mcg injected subcutaneously at bedtime, octreotide has been shown to significantly reduce nausea and emesis, bloating, and abdominal pain in scleroderma patients with CIP and small bowel bacterial overgrowth.

Antibiotics

Intestinal stasis may lead to the syndrome of small bowel bacterial overgrowth with resultant bloating, discomfort, nausea, and diarrhea. Occasionally, significant malabsorption with weight loss and the development of micronutrient deficiencies may occur. A program of cycling a rotating variety of broad-spectrum antibiotics for 1 or 2 weeks each month may improve symptoms and improve the nutritional status.

Pain Control

As noted previously, abdominal pain has been reported to be the most common symptom of CIP, at least in adults. Few medications have demonstrated benefit for pain relief in CIP, and, unfortunately, many patients with CIP eventually are treated with chronic opiates. Although lacking evidence to support their use, non-narcotic pain modulators such as tricyclic antidepressants, serotonin-norepinephrine reuptake inhibitors, and GABA analogues should be considered. Other considerations include octreotide which has been shown to reduce pain in placebo-controlled trials and tramadol, a mu-opioid receptor agonist that is less constipating than opiates. Recently, transdermal buprenorphine, a partial agonist at the μ-opioid receptor and an antagonist at the kappa- and delta-opioid receptors, was studied in children with idiopathic CIP, and three of four children reported adequate pain relief and none required further dose escalation.

Small Intestinal Transplantation

Small bowel transplantation has become an accepted therapy for patients with intestinal failure (mainly short bowel syndrome) and life-threatening PN-related complications. Patients with CIP account for approximately 9 % of the total intestinal transplants performed in both adults and children. In addition to general pre-transplant screening, patients with CIP should be evaluated for urological anomalies such as megacystis and vesicoureteric reflux, which may occur in up to 33 % of CIP patients. A multivisceral allograft consisting of stomach, duodenum, pancreas, and small intestine can be implanted when the disease involves the stomach; a liver can be implanted if there is irreversible liver disease. Recent UNOS data in children demonstrated comparable overall survival rates for patients with functional intestinal disorders compared to other indications for intestinal transplant.

Case Resolution

At her initial visit, a number of different serologic tests were performed and were normal. Esophageal manometry revealed severe ineffective esophageal motility bordering on motor failure with only 20 % of water swallows being transmitted. A 4-h solid-phase gastric emptying scan revealed delayed gastric emptying with 28 % retention at 4 h. Antroduodenal manometry revealed normal amplitude but decreased frequency of antral contractions and an absence of a migrating motor complex in the small intestine with no response to octreotide. The patient was diagnosed with a neuropathic form of chronic intestinal pseudo-obstruction and was started on parenteral nutrition due to her weight loss and documented nutritional compromise. A nonabsorbable antibiotic was used to empirically treat for presumed small bowel bacterial overgrowth. Gabapentin was used to treat her abdominal pain with some improvement. A scopolamine patch and ondansetron were used to treat nausea with moderate relief. Eventually, a jejunostomy tube was placed, and enteral feedings begun although the patient was unable to tolerate more than 40 ml/h secondary to abdominal discomfort. While the patient continues to have symptoms, her overall symptoms are less bothersome, and her weight has slowly returned to her baseline.

Key Clinical Teaching Points

- Chronic intestinal pseudo-obstruction (CIP) should be considered in patients with symptoms suggestive of obstruction and small bowel dilation but without mechanical obstruction on imaging.
- CIP may be due to either an intestinal neuropathy or myopathy. Esophageal or antroduodenal manometry may demonstrate disordered or absent peristalsis and aid in the determination of the diagnosis and prognosis.
- Treatment of CIP is directed at symptom management. In addition to antiemetics and prokinetics, octreotide 50 mcg subcutaneously at bedtime may improve symptoms.
- Patients with CIP should be followed by an experienced nutritionist and may require enteral or parenteral nutrition support.
- Small intestinal transplant is an option for CIP patients with intestinal failure and life-threatening PN-related complications.

Teaching Questions

1. An 18-year-old male presents with 2 years of nonprogressive chronic nausea, vomiting, distension, and abdominal pain. An upright abdominal X-ray is notable for dilated small intestine. Which one of the following is the best next step in the evaluation for CIP?

   (A) Celiac serologies
   (B) Upper endoscopy
   (C) Antinuclear antibody
   (D) MR enterography

2. A 45-year-old female with CIP and gastroparesis has lost 15 lb (10 % of body weight) over the past 6 months due to reduced oral intake resulting from chronic pain, nausea, and vomiting. Which one of the following is the next best step in nutrition management?

   (A) Placement of Hickman catheter to initiate parenteral nutrition
   (B) Endoscopic placement of a gastrostomy tube for venting
   (C) Trial of nasojejunal feeding
   (D) Partial gastrectomy

3. A 32-year-old male with CIP requiring parenteral nutrition for the past 3 years has suffered multiple central line infections and urinary tract infections over the past year. Which one of the following evaluations would not be required before undergoing small bowel transplantation?

   (A) Urology referral
   (B) Colonoscopy
   (C) Hepatic function testing
   (D) Gastric emptying scan

Key References

1. Amiot A, Joly F, Alves A, Panis Y, Bouhnik Y, Messing B. Long-term outcome of chronic intestinal pseudo-obstruction adult patients requiring home parenteral nutrition. Am J Gastroenterol. 2009;104:1262–70. In a large cohort of adult CIP patients requiring HPN, a higher survival probability than previously reported was found.
2. Amiot A, Joly F, Cazals-Hatem D, Merrouche M, Jouet P, Coffin B, Bouhnik Y. Prognostic yield of esophageal manometry in chronic intestinal pseudo-obstruction: a retrospective cohort of 116 adult patients. Neurogastroenterol Motil. 2012;24:1008–e542. Abnormal esophageal manometry was associated with lower survival and inability to maintain sufficient oral feeding in patients with CIP.
3. Bond GJ, Reyes JD. Intestinal transplantation for total/near-total aganglionosis and intestinal pseudo-obstruction. Semin Pediatr Surg. 2004;13:286–92. This study shows that children who undergo intestinal transplant for CIP have similar survival rates compared to children who undergo intestinal transplant for other causes.
4. Gabbard SL, Lacy BE. Chronic intestinal pseudo-obstruction. Nutr Clin Pract. 2013;28:307–16. Recent comprehensive review of CIP.
5. Lindberg G, Iwarzon M, Tornblom H. Clinical features and long-term survival in chronic intestinal pseudo-obstruction and enteric dysmotility. Scand J Gastroenterol. 2009;44:692–9. Found that CIP and ED, conditions with similar symptoms but differing radiologic findings, also differ with respect to severity of measurable physiological derangement, nutritional needs and long-term prognosis.
6. Soudah HC, Hasler WL, Owyang C. Effect of octreotide on intestinal motility and bacterial overgrowth in scleroderma. N Eng J Med. 1991;325:1461–7. Octreotide was shown to evoke phase 3 contractions and, more importantly, significantly reduce nausea, bloating and abdominal pain in patients with CIP due to scleroderma with associated SIBO.
7. Stanghellini V, Cogliandro R, Giorgio R, Barbara G, Morselli-Labate AM, Cogliandro L, Corinaldesi R. Natural history of chronic idiopathic intestinal pseudo-obstruction in adults: A single center study. Clin Gastro Hep. 2005;3:449–58. Patients were diagnosed with CIP an average of 8 years after symptom onset and underwent an average of 2.3 surgeries before diagnosis demonstrating the difficulty in diagnosing CIP.

Part IV
Gallbladder Disorders

Chapter 13
Functional Gallbladder Disorder

Stephanie L. Hansel

Case Study

A 45-year-old woman presents with a 6-month history of episodic right upper quadrant pain. There are no obvious triggers for the pain episodes; the episodes occur weekly on average, anytime throughout the day or night. The pain starts in the right upper quadrant as a dull pain that increases steadily to a moderate to severe level of pain. On a few occasions, the pain has radiated around to her back. After the pain starts, it can last for up to 2–3 h. In the past she has tried antacids, acetaminophen, ibuprofen, laxatives, and warm compresses to alleviate the pain without success. She denies other symptoms with these episodes and is asymptomatic between episodes. She has been to the emergency department twice in the past 6 months for this pain and has been told that her physical examination, liver and pancreatic enzymes, and right upper quadrant ultrasound were normal. She recently underwent an upper endoscopy which was normal. Despite the negative testing, she remains worried about a problem with her gallbladder or pancreas and questions you about whether any additional testing should be done. She also wonders if she should be seen by a surgeon to consider an exploratory laparotomy or cholecystectomy because she had a friend with similar symptoms that went away after a cholecystectomy.

S.L. Hansel, M.D., M.S. (✉)
Division of Gastroenterology and Hepatology, Mayo Clinic,
200 First Street SW, Rochester, MN 55905, USA
e-mail: hansel.stephanie@mayo.edu

B.E. Lacy et al. (eds.), *Functional and Motility Disorders of the Gastrointestinal Tract*, DOI 10.1007/978-1-4939-1498-2_13

Introduction

Functional gallbladder disorder refers to biliary-like pain in the absence of structural disease. It is a controversial condition and has many aliases including acalculous biliary disease, acalculous gallbladder dysfunction, biliary dyskinesia, chronic acalculous gallbladder dysfunction, and gallbladder dyskinesia. The multitude of names is likely a direct reflection of the difficulty defining this disorder and understanding its pathogenesis. In fact, there is not a specific ICD-9 code for functional gallbladder disorder. Despite these difficulties, this constellation of symptoms is very relevant as it is frequently encountered in medical and surgical practices. The Rome committee has attempted to standardize the definition of biliary pain and criteria for the diagnosis of functional gallbladder disorder (see Table 13.1); however, due to significant overlap with other functional gastrointestinal disorders, continued confusion persists.

Epidemiology

The incidence of functional gallbladder disorder is unknown. The best estimate of its prevalence comes from epidemiological studies in Italy performed in the 1980s. These studies found that approximately 21 % of women and 8 % of men report biliary-like pain but have normal ultrasounds of the gallbladder.

The natural history is also poorly understood. To date, there is only one prospective trial of 21 patients with a normal-appearing gallbladder and abnormal

Table 13.1 Rome III criteria for functional gallbladder disorder

Episodes of pain located in the epigastrium and/or right upper quadrant and all of the following:
1. Episodes lasting 30 min or longer
2. Recurrent symptoms occurring at different intervals (not daily)
3. The pain builds up to a steady level
4. The pain is moderate to severe enough to interrupt the patient's daily activities or lead to an emergency department visit
5. The pain is not relieved by bowel movements
6. The pain is not relieved by postural change
7. The pain is not relieved by antacids
8. Exclusion of other structural disease that would explain the symptoms
Supportive criteria:
The pain may present with one or more of the following:
1. Associated with nausea and vomiting
2. Radiates to the back and/or right infra subscapular region
3. Awakens from sleep in the middle of the night

gallbladder ejection fraction (GBEF). These patients were randomized to cholecystectomy versus no surgery and followed for up to 54 months. All ten patients in the no surgery group continued to report symptoms during the follow-up phase, whereas all patients offered surgery reported improvement in their symptoms following surgery. The published retrospective studies of patients with suspected functional gallbladder disorder are quite variable in their methods and outcome measures and report resolution of symptoms without cholecystectomy in 16–80 % of the patients. Importantly, a meta-analysis completed to determine whether patients with functional biliary pain and a low GBEF experience a better outcome after cholecystectomy in comparison to those with a normal GBEF failed to show an increased likelihood of improved symptoms after cholecystectomy in patients with suspected functional biliary pain and reduced GBEF compared to those with normal GBEF.

Pathophysiology

Normal gallbladder function is well understood and known to be quite complex. In contrast, the pathophysiology of functional gallbladder disorder is poorly understood. There are two main hypotheses to explain the cause of the pain in this disorder: (1) increased pressure from a structural or functional outflow obstruction and (2) visceral hypersensitivity. The first hypothesis postulates that functional gallbladder disorder is part of a spectrum of gallbladder disease whereby bile saturation and gallbladder dysmotility lead to crystal formation. The crystals may eventually develop into gallstones or infiltrate the gallbladder wall causing inflammation. Pain may occur from either gallstones (if present) or from inflammation of the gallbladder wall. Histologic studies have demonstrated conflicting findings and, therefore, have not universally supported this hypothesis. It remains unclear whether the histologic changes often seen in the gallbladder wall are a cause or effect of poor gallbladder motility.

Sphincter of Oddi dysfunction, another controversial disorder, has been studied as a potential cause of outflow obstruction in functional gallbladder disorder. There appears to be poor correlation, however, between GBEF and sphincter of Oddi pressures. Even though there are similarities in presentation, functional biliary sphincter of Oddi disorder and functional pancreatic sphincter of Oddi disorder seem to be distinct and separate disorders.

Finally, as in most functional gastrointestinal disorders, visceral hypersensitivity has also been implicated in the pathogenesis of functional gallbladder disorder. Visceral hypersensitivity refers to enhanced perception or responsiveness within the gut to even normal events and involves the cerebral and thalamic neural pathways communicating with the gut. This process may lead to abnormalities in the signaling pathways such as cholecystokinin which, in turn, could lead to abnormal messaging to the gallbladder and resultant pain.

Diagnosis and Evaluation

Rome III criteria have been developed to assist in the diagnosis of functional gallbladder disorder (see Table 13.1). To meet these criteria, a thorough history and physical examination must be performed and structural disease or other conditions that might explain the symptoms must be excluded (see Table 13.2). Common organic diseases can be excluded by obtaining the testing listed in Table 13.3. The utility of obtaining an upper endoscopic ultrasound or more extensive imaging of the abdomen is unknown and is not currently recommended.

Once structural causes have been eliminated, a functional assessment of gallbladder emptying should be considered. Although its clinical utility remains controversial, cholecystokinin-cholescintigraphy (CCK-CS), also known as a CCK-HIDA scan, has been recommended in this setting by the Rome committee. This test consists of the intravenous administration of ^{99m}technetium-labeled hepatoiminodiacetic acid which is taken up by the liver and excreted into the biliary system where it accumulates in the gallbladder. When CCK is given, it stimulates gallbladder emptying, and a gallbladder ejection fraction can be calculated. Recently, an interdisciplinary panel consisting of experts in the area of functional gallbladder disorder recommended the use of a single, standardized, recently described CCK-CS protocol that involves the slow infusion of CCK over 60 min with a normal GBEF defined as ≥ 38 %. A low GBEF < 38 % is supportive of the diagnosis in the proper clinical context but, importantly, is not specific for functional gallbladder disorder. A low GBEF can occur in asymptomatic patients or other medical conditions

Table 13.2 Differential diagnosis of functional gallbladder disorder

Cholelithiasis
Choledocholithiasis
Peptic ulcer disease
Functional dyspepsia
Gastroesophageal reflux disease
Functional biliary sphincter of Oddi disorder
Functional pancreatic sphincter of Oddi disorder
Irritable bowel syndrome
Abdominal wall pain
Pancreatitis
Gastroparesis

Table 13.3 Diagnostic testing in functional gallbladder disorder

Abdominal ultrasound
Liver tests
Amylase
Lipase
Esophagogastroduodenoscopy (EGD)
Cholecystokinin-cholescintigraphy (CCK-CS)

(i.e., diabetes, celiac disease, obesity) or be a result of medications (i.e., opiates, anticholinergic agents, calcium channel blockers, oral contraceptives). The interdisciplinary panel also discouraged the use of CCK provocation of pain to determine patient care decisions.

Treatment

Treatment of functional gallbladder disorder most commonly consists of cholecystectomy. Because surgical treatment is preferred only after objective determination of an abnormality, in this setting a decision to proceed with cholecystectomy is typically based upon the results of CCK-CS and calculation of the GBEF (see Table 13.4). Patients with classical symptoms and a low GBEF may benefit from a cholecystectomy. The evidence for this is, however, based on one small prospective trial and several retrospective studies using heterogeneous methodologies. Most of these studies found that up to 90 % of patients with classic symptoms and low GBEF reported improvement or resolution of symptoms following cholecystectomy.

Patients with atypical symptoms or normal GBEF should be offered medical management for their symptoms and follow-up appointment(s) to reassess their symptoms. Prokinetic agents, bile acid composition modifiers, anti-inflammatory agents, and agents to reduce visceral hyperalgesia have been suggested to be helpful but have not been subjected to rigorous study. Despite the lack of evidence to support their use, given the limitations mentioned regarding the diagnosis of this condition and the limited risk involved, consideration of a more conservative approach and a trial of these agents should be considered. Figure 13.1 shows a suggested approach to the evaluation and management of the patient with suspected functional gallbladder disorder.

Case Resolution

After completing a thorough history and examination and determining that the clinical scenario met the Rome criteria for functional gallbladder disorder, the patient underwent CCK-CS using a slow infusion of CCK. A GBEF of 16 % was found and the patient was referred to a surgeon for consideration of a cholecystectomy. Her symptoms resolved within 2 weeks of surgery and remain absent 6 months later.

Table 13.4 Treatment options in functional gallbladder disorder

If GBEF ≥ 38 %
Symptomatic treatments
Neuromodulators targeting visceral pain
If GBEF < 38 %
Trial of symptomatic treatments
Referral for cholecystectomy

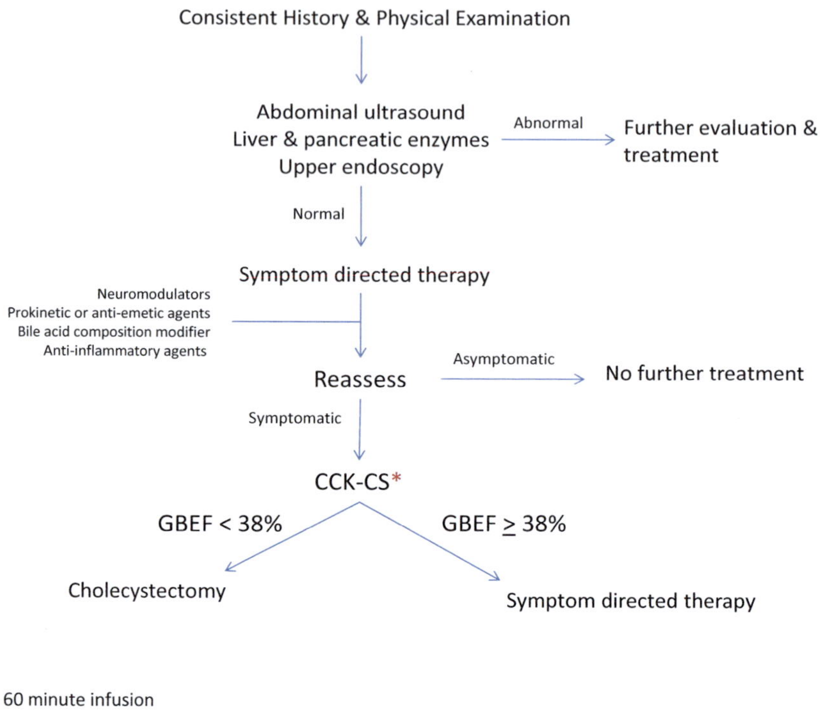

Fig. 13.1 Suggested evaluation and management approach for individuals with suspected functional gallbladder disorder. *GBEF* gallbladder ejection fraction, *CCK-CS* cholecystokinin-cholescintigraphy. See text for details

Key Clinical Teaching Points

- Although opinions remain divided regarding its utility, patients meeting the Rome diagnostic criteria for functional gallbladder disorder may benefit from CCK-CS with calculation of the GBEF to further determine who may benefit from cholecystectomy.
- A GBEF < 38 % using a slow infusion of CCK over 60 min may be a reasonable discriminator of successful outcome of cholecystectomy.
- Patients with biliary-like abdominal pain and a GBEF > 38 % may benefit from further testing and/or observation with medication trials targeting specific symptoms and/or visceral hypersensitivity.
- Medical therapy is limited in functional gallbladder disorder as none has been subjected to rigorous study in this disorder.
- Laparoscopic cholecystectomy remains the primary therapy for functional gallbladder disorder despite a lack of high-quality supportive evidence. Careful patient selection is essential to maximize the chance of successful outcome.

- Cholecystectomy should be considered only in patients with a normal GBEF who describe classical biliary pain and after a substantial period of observation as symptoms will spontaneously resolve in many of them.

Teaching Questions

1. A 35-year-old female is referred to you for evaluation of episodic right upper quadrant pain. The pain is intermittent without radiation. She is unaware of any triggers for the pain. There are no associated symptoms or weight loss. Which test is not necessary at this point?

   (A) Liver and pancreatic enzymes
   (B) Transcutaneous abdominal ultrasound
   (C) Esophagogastroduodenoscopy
   (D) CT scan abdomen and pelvis

2. Aside from functional gallbladder disorder, conditions that may lead to a decreased gallbladder ejection fraction include all of the following EXCEPT:

   (A) Celiac disease
   (B) Chronic narcotic use
   (C) Functional sphincter of Oddi disorder
   (D) Diabetes mellitus

3. Which of the following patients would seem to be the best candidate for referral for a laparoscopic cholecystectomy?

   (A) A 25-year-old female with severe bloating and nausea and constant right upper quadrant abdominal pain with a GBEF of 27 %
   (B) A 50-year-old female with severe intermittent right quadrant pain and a GBEF of 21 %
   (C) A 25 year-old male with severe intermittent right upper quadrant pain on chronic oxycodone with a GBEF of 35 %
   (D) A 35 year-old female with severe intermittent right upper quadrant pain and a GBEF of 78 % who has been seen in the emergency room on a repeated basis for pain control

Key References

1. Behar J, Corazziari E, Guelrud M, Hogan W, Sherman S, Toouli J. Functional gallbladder and sphincter of Oddi disorders. Gastroenterology. 2006;130(5):1498–509. Provides a description of the most recent Rome criteria for the diagnosis of functional gallbladder disorder.
2. Bielefeldt K. The rising tide of cholecystectomy for biliary dyskinesia. Aliment Pharmacol Ther. 2013;37(1):98–106. Recent article exploring trends in cholecystectomy use in the United States.

3. Delgado-Aros S, Cremonini F, Bredenoord AJ, Camilleri M. Systematic review and meta-analysis: does gallbladder ejection fraction on cholecystokinin cholescintigraphy predict outcome after cholecystectomy in suspected functional biliary pain? Aliment Pharmacol Ther. 2003;18:167–74. Systematic review and meta-analysis showing data that do not support the use of GBEF to select patients with suspected functional biliary pain for cholecystectomy.
4. DiBaise JK, Richmond BK, Ziessman HH, Everson GT, Fanelli RD, Maurer A, et al. Cholecystokinin-cholescintigraphy in adults: consensus recommendations of an interdisciplinary panel. Clin Gastroenterol Hepatol. 2011;9(5):376–84. Defines the optimal method for performing CCK-CS and addresses limitations of the test.
5. Gurusamy KS, Junnarkar S, Farouk M, Davidson BR. Cholecystectomy for suspected gallbladder dyskinesia. Cochrane Database Syst Rev. 2009;(1):CD007086. doi:10.1002/14651858.CD007086.pub2. Cochrane review highlighting that the evidence for the benefits and harms of cholecystectomy in gallbladder dyskinesia from randomized clinical trials is based on a single small trial at high risk of bias.
6. Yap L, Wycherly AG, Morphett AD, et al. Acalculous biliary pain: cholecystectomy alleviates symptoms in patients with abnormal cholescintigraphy. Gastroenterology. 1991;101(3):786–93. Only prospective, controlled study of cholecystectomy in patients with suspected functional gallbladder disorder.

Chapter 14
Right Upper Quadrant Pain After Cholecystectomy

Lincoln Eduardo Villela Vieira de Castro Ferreira, Fábio Heleno de Lima Pace, and Todd H. Baron

Case Study

A 38-year-old woman with a BMI of 28 kg/m^2 presents with a 4-month history of episodic, intermittent right upper abdominal and epigastric pain. The pain is of moderate to severe intensity and lasts approximately 40 min. The pain often begins after meals, especially after fatty foods, radiates to the back, and is occasionally associated with nausea and vomiting. The severity is mild in intensity at the onset and slowly increases in severity. It is not relieved with bowel movements or postural change, and the pain intensity and frequency have been stable. There have been no changes in bowel habits; the patient denies fevers or weight loss. The patient has two children. Her past surgical history is notable for cholecystectomy performed 10 months ago for similar symptoms. Pathology showed chronic cholecystitis. The pain seemed to resolve after the cholecystectomy but returned approximately 3 months later. Laboratory tests obtained during two attacks revealed serum aminotransferases and alkaline phosphatase levels approximately 3 times the upper limits of normal. Between these attacks laboratory tests were normal. Transabdominal ultrasound is performed and reveals a common bile duct diameter of 12 mm with a normal-appearing liver and pancreas. Upper endoscopy is normal. Abdominal computed tomography (CT), magnetic resonance cholangiopancreatography (MRCP),

L.E.V.V. de Castro Ferreira, M.D.
Universidade Federal de Juiz de Fora, Juiz de Fora, Brazil

F.H. de Lima Pace
Hepatology Reference Center, Gastroenterology Department,
Universidade Federal de Juiz de Fora, Juiz de Fora, Brazil

T.H. Baron, M.D., FASGE (✉)
Division of Gastroenterology and Hepatology, Mayo Clinic,
200 First St SW, Rochester, MN 55905, USA
e-mail: todd_baron@med.unc.edu

B.E. Lacy et al. (eds.), *Functional and Motility Disorders of the Gastrointestinal Tract*, DOI 10.1007/978-1-4939-1498-2_14

and endoscopic ultrasound (EUS) are also performed and are normal other than the dilated bile duct previously described. She is frustrated and wants to know what else can be done to find and eliminate the cause of her pain.

Introduction

The occurrence of right upper quadrant abdominal pain that resembles biliary-like pain in the absence of a gallbladder, known as postcholecystectomy syndrome (PCS), is clinically challenging. This term seems inadequate, as it includes biliary and non-biliary causes, possibly unrelated to cholecystectomy (see Table 14.1). Biliary causes include bile duct injury (leak and strictures), retained or recurrent stones, spillage of stones into the abdomen during cholecystectomy, gallbladder remnant, papillary stenosis, and sphincter of Oddi dysfunction (SOD). Non-biliary causes include irritable bowel syndrome, functional dyspepsia, acid-related disorders such as peptic ulcer disease and gastroesophageal reflux, pancreatic disease, hepatocellular disorders, coronary artery disease, and musculoskeletal disorders.

Clinical manifestation of PCS may occur early in the postoperative period, usually because of incomplete surgery (e.g., retained calculi in the cystic duct remnant or in the common bile duct) or operative complications (e.g., bile duct ligature or bile leakage). A later onset is commonly caused by inflammatory scarring, strictures involving the sphincter of Oddi or the common bile duct, recurrent calculi, or spillage of stones into the abdomen. Symptoms of SOD may happen any time after cholecystectomy, and because it is not associated with any structural abnormalities, the approach to patients with suspected SOD often requires more attention.

Table 14.1 Causes of right upper quadrant pain after cholecystectomy

Differential diagnosis
(a) Retained bile duct stone
(b) Recurrent bile duct stone
(c) Remnant gallbladder
(d) Remnant duct cystic
(e) Bile duct injury (leak, ligature, or stricture)
(f) Spillage of stones
(g) Papillary stenosis
(h) Sphincter of Oddi dysfunction
(i) Pancreatic disease
(j) Acid-related disorders
(k) Hepatocellular disorders
(l) Functional dyspepsia
(m) Ischemic heart disease
(n) Musculoskeletal disorders
(o) Irritable bowel syndrome

SOD is a benign acalculous obstruction to the flow of biliary secretions through the sphincter of Oddi (SO). The cause of SOD remains speculative, but it could be associated with hormonal or neurological disturbances of the SO, leading to its intermittent obstruction despite the absence of organic abnormalities. Sphincter of Oddi dyskinesia refers to a primary motor abnormality of the SO, which may result in a hypotonic or, more commonly, a hypertonic sphincter. In contrast, SO stenosis refers to a structural alteration of the sphincter, probably from an inflammatory process with subsequent fibrosis. Because it is often impossible to distinguish patients with SO dyskinesia from those with SO stenosis, the term SOD has been used to incorporate both groups. Importantly, SOD can involve abnormalities in the biliary sphincter, pancreatic sphincter, or both. Non-biliary causes of PCS should always be investigated simultaneously.

Epidemiology

Postcholecystectomy syndrome occurs in 10–40 % of patients. The time to the onset of symptoms can range from days to years depending on the cause. Women may be at higher risk, with symptoms recurring in 43 % compared to 28 % in men. In about 5 % of patients who undergo laparoscopic cholecystectomy, the reason for chronic abdominal pain remains unknown. Among all possible causes of PCS, retained calculi in the common bile duct or cystic duct remnant are the most frequent.

As a functional disorder, SOD may coexist with other functional GI disorders such as gallbladder dyskinesia (i.e., functional gallbladder disorder), functional dyspepsia, gastroparesis, and irritable bowel syndrome. The estimated prevalence of SOD in the general population is 1.5 %, affecting women more frequently than men (3:1) and usually occurring between the ages of 20 and 50 years. SOD results in work absenteeism, disability, and significant healthcare utilization. Though it may occur in patients with gallbladder in situ, SOD is most commonly considered in patients who have previously undergone cholecystectomy.

The primary symptom of the SOD is pain. Although pain is considered a subjective complaint, substantial information can be obtained after careful questioning in determining whether the pain is biliary-like. Completely defining the pain features is essential. Data about location, intensity, frequency, duration, and other symptom associations should be collected. The classic location of pain is right upper quadrant and/or epigastric. Pain often radiates to the back, particularly the right shoulder, and classically begins 1–2 h after ingestion of a fatty meal; however, the relationship to food intake is considered unreliable. Many patients report pain occurring at night with a peak occurrence around midnight. While pain is recurrent, it recurs at variable intervals (not daily) and may be associated with nausea and vomiting. The pain typically plateaus in less than an hour and is severe enough to interrupt daily activities or require consultation with a physician. Once it has reached its peak, the pain usually lasts at least 30 min and then slowly subsides over several hours, with the entire attack usually lasting less than 4–6 h. These pain characteristics have been codified

Table 14.2 Functional gallbladder and sphincter of Oddi disorders diagnostic criteria (Rome III)

Functional gallbladder and sphincter of Oddi disorders diagnostic criteria must include episodes of pain located in the epigastrium and/or right upper quadrant and all of the following:
(a) Episodes lasting 30 min or longer
(b) Recurrent symptoms occurring at different intervals (not daily)
(c) The pain builds up to a steady level
(d) The pain is moderate to severe enough to interrupt the patient's daily activities or lead to an emergency department visit
(e) The pain is not relieved by bowel movements
(f) The pain is not relieved by postural change
(g) The pain is not relieved by antacids
(h) Exclusion of other structural disease that would explain the symptoms
Supportive criteria: The pain may present with one or more of the following: associated with nausea and vomiting, radiates to the back and/or right infra-subscapular region, awakens from sleep in the middle of the night

in consensus guidelines of a Rome III committee in order to standardize the qualities associated with biliary-type pain and to help diagnose functional gallbladder disorder and SOD (see Table 14.2). It should be emphasized that continuous, daily abdominal pain is not consistent with SOD.

Pathophysiology

Choledocholithiasis after cholecystectomy may result from either a migrated gallbladder stone not detected in the perioperative period or a stone forming de novo in the common bile duct (secondary calculus), which develops as a result of biliary stasis often associated with strictures or papillary stenosis. When the symptoms of pain develop early, the possibility of bile duct stone should be investigated, even in the absence of jaundice or bile duct dilatation. Choledocholithiasis may be complicated by acute pancreatitis and cholangitis.

The mechanism by which the cystic duct stump is associated with PCS has been investigated. In one study of seven cases, retained gallbladder calculi and cystic duct remnant stones were found to be the cause of recurrent biliary symptoms. Some authors believe a long stump alone is not the cause of recurrent symptoms and the possibility of a remnant gallbladder must be kept in mind. The presence of a gallbladder remnant after cholecystectomy is very rare. The gallbladder remnant becomes symptomatic due to chronic inflammation or harboring gallstones. Other authors have suggested that PCS may arise from the cystic duct remnant or a neuroma of the cystic duct stump. In one series of three patients, pain was exacerbated during EUS with the patient lightly sedated by pushing on cystic duct surgical clips with an EUS-guided needle. The pain was temporarily alleviated by EUS-guided injection of bupivacaine and triamcinolone. In two patients, surgical resection of the cystic duct remnant was performed. Another consideration is neurogenic pain at the

Table 14.3 Hogan–Geenen sphincter of Oddi dysfunction modified classification system

	Typical pain	LFT > 2× normal		Bile duct > 10 mm
Type I	+	+		+
Type II	+	+	Or	+
Type III	+	–		–

site of cholecystectomy, particularly open cholecystectomy. This entity may be managed by pain specialists with local injection therapies.

Factors that have been associated with bile duct injury include surgeon experience, patient age, male sex, and acute cholecystitis. Bile duct injury may result in a leak, stricture, or bile duct disruption. The main causes of ductal injury are erroneous cutting of bile ducts, inadvertently placed clips or ligatures, periductal bile leakage resulting in fibrosis, and thermal injury owing to electrocautery.

Spillage of stones into the abdomen can occur during dissection of the gallbladder off the liver bed, tearing with grasping forceps, or during extraction of the gallbladder through one of the port sites. It may result in intra-abdominal abscess, subcutaneous abscess, and later discharge of stones through the abdominal wall or biliary tract. The abscess may be diagnosed as "simple" when the stones are radiolucent.

The role of dysfunction at the level of the sphincter of Oddi in patients with presumed functional gallbladder disorder remains unclear. Although similar gallbladder ejection fractions in patients with and without documented SOD have been described, other reports describe a similar frequency of SOD in patients with and without gallbladder dysfunction based on gallbladder ejection fraction. In a prospective study designed to evaluate the relationship between SOD and gallbladder dysfunction, 81 patients with biliary-type pain and an intact, sonographically normal gallbladder underwent both SO manometry and cholecystokinin-HIDA cholescintigraphy. In 41 patients with a normal gallbladder ejection fraction, 57 % had SOD, while 50 % had SOD in the 40 patients with an abnormal gallbladder ejection fraction suggesting that both SOD and functional gallbladder dysfunction are common in this group of patients and appear to occur independently of one another.

For patients without a gallbladder suspected to have SOD, a biliary classification system was initially developed (Hogan–Geenen SOD classification system) based on clinical history, laboratory tests, and endoscopic retrograde cholangiopancreatography (ERCP) bile duct drainage times. Subsequently, the classification was modified by removing the biliary drainage times given practical limitations in determining drainage times and evidence suggesting that drainage times do not correlate with findings on SO manometry. The current classification contains three categories (see Table 14.3). Type I SOD consists of the presence of typical biliary pain, abnormal aminotransferase levels > 2 times the upper limits of normal on more than two occasions, and a dilated common bile duct (>10 mm) on noninvasive imaging. Type II SOD comprises biliary pain plus one of the other two additional criteria, elevated liver tests or common bile duct dilation but not both. Finally, type III SOD consists of biliary pain only with no objective criteria.

Diagnosis and Evaluation

The diagnosis of PCS will depend on the patient's history, clinical symptoms, and laboratory and imaging exams. Biliary and non-biliary causes need to be considered. For instance, biliary duct injury may lead to bile leakage, intra-abdominal abscess, cholangitis, and secondary biliary cirrhosis due to chronic strictures. Early postcholecystectomy symptoms such as fever, abdominal pain, and jaundice may be associated with retained stones or bile duct injury (leak or ligature). The same symptoms 2 years after cholecystectomy may be secondary to recurrent stones or bile duct stricture. Patients with a gallbladder remnant complain primarily of pain and rarely develop jaundice. Papillary stenosis usually presents with biliary-type abdominal pain, significantly elevated liver enzymes, and a dilated common bile duct without evidence of stones. The symptoms of papillary stenosis more commonly have a later presentation. Retained or recurrent stones and bile duct injury may be complicated by acute cholangitis. SOD may be present prior to cholecystectomy or any time after cholecystectomy.

Blood tests and liver function tests (LFTs) in particular are essential to evaluate risk of infection and degree of hepatic dysfunction. Imaging tests such as transabdominal ultrasound, abdominal CT, MRCP, cholescintigraphy, percutaneous transhepatic cholangiography, and ERCP may help identify abnormality structural such as bile duct dilatation, strictures, stones, and bilomas.

The traditional imaging approach to PCS includes ultrasonography and/or abdominal CT. MRCP is a noninvasive method and reliable alternative to direct cholangiography for the evaluation of the biliary tract. EUS and ERCP should be reserved for those cases where the suspected structural lesions persist, although previous imaging tests have failed to demonstrate them, or when there are therapeutic purposes. Thus, EUS could be performed when retained small bile duct stones are suspected in the setting of a normal MRCP or when a rendezvous biliary drainage is desired. ERCP, for instance, could be performed to confirm and treat a bile leak.

Once structural abnormalities have been eliminated, the suspicion of SOD and non-biliary causes need to be investigated. The initial evaluation of all patients suspected to have SOD includes a detailed history and physical examination with special attention directed to the nature, quality, severity, and character of pain. Details of the pain should be investigated and compared with the criteria established in Rome III as previously described. It is common for SOD patients to have undergone cholecystectomy because of a gallbladder "problem" or "poorly functioning" gallbladder often in the absence of documented cholelithiasis. Chronic narcotic analgesic use is found not uncommonly in patients with SOD and can confuse the diagnosis with narcotic bowel syndrome.

During the evaluation of suspected SOD, it is recommended that serum LFTs (aminotransferases, serum bilirubin, alkaline phosphatase) and pancreatic enzymes be performed during episodes of pain. Classic findings include an elevation in aminotransferases > 2 times the upper limit of normal on at least two separate occasions. Importantly, lesser degrees of elevation are common in SOD, while more severe elevations are suggestive of CBD stones, biliary tumors, and parenchymal liver disease. Jaundice due to SOD is so uncommon that it essentially excludes a diagnosis of SOD. Special attention should be given to obese patients where persistently elevated liver tests may be seen even in the absence of pain and are related to fatty liver rather than SOD.

Transabdominal ultrasound, abdominal CT, MRCP, and EUS are useful to exclude structural biliary obstruction; however, the completion of all of these tests in every potential case is not generally needed. Bile duct stones are very rarely found when routine imaging tests such as transabdominal ultrasound and laboratory testing are normal. Occasionally a dilated bile duct may be found, particularly in patients with type I and II SOD. Upper endoscopy is useful to exclude upper gastrointestinal anatomic and mucosal abnormalities such as peptic ulcer disease, reflux esophagitis, and tumors. This is particularly important in the setting of alarm symptoms such as weight loss. The absence of underlying structural disease on imaging and the lack of response to a trial of proton pump inhibitors increase the likelihood that SOD is present.

In a healthy individual, after stimulating biliary secretion with a lipid-rich meal or cholecystokinin administration, the flow of bile increases, the SO relaxes, and a larger amount of bile enters the duodenum. In the setting of SOD, the common bile duct paradoxically dilates after administration of secretory agents. At present, there are few studies comparing these noninvasive tests with sphincter of Oddi manometry (SOM; the gold standard) and outcome after sphincterotomy.

Dynamic (quantitative) hepatobiliary scintigraphy (HBS) measures bile flow through the ampulla as determined by the duration of time required for the radionuclide to reach the duodenum. Dynamic HBS, however, remains poorly standardized. As a result, the precise criteria to define an abnormal study remain controversial; however, a duodenal arrival time > 20 min and hilum-to-duodenum time > 10 min are commonly used. Although some studies have shown good correlation between HBS and SOM, others have found a poor specificity in healthy volunteers and an increased number of normal exams in patients with SOD types II and III. In a retrospective study comparing HBS and fatty-meal sonography as potential predictors of SOD, 304 post-cholecystectomy patients with suspected SOD underwent SO manometry, fatty-meal stimulation (FMS), and scintigraphy (HBS). SOD was found in 73 patients (24 %) as determined by SO manometry. The sensitivity and specificity were 21 and 97 % for FMS and 49 and 78 % for HBS. Of importance, in patients with abnormal manometry who experienced a long-term response to endoscopic biliary sphincterotomy, 85 % (11/13) had both an abnormal FMS and HBS. Thus, while noninvasive tests are not able to reliably predict an abnormal SO manometry, they might be of assistance in predicting response to sphincterotomy in SOD patients.

SO manometry is considered the "gold standard" for diagnosis and determining the management of SOD. SO manometry is a complex endoscopic procedure that is not widely available. It is generally performed at tertiary referral medical centers at the time of ERCP. Patients with type I SOD usually have a fibrotic cause for sphincter dysfunction (true papillary stenosis; see Fig. 14.1). As the majority of type I SOD patients have been shown to have an abnormal SO manometry and a near-uniform

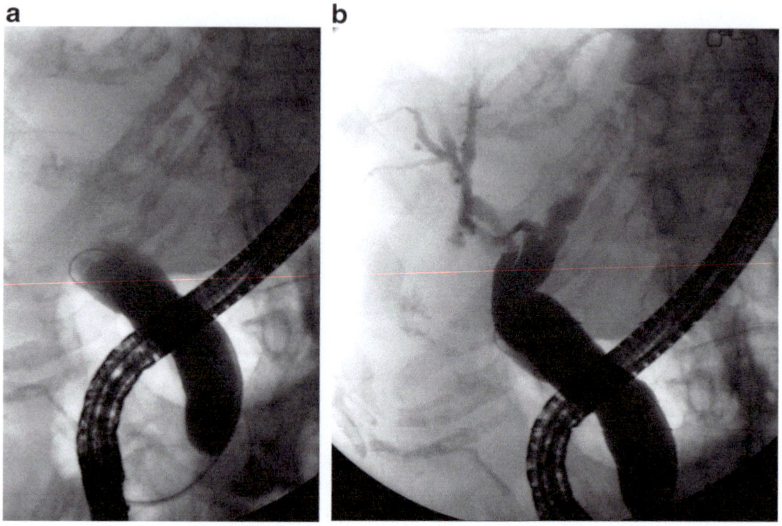

Fig. 14.1 Patient with type I SOD. (**a**) Distal CBD dilated down to level of ampulla. (**b**) Upper biliary tree also dilated. The patient responded to biliary sphincterotomy

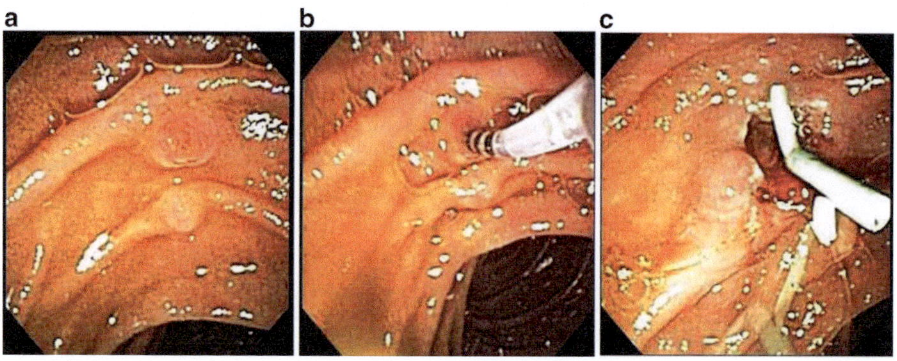

Fig. 14.2 Type II SOD. (**a**) Normal papilla. (**b**) Manometry catheter in bile duct. (**c**) Immediately after biliary sphincterotomy and placement of prophylactic pancreatic duct stent

long-term response to biliary sphincterotomy, manometry is not considered necessary in this group (see Fig. 14.1). For patients with type II SOD, however, SO manometry is generally recommended. Up to two-thirds of type II SOD patients have abnormal SO manometry. In this group of patients, sphincterotomy has been shown to be helpful in up to 85 % when SO manometry is abnormal (Fig. 14.2). Although controversial, some endoscopists offer empiric biliary sphincterotomy in type II patients. In patients with type III SOD, only 50 % of patients with abnormal SO manometry respond to sphincterotomy (see Table 14.4). Thus, given potential risks

Table 14.4 Hogan–Geenen sphincter of Oddi classification system related to the frequency of abnormal sphincter of Oddi manometry and pain relief by biliary sphincterotomy

Patient group classifications	Frequency of abnormal sphincter manometry	Probability of pain relief by sphincterotomy if manometry		Manometry before ES
		Abnormal	Normal	
Type I	75–90 %	90–95 %	90–95 %	Unnecessary
Type II	55–65 %	85 %	35 %	Highly recommended
Type III	25–60 %	55–65 %	<10 %	Mandatory

Table 14.5 Diagnostic tests to consider in patients with biliary-type pain and normal transabdominal ultrasound

Diagnostic tests
(a) Upper endoscopy
(b) Liver and pancreatic enzymes
(c) Abdominal CT
(d) MRCP
(e) Sphincter of Oddi manometry (selected cases)
(f) Endoscopic ultrasound of the gallbladder and biliary tree
(g) Cholecystokinin cholescintigraphy for GBEF determination

associated with SO manometry, the benefit of studying patients with type III SOD remains in doubt and is generally not recommended.

Several studies have demonstrated that post-ERCP pancreatitis (PEP) is the most common major adverse event after SO manometry, especially in patients with type III SOD. A microtransducer (non-perfused) manometry system, prophylactic pancreatic duct stent placement, and administration of rectal nonsteroidal anti-inflammatory drugs (NSAIDs) have been used to reduce the incidence of PEP in SOD patients. Purely diagnostic ERCP (i.e., without manometry) is not justified in these patients.

The diagnosis of SOD in patients with gallbladder in situ is challenging. The exact role of SO manometry in the setting of an intact gallbladder is not established. In 81 patients with typical biliary-type pain and a normal gallbladder ultrasound, approximately one-half of these patients were found to have SOD on SO manometry; however, the finding of SOD did not correlate with the gallbladder ejection fraction. All patients in the group with elevated sphincter pressures underwent biliary sphincterotomy, and most experienced pain relief at 1 year. During longer-term follow-up, however, most patients ultimately required cholecystectomy for pain control. The significance of SOD in the setting of an intact gallbladder remains controversial. Some prefer to avoid SO manometry in patients with gallbladder in situ, recommending laparoscopic cholecystectomy instead as the next step. ERCP with SO manometry may be reasonable where typical biliary pain is accompanied by transient elevations of liver enzymes. Table 14.5 lists tests that may be considered in patients with biliary-type pain and normal transabdominal ultrasound.

Treatment

The treatment of the PCS depends on the underlying etiology. The successful management of bile duct injuries is determined by the type of injury, the timing of its recognition, the presence of complicating factors, patient comorbidity, and surgical expertise. Depending on the type of injury, management may include endoscopic, percutaneous, and open surgical interventions.

Retained or recurrent common bile duct stones or cystic duct remnant stones are primarily treated with ERCP with endoscopic sphincterotomy, as well as papillary stenosis. Patients with a gallbladder remnant should undergo completion cholecystectomy, if they are good surgical candidates and the operation is technically feasible. This is considered definitive treatment and usually can be performed laparoscopically. The treatment of spilled stones is addressed when complications arise such as intra-abdominal or subcutaneous abscesses.

The aim of therapy for SOD is to reduce the resistance to flow of biliary secretions. The management of SOD is often difficult except in patients with type I SOD. Treatment options are shown in Table 14.6. Endoscopic biliary sphincterotomy for SOD I and biliary sphincterotomy with or without pancreatic sphincterotomy for SOD II and III patients reduce sphincter pressure and are the treatment of choice. Clinical improvement following endoscopic sphincterotomy has been reported to occur in 55–95 % of patients, depending on the type of SOD and the finding of abnormalities in SO manometry. There are scant data to support the use of a biliary stent as a short-term alternative to sphincterotomy (i.e., a therapeutic trial to predict response to sphincterotomy). Biliary stenting in this situation was associated with a rate of post-ERCP pancreatitis of 38 % in one study. Because of this, the placement of a pancreatic duct stent and/or administration of NSAIDs is strongly recommended when an empiric biliary stent is placed.

The surgical approach for SOD has largely been replaced by endoscopy therapy. At present, surgical therapy is reserved for patients with restenosis following endoscopic sphincterotomy and in the rare patient where endoscopic evaluation or therapy is not available or technically feasible.

Several agents designed to reduce sphincter pressure through relaxation of smooth muscle have been tried. Sublingual calcium channel blockers (e.g., nifedipine) and nitrates have been shown to reduce sphincter pressure in asymptomatic volunteers and symptomatic patients with SOD. Pain scores, emergency room visits, and use of oral analgesics were reduced in 75 % of patients with manometrically

Table 14.6 Treatment options in SOD

Treatment options
(a) Medical treatment (drugs such as nifedipine and nitrates)
(b) Endoscopic treatment (stent, botulinum toxin injection, and sphincterotomy)
(c) Surgical treatment

documented SOD in one study. In another 16-week double-blind crossover study using nifedipine in type II SOD patients, a reduction in the number of days with pain was seen. A slow-release form of nifedipine was tested in a small pilot study in patients with SOD with encouraging results. There are no controlled trials of nitrate therapy in patients with SOD. A case report described a patient treated with nitrates whose pain resolved and was associated with a decrease in both basal and phasic SO pressures. Relaxation of the SO muscle with nitrates is supported by the fact that topical application to the papilla of Vater during ERCP demonstrated a profound inhibition of SO motility. Botulinum toxin (Botox) injection into the SO has also been tried; however, its effect is usually transient. Furthermore, botulinum toxin injection for SOD has not been subjected to well-designed, randomized studies with sufficient follow-up to determine safety and efficacy. Other drugs including tricyclic antidepressants, selective serotonin reuptake inhibitors, and trimebutine, a spasmolytic agent, have also been tried but are limited by systemic side effects and short-lived, incomplete symptom improvement.

Case Resolution

The patient presented describes typical biliary pain, had abnormal LFTs during several episodes, and has a dilated common bile duct. Other imaging tests including CT and EUS showed only a dilated bile duct without structural lesions. These findings were felt to be consistent with the Rome III criteria for SOD. The patient was felt to have type I SOD. Sphincter of Oddi manometry was deemed unnecessary, and she underwent endoscopic biliary sphincterotomy with complete resolution of her symptoms shortly thereafter.

Key Clinical Teaching Points

- Right upper quadrant abdominal pain after cholecystectomy has a broad differential diagnosis including both biliary causes and non-biliary causes.
- Clinical manifestation of PCS may occur early in the postoperative period, usually because of incomplete surgery or operative complications, or later due to inflammatory scarring strictures involving the sphincter of Oddi or the common bile duct, recurrent calculi, or spillage of stones into the abdomen.
- Symptoms of SOD may happen any time after cholecystectomy. All SOD patients have abdominal pain; details about location, intensity, frequency, duration, and associations of pain should be collected in detail and compared with Rome III criteria to further classify as biliary-type pain.
- The exclusion of structural diseases that would explain the patient's symptoms is mandatory for the diagnosis of SOD.
- The treatment of the PCS depends on the underlying etiology. For patients with SOD, the options include medical therapy and endoscopic or surgical sphincterotomy.

Teaching Questions

1. A 52-year-old woman presents with biliary-type pain 3 months after cholecystectomy for cholelithiasis and has abnormal liver function tests but no fever or jaundice. Which one of the following is the most likely diagnosis?

   (A) Bile duct injury
   (B) Retained common bile duct stone
   (C) Spillage of stones into the abdomen
   (D) Sphincter of Oddi dysfunction (SOD)

2. Which one of the following tests should be considered first in the evaluation of the patient described above?

   (A) Endoscopic retrograde cholangiopancreatography (ERCP)
   (B) Transabdominal ultrasonography of the right upper quadrant
   (C) Magnetic resonance cholangiopancreatography (MRCP)
   (D) Upper gastrointestinal endoscopy

3. In a 37-year-old woman, laboratory tests were obtained during two attacks of upper abdominal pain and revealed serum aminotransferases and alkaline phosphatase levels approximately 3 times the upper limits of normal. Between these attacks, the labs were normal. Transabdominal ultrasound was performed revealing a common bile duct diameter of 12 mm with normal-appearing liver and pancreas. Upper endoscopy was also normal. Abdominal CT, MRCP, and endoscopic ultrasound (EUS) were also performed with the only abnormality being a dilated bile duct was found. Non-biliary causes were investigated and nothing was identified. The next step should be which one of the following?

   (A) Sphincter of Oddi manometry
   (B) ERCP with biliary sphincterotomy
   (C) Prescription of sublingual nifedipine
   (D) Surgical sphincterotomy

Key References

1. Behar J, Corazziari E, Guelrud M, Hogan W, Sherman S, Toouli J. Functional gallbladder and sphincter of Oddi disorders. Gastroenterology. 2006;130:1498–509. This paper defines the Rome III criteria for diagnosis of SOD.
2. Geenen JE, Hogan WJ, Dodds WJ, Toouli J, Venu RP. The efficacy of endoscopic sphincterotomy after cholecystectomy in patients with sphincter of Oddi dysfunction. N Engl J Med. 1989;320:82–7. This is considered a landmark study demonstrating that SO manometry predicted the outcome from endoscopic sphincterotomy and that endoscopic sphincterotomy offered long-term benefit in Type II biliary patients with SOD.
3. Girometti R, Brondani G, Cereser L, Como G, Del Pin M, Bazzocchi M, Zuiani C. Post-cholecystectomy syndrome: spectrum of biliary findings at magnetic resonance cholangiopancreatography. Br J Radiol. 2010;83:351–61. This paper discusses the possible biliary causes of PSC with focus on the role of MRCP.

4. Hogan W, Sherman S, Pasricha P, Carr-Locke D. Sphincter of Oddi manometry. Gastrointest Endosc. 1997;45:342–8. This was the first study that developed a biliary clinical classification for patients with suspected SOD (Hogan–Geenen SOD classification system) based on clinical history, laboratory results, and ERCP findings.
5. Jaunoo SS, Mohandas S, Almond LM. Postcholecystectomy syndrome (PCS). Int J Surg. 2010;8:15–7. This is review paper where possible etiologies are discussed.
6. Macaron C, Qadeer MA, Vargo JJ. Recurrent abdominal pain after laparoscopic cholecystectomy. Cleve Clin J Med. 2011;78:171–8. This is a paper where a case of stone in a duct cystic remnant is presented. The authors discuss the differential diagnosis and a step-by-step of how to approach the patient with PCS.

Part V
Colonic Disorders

Chapter 15
Chronic Constipation

Amy E. Foxx-Orenstein and Sarah Umar

Case Study

A 57-year-old woman with a 20-year history of constipation-predominant irritable bowel syndrome (IBS-C) presents with symptoms of worsening constipation. IBS symptoms had previously been well controlled on 20 mg of Lexapro daily and occasional milk of magnesia. Travel to Asia 9 months ago resulted in several days of no bowel movements, followed by hard, pebbly, and difficult to pass stools. Bowel movements now occur 2–3 times a day, although she never feels completely empty. There is no blood or pain with defecation. She feels that she has to strain excessively to evacuate the stool. The addition of supplemental fiber to her diet caused uncomfortable abdominal bloating. She is gravida 3, para 2; both were vaginal deliveries without complications. A screening colonoscopy 2 years ago was normal. Her symptoms are very bothersome, causing her to miss 2–3 workdays a month and occasional social engagements. Her family history is unremarkable. Her only medications include Lexapro and milk of magnesia as needed; these have not changed over the past 9 months. Physical examination reveals a healthy appearing woman with a BMI of 20 kg/m^2. Abdominal examination is normal. Anal inspection identified small, non-thrombosed external hemorrhoids, minimal perineal descent, and no evidence of prolapse. Digital examination identified high anal sphincter tone with hard, brown stool in the rectal vault. She feels consumed by her discomfort and hopes you can help her.

Conflict of interest: Dr. Foxx-Orenstein is a consultant and speaker for Ironwood and Forest Pharmaceutical.

A.E. Foxx-Orenstein, D.O. (✉) • S. Umar, M.D. (✉)
Division of Gastroenterology and Hepatology, Mayo Clinic, 13400 E Shea Blvd, Scottsdale, AZ 85259, USA
e-mail: foxx-orenstein.amy@mayo.edu; Umar.sarah@mayo.edu

B.E. Lacy et al. (eds.), *Functional and Motility Disorders of the Gastrointestinal Tract*, DOI 10.1007/978-1-4939-1498-2_15

Introduction

Chronic constipation is a common disorder encountered in gastroenterology and primary care clinical practices. It affects 2–27 % of the population, which represents 4–56 million adults in the United States alone. While only a minority of patients with constipation symptoms seek medical treatment, it accounts for nearly 2.5 million physician visits annually and 100,000 referrals to gastroenterologists, with nearly every visit resulting in a prescription for a laxative. Constipation is more common in women, the elderly, those of lower socioeconomic background, and also in those reporting symptoms of irritable bowel syndrome (IBS). Constipation has been shown to have a deleterious impact on health-related quality of life, and there is an association with somatic disorders, psychological distress, environmental stress, and depression. The burden of constipation extends to loss of work and school productivity, high absenteeism, and impaired daily activity performance. Patients with chronic constipation often have coexisting dyspepsia and gastroesophageal reflux symptoms. Frequent and severe abdominal pain is reported more often in those patients with episodic constipation who do not meet IBS criteria. This suggests a potential pathophysiologic overlap with IBS, which has implications for management.

Epidemiology

The wide range in the prevalence of constipation relates to different definitions used to survey constipation and differences in patients' perceptions of what constipation entails. The pooled prevalence of chronic constipation is 14 %, which is similar across geographic regions. There are age-related differences in the prevalence of constipation, becoming more prevalent after the age of 60, with the largest increase after age 70. The higher prevalence with age may be due to secondary causes of constipation such as polypharmacy, decreased mobility, comorbidities, and neurological disorders. Institutionalized patients are at high risk to develop constipation when compared with community-living elderly patients. Women are more likely to seek health care for their constipation and to use laxatives compared to men.

Pathophysiology

Constipation is categorized into either primary or secondary causes. Secondary causes (see Table 15.1) are often discovered by taking a thorough history. Primary types of constipation include normal transit (the most common), outlet dysfunction, and slow transit. There is often overlap of primary types and secondary causes of constipation in an individual.

Normal transit includes chronic functional (idiopathic) constipation (see Table 15.2) and IBS-C (see Table 15.3; also see Chap. 16). Patients experience constipation without abnormalities in diagnostic tests.

Table 15.1 Secondary causes of constipation

Drugs: opiates, nonsteroidal anti-inflammatory, anticholinergic, antidepressant, antihistamine, anti-Parkinsonian, iron, calcium
Neurogenic: autonomic neuropathy, Parkinson's disease, multiple sclerosis, CNS and spinal cord lesions, pseudo-obstruction, diabetes mellitus, pelvic nerve damage
Myogenic: connective tissue disorders, amyloidosis, diabetes mellitus, dermatomyositis, pseudo-obstruction
Lifestyle: low fiber, very high fiber, dehydration, institutional living, low physical activity
Miscellaneous: pregnancy, anal and colon cancer, psychological disorders, intestinal radiation, long-distance travel

Table 15.2 Diagnostic criteria for chronic functional idiopathic constipation

Criteria to be fulfilled for the last 3 months and symptom onset at least 6 months prior to diagnosis[a]
1. Must include two or more of the following:
(a) Straining during 25 % of defecations
(b) Lumpy or hard stools in at least 25 % of defecations
(c) Sensation of incomplete evacuation for at least 25 % of defecations
(d) Sensation of outlet obstruction for at least 25 % of defecations
(e) Manual maneuvers (digital extraction, perineal support) to facilitate at least 25 % of evacuations
(f) Fewer than 3 defecations per week
2. Looser stools are rarely present without the use of laxatives
3. There are insufficient criteria for IBS

Adapted from Longstreth GF, Thompson WG, Chey WD, et al. Functional bowel disorders. Gastroenterology. 2006;130:1480–91
[a]Criterion fulfilled for the last 3 months with symptom onset at least 6 months to diagnosis

Table 15.3 Rome III irritable bowel syndrome, constipation predominant

Recurrent abdominal pain or discomfort (uncomfortable sensation not described as pain) at least 3 days/month in the last 3 months associated with two or more of the following:[a]
1. Improvement with defecation
2. Onset associated with a change infrequency of stool
3. Onset associated with a change in form (appearance) of stool
4. <25 % of bowel movements were loose stools

Adapted from Longstreth GF, Thompson WG, Chey WD, et al. Functional bowel disorders. Gastroenterology. 2006;130:1480–91
[a]Criterion fulfilled for the last 3 months with symptom onset at least 6 months to diagnosis

Outlet dysfunction (defecation disorders, pelvic floor dysfunction) can be due to a number of conditions, including dyssynergia, excessive or inadequate perineal descent, rectal prolapse, anal stricture or fissure, hyposensitivity, rectocele or, rarely, intussusception or enterocele.

Slow-transit constipation is associated with a reduction in both the number and strength of high-amplitude propagating contractions (HAPC), which normally occur upon awakening and after meals. The pathogenesis may relate to a reduced number of neurons within the myenteric plexus and/or interstitial cells of Cajal and increased intestinal collagen deposition.

Diagnosis and Evaluation

The diagnosis of constipation tends to be subjective for patients being based on social and cultural norms. There is often a lack of agreement between "physicians" and patients' perceptions of constipation, with physicians perceiving constipation as fewer than three stools per week and patients more concerned with stool consistency, sense of complete evacuation, and ease and of passage. Many people with fewer than three stools per week do not consider themselves constipated, while others ardently strive for "a healthful" one movement daily. This perception of constipation has been linked to the expenditure of millions of healthcare dollars.

The evaluation of constipation needs to be individualized to a patient's medical needs and symptoms. Not all patients require the same diagnostic approach. The first step in the evaluation of constipation is a detailed history (see Table 15.4) and physical examination. A medication history is important as many drugs and supplements can cause constipation (see Table 15.1). The presence of alarm symptoms (see Table 15.5) or an abdominal mass requires additional evaluation which may include laboratory tests, a colonoscopy or a CT scan of the abdomen and pelvis. Laboratory evaluation including chemistries, complete blood count, and thyroid-stimulating hormone are commonly performed. The physical examination requires careful visual examination of the perineum to assess symmetry and inspection for a fistula, fissure or hemorrhoid, and the degree of perineal descent and prolapse with bearing down.

Table 15.4 Key bowel history questions

Duration of symptoms
Alarm symptoms
Number of bowel movements per day or week
Sense of complete evacuation
Stool size and consistency (small to medium to large, hard to firm to mushy to watery)
Straining and how severe
Use of manual maneuvers (perineal support, digitization, vaginal splinting)
Ability to sense the urge
Average time attempting to evacuate
Rectal prolapse and ease of reduction
History of rectocele, cystocele
Pelvic, obstetric, abdominal surgery
Number of vaginal/caesarian pregnancies and complications, duration of labor
Fecal soiling or incontinence (think constipation with overflow incontinence)

Table 15.5 Alarm symptoms

Age > 50
Gastrointestinal bleeding
Anemia
Unintentional weight loss
Acute onset or sudden change in symptoms
Personal or family history of inflammatory bowel disease or colorectal cancer
Nocturnal symptoms

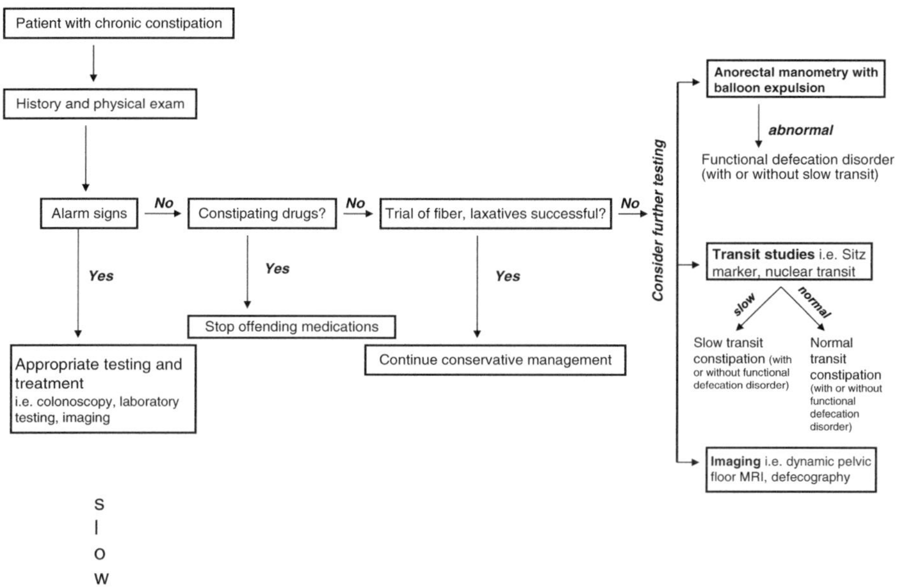

Fig. 15.1 Evaluation of chronic constipation

The digital examination determines the presence of anal pain, sphincter length, symmetry, and tone (scale 0–5, least to greatest) at rest/with squeeze/with bearing down and may detect a band-like contraction of the puborectalis muscle anteriorly with bearing down, if dyssynergia is present. When asked to simulate defecation, abdominal muscles should contract together with relaxation of the anal sphincter complex. The absence of a failure to contract the abdominal muscles, absence of perineal descent, and/or a failure to relax or a paradoxical contraction of the anal sphincter is predictive of a diagnosis of dyssynergia.

Diagnostic Testing

Anorectal manometry quantifies internal and external anal sphincter function at rest and with defecatory maneuvers, rectal compliance, and sensation (see Fig. 15.1). For symptoms of outlet dysfunction, balloon expulsion has been shown to be highly sensitive and predictive of dyssynergic defecation. Additionally, dynamic pelvic floor magnetic resonance defecography (dynamic MRI) and conventional defecography can provide supportive information. Dynamic MRI can also identify functional and structural abnormalities in the pelvis and objectively assess the relationship of defecation difficulties to other pelvic organs, all without exposure to radiation. Colonic transit studies objectively measure the speed of stool movement through the colon. Methods to measure transit include scintigraphy, radiopaque markers, and the recently available wireless motility capsule (WMC). The WMC measures intestinal pH, temperature, and pressure and allows for the determination of transit times of the stomach, small intestine, and colon. Similar to whole gut scintigraphy, the WMC can be used to evaluate for a generalized disturbance in gut motility. Importantly, in patients with dyssynergia, colon transit time can also be delayed, and this may normalize after treatment.

Treatment

There are many treatments, both pharmacologic and nonpharmacologic, for constipation. In the United States, nearly a billion dollars is spent annually on the management of constipation, with over 800 million dollars spent on medications, a number that likely underestimates the true cost as it does not include over-the-counter laxative purchases.

Most patients with constipation are initially managed with lifestyle changes including regular exercise, avoidance of constipating medications, and access to toileting. The use of dietary fiber and hydration has been the mainstay of therapy in chronic constipation. Most Americans consume far less than the daily recommended dose of 25–30 g. Studies have demonstrated that fiber may be more effective in certain subtypes of constipation such as functional constipation, rather than in patients with dyssynergic defecation or refractory, slow-transit constipation. Fiber supplements can be an effective way to reach the recommended daily dose. While fiber may exacerbate bloating and abdominal distension, given that it may be beneficial, is inexpensive, and is low risk, it is reasonable to consider this as first-line therapy in patients with mild constipation symptoms. When recommended, a soluble fiber supplement such as ispaghula/psyllium or synthetic fiber such as methylcellulose can be used, starting at a low dose to minimize potential side effects (e.g., bloating) with a target total daily fiber intake of 25–30 g.

Osmotic laxatives contain poorly absorbed molecules that create an osmotic gradient within the colon and, hence, draw water into the colon and the stool. Examples of osmotic laxatives include polyethylene glycol (PEG), lactulose, sorbitol, milk of magnesia, and magnesium citrate. There is good evidence supporting the use of PEG in chronic constipation, and side effects from this medication are exceptionally rare.

Stimulant laxatives increase intestinal motility by directly stimulating the lining of the colon. Senna, cascara, aloe, and bisacodyl are examples of stimulant laxatives. There is limited evidence to support their use as first-line treatments for chronic constipation. Stimulant laxatives can cause abdominal cramping and electrolyte abnormalities, and some are associated with the development of melanosis coli, which is of no clinical significance other than being a marker of chronic laxative use. Stool softeners are of unclear benefit and are not routinely recommended in the management of chronic constipation.

Lubiprostone is a chloride channel activator available by prescription that acts to increase luminal water. The sum effect is an increase in stool water, bowel distention, peristalsis, and laxation. It has been shown to increase the frequency of spontaneous bowel movements; however, its use may be limited by the adverse effect of nausea, so it is recommended to be taken with food.

Linaclotide is a guanylate cyclase type C (GC-C) receptor agonist available by prescription that causes secretion of chloride and bicarbonate into the intestinal lumen followed by increased fluid secretion and accelerated stool transit. It has low bioavailability and is undetectable in the systemic circulation when administered at therapeutic doses. It is helpful in patients with constipation and in patients with abdominal pain and bowel symptoms associated with constipation-predominant IBS. It has been shown to improve spontaneous bowel movements within the first week of treatment and improve pain within 6–9 weeks in patients with IBS symptoms.

Prucalopride is a selective 5-hydroxytryptamine $(5\text{-HT})_4$ receptor agonist that has been shown to increase the number of spontaneous, complete bowel movements. Prucalopride is considered safe and well-tolerated with the most common side effect being diarrhea; however, it is not currently available in the United States.

In patients with outlet dysfunction, and notably dyssynergic defecation, biofeedback therapy has been shown to have significant benefits and should be the first-line therapy once this diagnosis is made. Biofeedback appears to be more effective than conventional pharmacologic management in the treatment of dyssynergic defecation and is noninvasive and without side effects; however, it is not widely available.

Surgical intervention is usually reserved for those patients with refractory symptoms despite optimal medical management. Sacral nerve stimulation (SNS) is an emerging surgical intervention in patients with fecal incontinence but has also been shown to be beneficial in those with slow-transit constipation. Sacral nerve stimulation is thought to increase the frequency of bowel movements by increasing colonic propagating sequences. Although subtotal colectomy with ileorectal anastomosis in patients with refractory slow-transit constipation may result in substantial improvement in stool frequency, in those patients with abdominal pain or discomfort, it often persists. Furthermore, subtotal colectomy is associated with high morbidity requiring careful patient selection. Segmental colon resection is not recommended as a surgical option in refractory chronic constipation. Finally, a diverting colostomy may be considered in those with refractory dyssynergic defecation.

Case Resolution

Several tests were performed. A balloon expulsion test was abnormal; she could not expel the 50 mL rectal balloon in <2 min. Anorectal manometry showed simulated defecation and normal sensation, while defecography showed minimal perineal descent and a small anterior rectocele that emptied completely. Thus, testing confirmed the suspected diagnosis of dyssynergic defecation. Slow-transit constipation was not considered a primary cause of the patient's symptoms due to the patient's report of daily bowel movements and the rectocele was felt to be clinically insignificant. She subsequently underwent biofeedback training over three sessions with substantial benefit in terms of ease of passage of formed stools and much less dyschezia. She also made a commitment to increase exercise, to consume more fluid and high-fiber foods, and to continue her current medications for C-IBS.

Key Clinical Teaching Points

- While only a minority of patients with constipation seeks medical treatment, constipation symptoms account for 2.5 million physician visits and an estimated 800 million dollars spent on medications annually.
- The increase in prevalence with age is due in part to polypharmacy, decreased mobility, comorbidities, and neurological disorders.
- There are three primary types of constipation, normal transit, outlet dysfunction, and slow transit, and many secondary causes that can be discovered in the history and physical.
- Pharmacologic options to treat constipation are many and variably effective requiring a systematic approach to their use.
- Biofeedback is the most effective treatment for pelvic floor dyssynergia.

Teaching Questions

1. RB, an 80-year-old woman accompanied by her daughter, is being seen for new-onset constipation. RB has progressive dementia requiring nursing home care, but stays with her family on some weekends. RB rarely has a bowel movement during those visits, and the time she did it stopped up the toilet. RB takes verapamil, hydrochlorothiazide, a fiber tablet, calcium, and Lexapro. You ask about episodes of incontinence, and the daughter confirms your suspicion. Given the history, which one of the following is the most likely cause of her fecal incontinence?

   (A) Polypharmacy
   (B) Bacterial overgrowth due to slow transit
   (C) Excessive perineal descent
   (D) Overflow incontinence

2. DG is a 39-year-old forest fire fighter who comes to see you for pain when passing stool and blood on the toilet tissue. He has worked long hours in the forests of Idaho where there is limited access to a toilet, sometimes needing to hold in

stool for hours. The appearance changed from soft torpedo to small hard balls to thin ribbon over the past few months, and he strains hard to go. He takes no medications, appetite is good, weight is stable, has no nighttime symptoms, and otherwise feels well. Family history is negative for colon cancer and inflammatory bowel disease. His abdomen and anorectal exam are normal. Hemoglobin is 11. He talked with his buddies and thinks he has a fissure. Which one of the following diagnostic tests should be done first before prescribing a treatment?

(A) Balloon expulsion test as he clearly has pelvic floor dyssynergy
(B) Defecography as it would show a rectosigmoid mass if present and evidence of dyssynergia
(C) Colonoscopy
(D) Anoscopy to evaluate for hemorrhoids and fissure

3. RM is a 28-year-old female with systemic sclerosis of 7 years' duration. Constipation symptoms have been present since her teenage years but have recently changed. She now has a bowel movement once a week, described as soft brown, never hard. She hardly gets the urge to go to the bathroom, feeling more abdominal fullness and cramping than an urge before a movement. She never strains. Store-bought laxatives did not help and fiber tablets worsened bloating and constipation. Bloating and distention is worse after meals, so much so that she is avoiding food, losing 5 lb. over the last month. Which one of the following diagnostic tests will give the most useful information about her gastrointestinal function?

(A) Sitzmark test
(B) Wireless motility capsule (WMC)
(C) Magnetic resonance defecography (MRD)
(D) Anorectal manometry

Key References

1. American College of Gastroenterology Chronic Constipation Task Force. An evidence-based approach to the management of chronic constipation in North America. Am J Gastroenterol. 2005;100 Suppl 1:S1–4. Excellent evidence-based review of the management of chronic constipation.
2. Drossman DA, Li Z, Andruzzi E, Temple RD, Talley NJ, Thompson WG, et al. U.S. Householder survey of functional gastrointestinal disorders. Prevalence, sociodemography, and health impact. Dig Dis Sci. 1993;38:1569–80. Landmark paper on the sociodemographics and health impact of functional gastrointestinal disorders.
3. Gallegos-Orozco JF, Foxx-Orenstein AE, Sterler SA, Stoa J. Chronic constipation in the elderly. Am J Gastroenterol. 2012;107:18–25. Recent comprehensive review of constipation in the elderly.
4. Longstreth GF, Thompson WG, Chey WD, Houghton LA, Mearin F, Spiller RC. Functional bowel disorders. Gastroenterology. 2006;130:1480–91. Key text of Rome III definitions of functional disorders.
5. Sonnenberg A, Koch TR. Physician visits in the United States for constipation: 1958-1986. Dig Dis Sci. 1989;34:606–11. An older paper that has stood the test of time as it details physician visits for constipation over a 28 year period.

6. Suares NC, Ford AC. Prevalence of, and risk factors for, chronic idiopathic constipation in the community: a systematic review and meta-analysis. Am J Gastroenterol. 2011;106:1582–91. Excellent meta-analysis on prevalence and risk factors of constipation in a community population.
7. Wald A, Scarpignato C, Kamm MA, Mueller-Lissner S, Helfrich I, Schuijt C, et al. The burden of constipation on quality of life: results of a multinational study. Aliment Pharmacol Ther. 2007;26:227–36. A nice article on how chronic constipation affects patients' quality of life.

Chapter 16
Irritable Bowel Syndrome

Lucinda Harris and Sarah Umar

Case Study

A 32-year-old nurse is referred by her primary care provider (PCP) for further evaluation of symptoms thought compatible with the diagnosis of irritable bowel syndrome (IBS). She states that she has diarrhea (type 6–7 on the Bristol stool scale) three to five times each day. Her symptoms are extremely distressing because of frequent bathroom visits. The diarrhea occurs at least 4–5 days out of 7 for the past 5 years and, because it is often unpredictable, has made her anxious at work and stopped her from attending events outside of work. She has occasional nocturnal awakening, and the diarrhea is accompanied by fecal urgency, abdominal bloating, and lower abdominal cramping that is generally relieved by having a bowel movement. She denies any constitutional symptoms, fever, chills, fecal incontinence, or rectal bleeding. The diarrhea stops if she doesn't eat and if she takes loperamide. She reports that fruit, beef, sodas, and anxiety seem to trigger her symptoms. She had tried psyllium in the past, but this makes her feel more bloated. She currently takes dicyclomine 10 mg four times a day, and, although it helps with her sensation of fecal urgency, it gives her a dry mouth and makes her a little sleepy. She is frustrated by her symptoms, as finding a bathroom controls her leisure activities and also creates distress at work.

Her past medical history is notable for rare migraine headaches. She is married with two children. She doesn't smoke, and alcohol intake is minimal. Family history is notable for colon polyps in her father at age 55. There is no family history of IBD or celiac disease.

Her PCP had performed blood work revealing a normal CBC, sedimentation rate, TSH, and serologic tests for celiac disease (serum tissue transglutaminase [tTG] antibody and serum immunoglobulin A [IgA]).

L. Harris, M.D. • S. Umar, M.D. (✉)
Division of Gastroenterology and Hepatology, Mayo Clinic, 13400 E Shea Blvd, Scottsdale, AZ 85259, USA
e-mail: Umar.sarah@mayo.edu

B.E. Lacy et al. (eds.), *Functional and Motility Disorders of the Gastrointestinal Tract*, DOI 10.1007/978-1-4939-1498-2_16

On physical exam, she is visibly anxious. Vital signs and a careful physical examination, including a rectal examination, are normal. She asks whether her diagnosis is correct and whether she needs any further tests and wonders whether other treatment options are available.

Introduction

Irritable bowel syndrome is one of the most common medical conditions seen and managed by both primary care and gastroenterology providers. This disorder, characterized by abdominal pain with altered bowel habits and without structural or biochemical abnormalities to explain symptoms, has diverse etiologies. The severity of the disease can range from mild and intermittent to severe and constant. Previously, mild to moderate disease was thought to predominate, but more recent data suggest that the number of patients with severe disease may be substantially higher than once thought, with prevalence rates of severe disease as high as 69 % reported in tertiary care settings.

Recent research has also demonstrated that quality of life (QoL) and the functional status of IBS patients can be significantly impaired. The troublesomeness of symptoms is reflected in the fact that suicidal ideation among IBS patients ranges from 4 % in the primary care setting to 38 % in a tertiary clinic. Many patients have seen multiple providers who have done little more than tell them they have a disorder of stress or anxiety.

IBS is costly to the healthcare system and to the economy as a whole, resulting in annual costs of up to 30 billion dollars. Patients with IBS have been shown to utilize the healthcare system for both gastrointestinal (GI) and non-GI complaints more than patients without IBS. This negatively impacts the productivity of patients with IBS, and in fact, their absenteeism from work or school is three times higher than that of patients without IBS.

Finally, IBS creates challenges because even though this disorder now has definite symptom-based diagnostic criteria, patients often have overlapping symptoms such as gastroesophageal disease (GERD) and functional dyspepsia that must also be treated. A recent meta-analysis found that the prevalence of GERD symptoms was four times higher in IBS patients. Patients with moderate to severe disease therefore present unique challenges to the clinician in terms of efficient and effective diagnosis and treatment.

Epidemiology

Despite once being thought of as a disease limited only to the Western world, recent studies have shown that IBS can be identified worldwide. The prevalence of IBS ranges from 5 to 15 % in the Western world, while limited community studies from

Asia, Africa, and Latin America have found prevalence rates varying from 4 to 25 % with the majority being in the 10–15 % range. IBS is more likely to occur in women than in men, and epidemiologic studies consistently demonstrated that women outnumber men by two- to fourfold, depending on where the survey was performed. It should be recognized, however, that IBS does not solely affect women. It has also been described as a component of the Gulf War syndrome, a multisystem complex that affects primarily male soldiers who have served in the Gulf War. Overall, IBS accounts for 12 % of primary care visits and at least 28 % of all gastroenterology consultations.

Pathophysiology

The primary pathophysiologic mechanism thought to underlie IBS symptoms is dysregulation of brain–gut interactions. There are a variety of central and peripheral factors (e.g., genetic predisposition, environmental factors, chronic stress, inflammation or infection, altered intestinal flora) that may contribute to an altered brain–gut axis. These alterations may eventually cause disturbances of mucosal immune response, intestinal motility and permeability, and visceral sensitivity, all of which may contribute to symptoms of abdominal pain or discomfort and compromised bowel function.

A role for a genetic predisposition in the pathophysiology of IBS has been supported by familial clustering and twin studies; however, these data continue to evolve, and environmental factors, such as how abdominal pain is treated by parents when the child is growing up, may have even more of an impact on the development of IBS.

Altered gastrointestinal motility and visceral sensitivity are key concepts in the understanding of the pathogenesis of IBS. Mechanisms associated with visceral hypersensitivity in IBS involve hypervigilance to expected aversive visceral events and hyperalgesia induced by sustained noxious visceral stimulation. Using various paradigms of balloon distension, studies have shown that IBS patients generally demonstrate lowered sensory thresholds to balloon distension and increased sensory ratings, when compared with healthy individuals.

Functional differences in the central nervous system have also been demonstrated in IBS. Using neuroimaging studies such as positron emission tomography and functional magnetic resonance imaging of the brain, it has been demonstrated that several regions of the brain are part of a central pain-processing circuitry ("central pain matrix") that includes the insula and the anterior cingulate cortex, as well as other regions belonging to the corticopontine area. These pain processing areas have been shown to have altered activation in response to rectosigmoid stimulation in IBS patients compared with healthy controls. Furthermore, in patients with IBS, the central nervous system may fail to activate pain inhibition or increase activation of pain facilitatory pathways, in response to incoming or anticipated visceral pain.

In terms of GI tract motility, serotonin (5-hydroxytryptamine, 5-HT) is a key potentiator of gastrointestinal (GI) motility (e.g., stimulating peristalsis) as well as

GI sensation and secretion. Ninety-five percent of serotonin is found in the gut; 90 % is localized within the enterochromaffin cells, and 10 % is found within the enteric neurons. Altered serotonin signaling mechanisms have been reported in IBS, particularly a decreased level of the serotonin reuptake transporter protein. This transporter protein is thought to be the mechanism by which the body regulates the amount of serotonin in the extracellular space and is genetically predetermined. Serotonin reuptake transporter gene polymorphisms may influence the response to serotonergic agents employed in the treatment of IBS. A number of these agents have been found to be efficacious in the treatment of IBS and are discussed below. Although serotonin is a key modulator of GI function, there are also other neurotransmitters and hormones involved in gut motility, sensation, and secretion that are potentially important targets for current and future drug development.

Stress seems particularly important in altering brain–gut interactions, as evidenced clinically as an exacerbation of IBS symptoms. Rectal distension studies in IBS patients have shown altered visceral perception and neuroendocrine responses to a stressor compared with healthy controls. Although stress affects the gut in both healthy individuals and IBS patients, recent evidence suggests there may be greater reactivity in IBS patients in the major mediator of stress in the brain–gut axis, corticotrophin-releasing factor (CRF). Therapeutic agents targeted at CRF receptors have been studied in the treatment of IBS, but have not yet yielded any commercially available treatments to date.

Recently, the role of infection, inflammation, and alterations in the gut flora has been investigated in the pathophysiology of IBS. Post-infectious IBS has been identified in 7–30 % of patients with a recent history of established bacterial gastroenteritis. A variety of mechanisms on the mucosal and cellular level are currently being investigated for their potential role in post-infectious IBS. Decreased ability to downregulate the inflammatory response to infection may result in increased proinflammatory cytokines and/or enterochromaffin cells. Researchers are also exploring the use of probiotics and antibiotics as possible immune modulators and small bowel intestinal overgrowth as a potentially pathogenetic mechanism in IBS.

Diagnosis and Evaluation

IBS is a clinical diagnosis, and, as there are neither stereotypical endoscopic findings nor biomarkers which confirm or disprove the diagnosis, the cornerstone of IBS diagnosis is the Rome criteria (Table 16.1). The Rome criteria is a symptom-based classification of the functional bowel disorders that has undergone multiple evolutions since its inception in 1988 with the most current version being Rome III (published in 2006). IBS, according to the Rome III definition, is a functional bowel disorder in which abdominal pain or discomfort is associated with a change in bowel habit. Patients need to have had recurrent abdominal pain or discomfort for at least 3 days per month in the last 3 months. This has to have been associated with two or more of the following: improvement with defecation, onset associated

Table 16.1 Definition of IBS—Rome III criteria

Rome III IBS diagnostic criteria and IBS subtypes
Criteria need to be fulfilled for the last 3 months with symptom onset at least 6 months prior to diagnosis
IBS is defined as recurrent abdominal pain or discomfort (uncomfortable sensation not described as pain) at least 3 days per month in the last 3 months associated with 2 or more of the following:
1. Improvement with defecation
2. Onset associated with a change in frequency of stool
3. Onset associated with a change in form (appearance) of stool
IBS can be further subtyped by predominant stool pattern:
IBS with constipation (hard or lumpy stools ≥25 %/loose or watery stools <25 % of bowel movements)
IBS with diarrhea (loose or water stools ≥25 %/hard or lumpy stools <5 % of bowel movements)
Mixed IBS (hard or lumpy stools ≥25 %/loose or watery stools ≥25 % of bowel movements)
Unsubtyped IBS (insufficient abnormality of stool consistency to meet the above subtypes)

with a change in frequency of stool, or onset associated with a change in form or appearance of stool. There are four subtypes of IBS (Table 16.1).

The American Gastroenterological Association position statement on IBS states that the diagnosis is based on identifying positive symptoms (e.g., Rome criteria) consistent with the condition while excluding other conditions with similar clinical presentations in a cost-effective manner. Spiller and colleagues formulated an algorithm for the evaluation of patients with abdominal pain and deranged bowel habits. This allows the clinician to evaluate for potential alarm symptoms via diagnostic testing and, in the absence of significant findings, to classify the patient into one of the subtypes of IBS (Fig. 16.1).

A careful history and physical should be taken. One should obtain information about the character and frequency of bowel movements, presence and characteristics of abdominal discomfort, duration of symptoms, and inquiry into alarm symptoms. In patients complaining of "diarrhea," one should ask about fecal incontinence as often patients complain of diarrhea when they are actually describing symptoms of incontinence. In patients with complaints of "constipation," one should ascertain whether it is an infrequent urge to defecate or whether it is more of difficulty with evacuation of stool which suggests pelvic floor abnormalities such as rectal prolapse or dyssynergic defecation. Important considerations in the differential diagnosis according to bowel habit are outlined in Table 16.2.

It is also important to obtain a social and psychosocial history, as there is a well-known association between IBS and a history of abuse and psychiatric illness. Furthermore, it is important to understand how the symptoms are affecting the patient's quality of life. As mentioned in the case study, IBS symptoms were affecting both the patient's functioning at work and her ability to participate in social activities. The physical exam should include a rectal exam to evaluate the

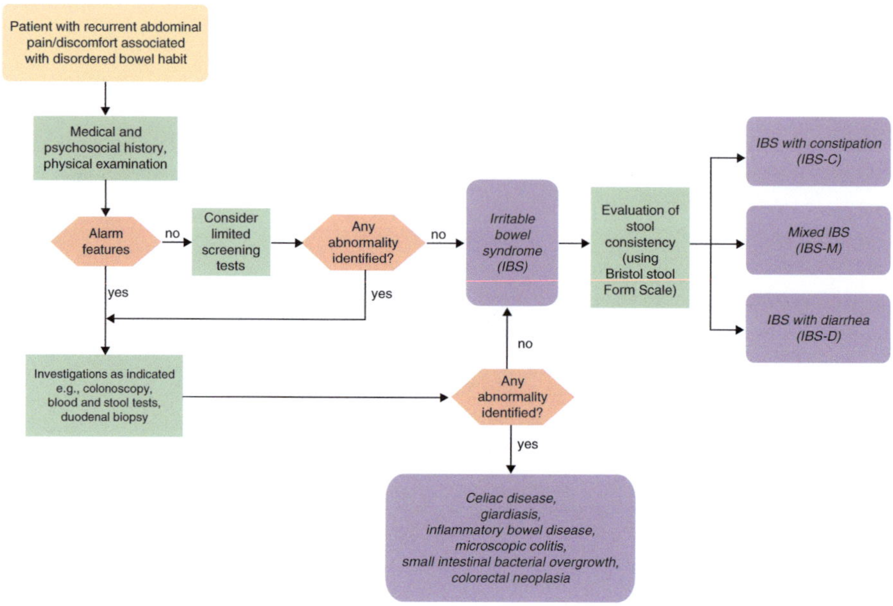

Fig. 16.1 Algorithm for diagnosis of IBS. From Spiller RC, Thompson WG. Bowel disorders. Am J Gastroenterol. 2010;105(4):775–85

perianal area and assess for stool character, rectal tone, presence of blood, and evidence of dyssynergia.

In patients who demonstrate "red flag" alarm symptoms (see Table 16.3), further investigations such as upper endoscopy and colonoscopy, a complete blood count, thyroid-stimulating hormone (TSH), inflammatory markers such as C-reactive protein, celiac serologies (serum IgA and tissue transglutaminase (tTG) antibody), and stool studies to rule out infection, such as *Clostridium difficile* and *Giardia*, should be considered on a case-by-case basis. Table 16.4 outlines the American College of Gastroenterology diagnostic recommendations for IBS. Interestingly, a recent study of 200 patients seen in an academic medical facility who met IBS criteria revealed that 70 % of patients endorsed a red flag symptom. It was found that in patients endorsing alarm symptoms, many were not tested further, and, in those who were, the yield of testing was low. This study suggests that in patients who meet criteria for IBS, further testing, even in the presence of alarm symptoms, may be of low yield.

Treatment

The management of IBS differs based on the patient's symptoms and the IBS subtype. One of the most important points to remember in treating a patient with IBS, regardless of subtype, is that developing a trusting relationship with the healthcare provider is important—this requires establishment of mutual respect and good rapport.

Table 16.2 Differential diagnosis of IBS based on symptom type[a]

Symptom	Differential diagnosis
Diarrhea	
Infectious	Viral
	Bacterial
	Parasites (e.g., *Giardia*)
	HIV-associated conditions
Inflammatory bowel disease	Ulcerative colitis
	Crohn's disease
	Microscopic colitis
Malabsorption	Intestinal disorders
	Pancreatic insufficiency
	Postsurgical (e.g., Roux-en-Y-gastrojejunostomy)
Diet	Wheat
	Alcohol
	Caffeine
	Carbohydrate malabsorption (e.g., fructose or lactose)
	Sorbitol
Medications	Chemotherapy
	Antibiotics
	SSRIs
	NSAIDs
Malignancy	Colon cancer
	Neuroendocrine tumor
Constipation	
Neurologic	Parkinson's disease
	Multiple sclerosis
	Spinal cord lesion
Endocrine disorder	Hyperparathyroidism
	Hypothyroidism
Malignancy	Colon cancer
Medications	Calcium channel blockers
	Opiates
	Chemotherapy
	TCAs
Abdominal pain/bloat	
Gynecologic	Endometriosis
	Dysmenorrhea
	Ovarian cancer
Psychiatric	Depression
	Anxiety
	Somatization

(a) *Giardia* may cause symptoms of alternating constipation and diarrhea
(b) Crohn's disease may cause obstructive symptoms of constipation, pain, or bloating
SSRIs selective serotonin reuptake inhibitor, *NSAIDs* nonsteroidal anti-inflammatory drugs, *TCAs* tricyclic antidepressants
[a]Not an all-inclusive list

Table 16.3 Alarm signs and symptoms requiring further investigation

Medical history	Physical examination
Age of onset > age 50	Oral ulcers (e.g., aphthous ulcers)
Nocturnal or refractory diarrhea	Fever
Weight loss of >10 lb.	Guaiac + stool
Rectal bleeding	Abdominal or rectal mass
Rashes/arthritis suggestive of IBD	Rectal bleeding
Travel history to area suggestive of GI infection	Rash suggestive of IBD or celiac disease (e.g., dermatitis herpetiformis, erythema nodosum)
Severe constipation/diarrhea	
Family history	**Laboratory data**
Celiac disease	Anemia
Colon cancer/polyps	Increased white blood cell count
Inflammatory bowel disease	Elevated sedimentation rate or C-reactive protein
	Abnormal blood chemistries

IBD inflammatory bowel disease

Table 16.4 ACG diagnostic recommendations for IBS

Diagnostic test	Recommendation
CBC	Not routinely recommended
Chemistries/thyroid function tests	Not routinely recommended
Stool for ova and parasites	Not routinely recommended
Abdominal imaging	Not routinely recommended
Serologic screening for celiac sprue	Pursue in patients with IBS-D or IBS-M
Lactose breath testing	Consider if symptoms persist after dietary modification
Breath testing for SIBO	Insufficient data to recommend
Colonoscopy	Perform in patients with alarm features[a] and in those aged >50: consider random colonic biopsies in patients with diarrhea

SIBO small intestinal bacterial overgrowth

Brandt LJ, et al. Am J Gastroenterol. 2009;104 Suppl 1:S1–35

[a]Alarm features—see Table 16.3

Multiple clinic visits with the healthcare provider are also helpful to not only set expectations but also understand that there are many ways, both pharmacologic and nonpharmacologic, to treat this condition. Providing reassurance that their symptoms are of a benign nature and that you will continue to work with them to find what works best to alleviate their symptoms are also important.

Table 16.5 outlines the various agents that have been used in the treatment of IBS according to predominant bowel symptom. For patients with constipation-predominant IBS (IBS-C), the use of fiber has long been a cornerstone of therapy; however, data regarding the efficacy of fiber supplementation are in conflict. Some studies have shown benefit, while others have not, likely due to small sample sizes and overall poor study design. Laxatives, both stimulant and osmotic, have also

Table 16.5 Treatment options for IBS

For all subtypes			
Lifestyle			
Diet	Assess for carbohydrate intolerance—lactose, FODMAPs, gluten		
Exercise	20–60 min of aerobic activity 3–5×/week decreases IBS symptom severity		
Sleep	Poor sleep habits are associated with increased severity of IBS symptoms		
Psychological therapies	Cognitive behavioral therapy, hypnotherapy, and multicomponent psychological therapy show greater efficacy than usual care		
Diarrhea			
Drug class	Drug name	Dose	Guidelines for use
Antispasmodics	Dicyclomine	10–20 mg AC and qHS	May be helpful for meal-related urgency
	Hyoscyamine	0.125 mg AC and qHS	
Antidiarrheals	Loperamide	1–2 mg 4×/day	Do not provide global relief of symptoms; can be titrated to desired effect
	Diphenoxylate–atropine	5 mg up to 4×/day	
Antibiotics	Rifaximin	400–550 mg 3×/day for 10–14 days	Global symptom improvement seen in non-constipated IBS; not yet FDA approved
5HT3 antagonist	Alosetron	0.5–1.0 mg 2×/day	Titrate to lowest effective dose for IBS-D Only available for women with severe IBS-D under risk management program Can cause significant constipation or ischemic colitis
Tricyclic antidepressants	Amitriptyline Desipramine Imipramine Nortriptyline	10–150 mg at bedtime	Used at lower doses than for mood disorders; titrate to lowest effective dose; may have greater efficacy for IBS-D, may be effective for pain
Constipation			
Laxatives			
Bulking agents	Psyllium	2.5–30 mg/day in divided doses	Benefit demonstrated for psyllium May be helpful in patients with looser stool as well as in fecal incontinence; May cause increased bloating and flatulence
	Calcium carboxyphil	1.250 mg 2–4×/day	
	Methylcellulose	500 mg, 1–2 tbsp daily to 3×/day	
Emollient laxatives	Docusate	1–3 tabs daily, 100 mg/tab	Efficacy in IBS-C not well established
	Mineral oil	5–10 cc/day	
Osmotic laxatives	Milk of magnesia	10–20 cc up to 4×/day (400 mg/5 cc)	Efficacy in IBS-C not well established Lactulose and polyethylene glycol may cause increased bloating
	Lactulose	15–30 cc daily (10–20 g/day)	
	Polyethylene glycol (PEG)	17 g in 8 oz fluid daily	

(continued)

Table 16.5 (continued)

Constipation			
Stimulant laxatives	Senna	15 mg	Efficacy in IBS-C not well established
	Bisacodyl	10 mg, 1–2 tabs orally/day	
5HT4 agonists	Prucalopride	1–2 mg daily	Currently available in Canada and some European countries for women for the treatment of chronic constipation
	Tegaserod	2–6 mg twice daily	Taken off market in 2007 because of possible cardiovascular side effects. Currently only available for emergency use
Chloride channel activator	Lubiprostone	8 μg twice daily with food	Only for women with IBS-C can increase to dose for chronic constipation at 24 μg twice (approved for men and women, also for opioid induced constipation)
Guanylate-C agonist	Linaclotide	290 mcg daily ½ h before food in the morning 145 mcg dose is for chronic constipation	Approved for both men and women for the treatment of IBS-C and chronic constipation

Johannesson E, Simren M, Strid H, et al. Physical activity improves symptoms in irritable bowel syndrome: a randomized controlled trial. Am J Gastroenterol. 2011;106:915–22

been used. PEG 3350 is a commonly used, safe, well-tolerated osmotic laxative that has had documented success in the treatment of chronic constipation and for symptoms of constipation in patients with IBS-C. These agents may exacerbate bloating and rarely improve the associated abdominal discomfort.

At present, two agents are FDA approved for the treatment of IBS-C. Lubiprostone (8 μg twice daily) is a chloride channel activator which acts to increase luminal water secretion. This, in turn, results in an increase in fluid in the GI tract, which is thought to promote peristalsis. It is also approved at a higher dose of 24 μg bid to treat chronic idiopathic constipation. Lubiprostone's most common adverse effects include nausea, diarrhea, and headache. Nausea may be ameliorated by advising the patient that the medication be taken with a meal. A more recently approved agent, linaclotide, is a guanylate cyclase type C (GC-C) receptor agonist which has been shown to be of benefit in patients with functional constipation and those with IBS-C. The data in the IBS-C trials (290 μg daily) demonstrated an improvement in complete spontaneous bowel movements within 1 week of therapy; however, many patients did not notice an improvement in abdominal pain until after taking the medication for several weeks. Diarrhea was the chief side effect. Prucalopride

(1 or 2 mg daily) is a highly selective 5-HT_4 receptor agonist (i.e., a serotonin receptor stimulating agent) that is approved in Canada and Europe for the treatment of chronic idiopathic constipation, but is not yet FDA approved for the treatment of IBS or chronic constipation the United States. It has been shown to be safe and well tolerated with the most common side effect being diarrhea. Extensive testing has been done with regard to electrocardiogram side effects, and it has not been shown, like its predecessor tegaserod (another 5-HT_4 agonist), to increase myocardial infarction or stroke.

In patients suffering from diarrhea-predominant IBS (IBS-D), fiber is commonly used as a bulking agent and to absorb excess water from the stool, but as in the case presentation, it frequently causes bloating. Although smooth muscle antispasmodics (e.g., dicyclomine) are used primarily for pain and spasm, these agents are occasionally used to decrease meal-related diarrhea. Anticholinergic side effects often limit their use. Other commonly used treatments for IBS-D include the antidiarrheal agents diphenoxylate–atropine and loperamide. In patients who do not respond well to the above, the use of tricyclic antidepressants may be considered. These agents have been shown in multiple trials to be effective for both bowel symptoms and abdominal pain, and they play a role in the modification of visceral hypersensitivity. In female patients who have failed other agents and who have at least a 6-month history of IBS, the 5-HT_3 antagonist, alosetron, has been approved for the treatment of IBS-D. The medication is in a special prescribing program because it has been associated with the development of ischemic colitis (prevalence rate of 0.2 %) and severe constipation (prevalence rate of 0.1 %). To prescribe the medication, practitioners must go to the drug manufacturer's website and attest to their comfort in diagnosing IBS. A discussion about the side effects of the medication and the symptoms of ischemic colitis and severe constipation needs to take place with the patient, and the patient fills out an attestation form that both the patient and the provider sign as an acknowledgment of the information provided.

The use of antibiotics in the treatment of IBS is controversial. Although they can be used to treat patients with all types of IBS, studies demonstrating their benefit have been done primarily in non-constipated patients. Their use is driven by the hypothesis that patients with IBS have small intestinal bacterial overgrowth or altered gut flora (i.e., dysbiosis) and that this alteration in the luminal microbial environment may lead to IBS symptoms possibly via effects on intestinal permeability and inflammation. Pimentel and colleagues have demonstrated that a significant proportion of IBS patients, particularly non-constipated patients, have abnormal breath tests indicating small bowel bacterial overgrowth and that IBS symptoms improve after normalization of breath test results following antibiotic administration. In contrast, other investigators have found little benefit with this treatment approach. Our practice is to perform testing for small intestinal bacterial overgrowth in patients with IBS symptoms especially diarrhea and bloating. If testing is positive, then it is reasonable to proceed with antibiotic treatment.

Probiotics have also been used in all subtypes of IBS. Probiotics are thought to have multiple mechanisms of action that include enhancing mucosal barrier function, modulation of inflammatory response, and competitive interactions with other pathogens. Although there have been a number of studies of probiotics, the only high-quality probiotic trials that have shown repeated efficacy are those using *Bifidobacterium infantis* 35624. Most studies evaluating the use of probiotics in IBS are plagued by insufficient sample size or other flaws in study design. Multiple meta-analyses, however, have been published, and many have shown benefit in abdominal pain/discomfort, bloating, and/or bowel habit derangements in IBS patients using probiotics. It general, it appears that probiotics are safe for most patients (although they should not be used in immunocompromised patients), but these medications are not subject to the same scrutiny as prescription medications so further data is needed regarding their safety and efficacy.

Finally, there are nonpharmacologic interventions such as diet, biofeedback, cognitive behavioral therapy, and acupuncture that are also successful and attractive to patients who are reluctant to take medications. Exercise and good sleep hygiene are also other potentially important lifestyle habits to encourage. Targeting lactose intolerance does not seem to have long-term effects, but emerging data suggest that a diet low in fermentable oligo-, di-, and monosaccharides and polyols (FODMAPs) may be helpful. This diet aims to decrease ingestion of fermentable substances that may trigger IBS symptoms and has found to be beneficial in many patients to control symptoms of pain, bloating, gas, and diarrhea.

Case Resolution

A global approach with active listening revealed that there were not only dietary triggers but a strong anxiety component as well with regard to IBS symptom generation. Setting realistic expectations was discussed with the patient. She was informed that we would indeed work to identify treatments to improve her symptoms, but that "fixing it" might not be entirely possible. Because of the association of her symptoms with fruit, a fructose breath test was performed and was positive. Although a low FODMAP diet was implemented, the patient reported that this resulted in only a partial improvement of her symptoms.

A tricyclic antidepressant and a low-dose as-needed anxiolytics were then initiated; however, side effects limited increasing the dose on the tricyclic antidepressant. After discussion of the potential benefit, the patient agreed to undergo a psychiatric consultation in an attempt to help her control her anxiety. Citalopram 10 mg daily was initiated, and she agreed to a course of cognitive behavioral therapy. Finally, following a discussion about alosetron and its side effects, the patient and physician signed the attestation form. In follow-up, her diarrhea symptoms responded to alosetron 0.5 mg once to twice daily, her abdominal pain was reduced, and her anxiety was much improved.

Key Clinical Teaching Points

- With respect to the diagnosis, it is important to utilize a symptom-based approach, determine the predominant symptoms that concern the patient, and rule out red flags.
- When evaluating a patient with suspected IBS, testing should be guided by the predominant symptom(s) and presence or absence of red flags.
- Treatment should incorporate a global approach targeting sleep, diet, exercise and quality of life, psychological well-being, and predominant gastrointestinal symptom(s).

Teaching Questions

1. Rome criteria for defining irritable bowel syndrome include all of the following except

    (A) Abdominal pain or discomfort
    (B) Change in stool consistency
    (C) Nocturnal bowel symptoms
    (D) Change in stool frequency

2. All of the following are postulated to be possible mechanisms for the pathophysiology of IBS except

    (A) Visceral hypersensitivity
    (B) Stress
    (C) Post-infectious
    (D) Altered gastrointestinal motility
    (E) Immunoglobulin deficiency

3. All of the following medications may be used for the treatment of diarrhea-predominant IBS except

    (A) Lubiprostone
    (B) Alosetron
    (C) Loperamide
    (D) Fiber
    (E) Amitriptyline (tricyclic anti-depressants)

4. What life style therapy may be helpful in the treatment of IBS

    (A) Low cholesterol diet
    (B) FODMAP diet
    (C) Lactose free diet
    (D) Large infrequent meals
    (E) Late night snacking

Key References

1. Ford AC, Moayyedi P, Lacy BE, et al. American College of Gastroenterology monograph on the management of irritable bowel syndrome and chronic idiopathic constipation. Am J Gastroenterology 2014;109: Suppl 1:S2–26.
2. Harris LA, Heitkemper MM. Practical considerations for recognizing and managing severe irritable bowel syndrome. Gastroenterol Nurs. 2012;35:12–21. A practical guide to managing challenging severe IBS patients.
3. Longstreth GF, Thompson WG, Chey WD, Houghton LA, Mearin F, Spiller RC. Functional bowel disorders. Gastroenterology. 2006;130(5):1480–91. A discussion of the current Rome III criteria.

Chapter 17
Colonic Inertia

Adil E. Bharucha and Michael Camilleri

Case Study

A 47-year-old woman was referred for further evaluation and management of chronic constipation. Her history was notable for symptoms of constipation-predominant irritable bowel since childhood. When first evaluated, she had a bowel movement once weekly, induced by oral laxatives and/or an enema, with no spontaneous bowel movements. Scintigraphy disclosed normal gastric emptying and small bowel transit but delayed colonic transit. Anorectal manometry and balloon expulsion tests were normal. At that time, her laxative regimen was adjusted.

Five years later, she returned with severe constipation. After no bowel movement for several days, she consumes a large amount of milk of magnesia and bisacodyl. These agents induce severe abdominal cramps and diarrhea followed by temporary relief of constipation. While enemas do not result in passage of stool, she is able to evacuate the enema fluid fairly easily. She denies straining excessively and does not need to use unusual positions on the toilet, has no sense of incomplete evacuation, and does not digitate the rectum or vagina to help evacuate the stool. She also describes right and left lower quadrant abdominal pain that are constant and not always relieved after defecation. Her appetite is fair and her weight has increased 10 lb. in the last 2 years. A colonic motility study with a barostat-manometry assembly was consistent with colonic inertia (see Figs. 17.1 and 17.2). She subsequently underwent laparoscopic colectomy with ileorectostomy. After surgery, she was doing well without laxatives, passing four semi-formed bowel movements daily and having minimal abdominal discomfort.

A.E. Bharucha, M.B.B.S., M.D., FAGA (✉) • M. Camilleri, M.D.
Division of Gastroenterology and Hepatology, Mayo Clinic, Charlton 8, 200 First Street SW, Rochester, MN 55905, USA

B.E. Lacy et al. (eds.), *Functional and Motility Disorders of the Gastrointestinal Tract*, DOI 10.1007/978-1-4939-1498-2_17

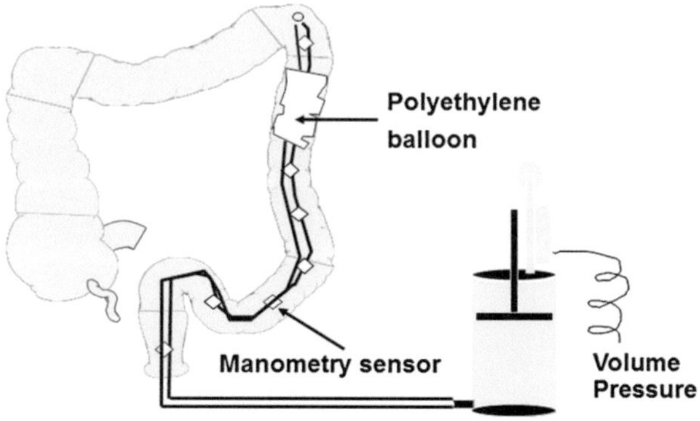

Fig. 17.1 Barostat-manometry assembly positioned in the descending colon with polyethylene balloon in apposition with colonic mucosa

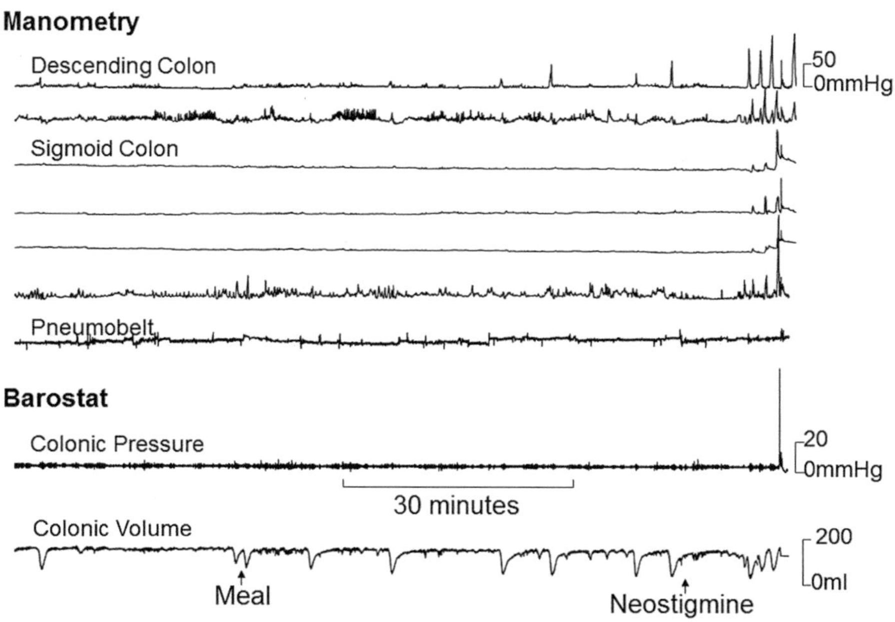

Fig. 17.2 Representative colonic barostat-manometry tracing of colonic inertia. The manometry sensors disclosed increased phasic pressure activity after neostigmine, but not after a meal. There was no change in the baseline volume of a colonic balloon inflated to a fixed pressure after a meal or neostigmine. Taken together, these features indicate colonic inertia

Introduction

Constipation is defined by bowel symptoms, and slow colonic transit is identified by assessing colonic transit time. The Oxford Dictionary defines inertia as "a tendency to do nothing or to remain unchanged." Colonic inertia refers to markedly reduced or absent colonic contractile responses to physiological (i.e., a meal) and pharmacological stimuli (e.g., bisacodyl or neostigmine) in patients with slow transit constipation. To emphasize, colonic inertia should only be identified by evaluating the colonic contractile response to a meal and a pharmacological stimulus. While slow colonic transit and colonic inertia are often used interchangeably, these terms are not synonymous. Currently, inertia should only be identified by evaluating the colonic contractile response to a meal or neostigmine with intraluminal sensors.

Epidemiology

The incidence, prevalence, and natural history of colonic inertia are unknown. A review of the literature observed that the median prevalence of constipation was 16 % (range 0.7–79 %) in adults overall and 33.5 % in adults aged 60–101 years. There are no reliable population-based estimates of the prevalence of colonic inertia. In a tertiary referral series of 1,411 patients with constipation managed by one gastroenterologist, the proportions of constipated patients who had normal transit constipation (NTC) were ~70 %, slow transit constipation (STC) ~5 %, and pelvic floor dysfunction or defecatory disorders (DD) ~25 %. Even in tertiary centers, only a minority of constipated patients undergoes intraluminal colonic testing; hence, the proportion of constipated patients who truly have colonic inertia is unknown. However, clinical observations and indirect estimates suggest that only a small fraction of patients with chronic constipation have colonic inertia. For example, among 1,009 constipated patients who underwent assessment of colonic transit and anorectal functions, only 52 (5 %) had an abdominal colectomy and ileorectal anastomosis (IRA) for medically refractory slow transit constipation. While colonic motor functions were not evaluated by intraluminal techniques in this study, these 52 patients presumably had severe colonic motor dysfunction refractory to medical management and, possibly, colonic inertia. Our clinical experience suggests that, similar to chronic constipation, the prevalence of colonic inertia is higher in women than in men.

Pathophysiology

Current concepts suggest that the colonic motor dysfunction in colonic inertia may be explained by a marked reduction in colonic intrinsic nerves and interstitial cells of Cajal (ICC), as documented by histopathology. While this is a plausible hypothesis, it must be noted that these histopathological abnormalities were documented in patients with severe chronic constipation or megacolon who did not have intraluminal assessment of colonic motor functions (i.e., with manometry and/or barostat); hence, whether they had colonic inertia is unknown. Moreover, the precise contribution of ICC loss to colonic sensorimotor dysfunction is unclear since other enteric neurons are also depleted or even increased in these conditions. The extent of ICC loss necessary to cause colonic motor dysfunction also remains unknown.

ICC loss can impair colonic motility since these cells regulate gut motility via several mechanisms: they generate electrical slow waves which then propagate through smooth muscle cells via gap junctions; they influence the smooth muscle membrane potential and membrane potential gradient; they convey electrical effects of motor neuron input to smooth muscle; and they mediate some of the mechanosensitivity of smooth muscle. ICC-generated slow waves are triggered by pacemaker currents which evolve into a rapid upstroke when they exceed a depolarization threshold. Slow waves from ICCs spread into smooth muscle via gap junctions and activate a variety of smooth muscle ion channels, including L-type calcium channels, contributing powerfully to the contractile response.

Diagnosis and Evaluation

Intraluminal assessment of colonic motility should be considered in patients with medically refractory slow transit constipation who do not have a defecatory disorder (see Chap. 15). These assessments may reveal colonic motor dysfunction in some patients with slow transit constipation. Manometric disturbances include fewer high amplitude propagated contractions (HAPCs), reduced phasic contractile responses to a meal and/or to pharmacological stimuli (e.g., bisacodyl or neostigmine). A barostat-based evaluation of colonic motor function may reveal reduced fasting tone and/or reduced tonic contractile responses to a meal and/or to pharmacological stimuli (e.g., bisacodyl or neostigmine). In patients with megacolon, compliance of the colon is increased; however, this is not usually observed in colonic inertia in the absence of megacolon. In general, colonic inertia is defined by reduced contractile responses to a meal and a pharmacological stimulus. However, the reduction required to define inertia has not been characterized. Healthy subjects have 1–15 HAPCs daily. Therefore, only patients who have no HAPCs over a 24-h period are truly abnormal.

Underscoring the need for intraluminal assessments to diagnose colonic inertia, barostat measurements revealed reduced fasting and/or postprandial colonic tone and/or compliance in 40 % with normal transit constipation, 47 % with slow transit constipation, 53 % with a defecatory disorder and normal transit, and 42 % with defecatory disorder and slow transit. In another study, 43 % of patients with slow transit constipation had normal fasting colonic motility and motor responses to a meal and bisacodyl. Together, these observations suggest that normal and slow colonic transit are imperfect surrogate markers for normal and abnormal colonic motor function, respectively. Again, slow transit constipation is not synonymous with colonic inertia.

Defecatory disorders and separately reduced caloric intake can also delay colonic transit. Indeed, up to 50 % of patients with defecatory disorders exhibit slow colonic transit. Hence, these conditions and other causes of colonic motor dysfunction (e.g., medications, metabolic disorders) should be excluded before concluding that delayed colonic transit is caused by primary colonic motor dysfunction.

Treatment

There are no therapeutic studies, even uncontrolled, in patients with colonic inertia. While over-the-counter laxative osmotic agents (e.g., polyethylene glycol, milk of magnesia), which are first-line agents for managing chronic constipation may be tried, clinical experience suggests that most patients with inertia do not achieve adequate relief with these agents. The efficacy of newer secretagogues (i.e., lubiprostone and linaclotide) in patients with colonic inertia is unknown. These agents increase intestinal chloride secretion by activating channels on the apical (luminal) enterocyte surface and are approved for treating chronic constipation. Stimulant laxatives (e.g., bisacodyl or glycerin suppositories) may be useful "rescue measures" such as when patients have not had a bowel movement for several days. Other stimulant agents include the 5-HT_4 agonist prucalopride and the cholinesterase inhibitor pyridostigmine, both of which are safe and well tolerated. These agents have been shown to accelerate colonic transit in patients with chronic idiopathic constipation and constipation due to diabetes mellitus, respectively.

Total abdominal colectomy with ileorectal anastomosis (IRA) should be strongly considered in patients with medically refractory slow transit constipation who do not have pelvic floor dysfunction or a diffuse upper GI dysmotility. This procedure treats the primary symptoms of constipation (infrequent and difficult evacuation), but may not improve other symptoms such as abdominal pain and bloating, which patients associate with constipation. This observation may at least partly explain the variable outcomes after IRA in the 1980s and 1990s. However, it is noteworthy that earlier studies may not have assessed pelvic floor function or colonic transit and patient selection for surgery may have been suboptimal.

During surgery, the colon is removed to the level of the sacral promontory; the rectum is carefully elevated to preserve the presacral nerves, and the anastomosis is made to the highest third of the rectum. Anastomosis to the sigmoid colon invariably results in persistent or recurrent constipation. Conversely, an anastomosis to the middle or lower third of the rectum may result in high stool frequency and sometimes fecal incontinence. In properly selected patients, IRA can achieve prompt and sustained relief of slow transit constipation and improve quality of life. Several series have established the safety and efficacy of performing abdominal colectomy and ileorectostomy using either purely laparoscopic or hand-assisted techniques. Complications occur in patients undergoing IRA for constipation just as they can occur in any patient undergoing abdominal surgery; ileus, small bowel obstruction, anastomotic leakage, and wound infections all occur but not at rates any higher than expected. Small bowel obstruction is the most common complication after IRA. This occurs in between 10 and 70 % of patients and can affect patients either early or late in their postoperative course. Most such episodes are managed conservatively and do not require reoperation. Finally, there have been no objective predictors of success identified in STC patients undergoing IRA although outcomes in properly selected patients have been predictably good.

Key Clinical Teaching Points

- Colonic inertia refers to markedly reduced or absent colonic contractile responses to physiological (i.e., a meal) and pharmacological stimuli (e.g., bisacodyl or neostigmine) in patients with slow transit constipation. Slow transit constipation is not synonymous with colonic inertia.
- Colonic motor dysfunction in colonic inertia may be explained by a marked reduction in colonic intrinsic nerves and interstitial cells of Cajal.
- Colectomy with ileorectostomy may be considered in patients with medically refractory slow transit constipation who do not have a defecatory disorder.

Teaching Questions

1. You are asked to evaluate a 55-year-old woman with complaints of chronic constipation since childhood who has persistent symptoms despite treatment with a variety of osmotic and stimulant laxatives. She denies alarm symptoms and has demonstrated slow colonic transit. A screening colonoscopy was normal 5 years ago. Which one of the following statements regarding this patient is true?

   (A) Colonic motility study (with manometry and/or a barostat) is necessary to diagnose colonic inertia
   (B) Slow colonic transit occurs exclusively in slow transit constipation
   (C) There is no role for colectomy
   (D) It is essential to repeat a colonoscopy

2. The major mechanism of action of ICC (interstitial cells of Cajal) in the colon is:

   (A) They generate electrical slow waves
   (B) They influence the smooth muscle membrane potential and membrane potential gradient
   (C) They convey electrical effects of motor neuron input to smooth muscle
   (D) All of the above
   (E) None of the above

3. In a patient with medically refractory constipation who has documented colonic inertia by manometry, which one of the disorders listed below is essential to exclude prior to referring the patient to a colorectal surgeon to discuss total abdominal colectomy with ileorectostomy?

   (A) Celiac disease
   (B) A defecatory disorder
   (C) Functional dyspepsia
   (D) Gastroesophageal reflux disease

Key References

1. Bharucha AE, Dorn SD, Lembo A, Pressman A, American Gastroenterological Association. American gastroenterological association medical position statement on constipation. Gastroenterology. 2013;144:211–7. A current review on the evaluation and treatment of constipation.
2. Bharucha AE, Pemberton JH, Locke 3rd GR. American gastroenterological association technical review on constipation. Gastroenterology. 2013;144:218–38. A state of the art review on constipation.
3. Camilleri M, Bharucha AE, di Lorenzo C, Hasler WL, Prather CM, Rao SS, Wald A. American Neurogastroenterology and Motility Society consensus statement on intraluminal measurement of gastrointestinal and colonic motility in clinical practice. Neurogastroenterol Motil. 2008;20:1269–82. A nice review of diagnostic tests available to measure colonic motility and transit.
4. De Giorgio R, Camilleri M. Human enteric neuropathies: morphology and molecular pathology. Neurogastroenterol Motil. 2004;16:515–31. A nice review article on enteric nervous system dysfunction with reference to its impact on colonic transit.
5. Hassan I, Pemberton JH, Young-Fadok TM, You YN, Drelichman ER, Rath-Harvey D, Schleck CD, Larson DR. Ileorectal anastomosis for slow transit constipation: long-term functional and quality of life results. J Gastrointest Surg. 2006;10:1330–6. Discussion 1336–7. A well-written article describing long term outcomes after colectomy and ileorectal anastomosis for slow transit constipation.
6. Nullens S, Nelsen T, Camilleri M, Burton D, Eckert D, Iturrino J, Vazquez-Roque M, Zinsmeister AR. Regional colon transit in patients with dys-synergic defaecation or slow transit in patients with constipation. Gut. 2012;61:1132–9. A study identifying how colon transit varies in patients with different forms of constipation.
7. Ravi K, Bharucha AE, Camilleri M, Rhoten D, Bakken T, Zinsmeister AR. Phenotypic variation of colonic motor functions in chronic constipation. Gastroenterology. 2010;138:89–97. An interesting article highlighting the fact that colonic transit may not predict colonic motor function.

Chapter 18
Chronic Diarrhea

Amy S. Oxentenko and Darrell S. Pardi

Case Study

A 58-year-old woman presents to clinic for the evaluation of a 4-month history of progressive diarrhea. She describes 6–8 watery bowel movements each day without abdominal pain. She notes urgency, occasional incontinence, and nocturnal stools at least twice weekly. She denies symptoms of hematochezia, melena, weight loss, or fever. She has not had any recent hospitalizations, medication changes, foreign travel, or exposure to antibiotics or sick contacts. Her past medical history is significant for Hashimoto's thyroiditis, depression, and osteoarthritis. She has had a cholecystectomy. Medications include levothyroxine, fluoxetine, and ibuprofen as needed. There is no family history of inflammatory bowel disease, celiac disease, or gastrointestinal neoplasia. She consumes one glass of wine daily. Review of systems is negative for ocular complaints, arthralgias, back pain, or skin rashes. A screening colonoscopy at age 50 was normal.

On examination, she is afebrile, with normal blood pressure and pulse and without orthostatic changes. Oral mucous membranes are moist, while a skin exam is negative for rashes or lesions. Her thyroid is normal size on palpation. Her cardiopulmonary exam is within normal limits, while examination of her abdomen reveals a scar, but is otherwise soft and non-tender. Rectal examination is notable for normal perineal sensation, resting tone, and squeeze tone, with no palpable masses or impacted stool. The remainder of the examination is normal.

A.S. Oxentenko, M.D. (✉)
Division of Gastroenterology and Hepatology, Mayo Clinic,
200 First Street SW, Rochester, MN 55905, USA
e-mail: Oxentenko.amy@mayo.edu

D.S. Pardi, M.D.
Division of Gastroenterology and Hepatology, Mayo Clinic,
200 First Street SW, Rochester, MN 55905, USA

B.E. Lacy et al. (eds.), *Functional and Motility Disorders of the Gastrointestinal Tract*, DOI 10.1007/978-1-4939-1498-2_18

Laboratory studies reveal a normal complete blood count, thyroid-stimulating hormone, IgA tissue transglutaminase antibody, and C-reactive protein. Stool studies, including bacterial cultures and ova and parasite exam, are negative. Colonoscopy shows normal colonic mucosa, with random biopsies noting increased intraepithelial and lamina propria lymphocytes, with a thickened subepithelial collagen band.

Introduction

Diarrhea is common in clinical practice, and the ability to evaluate a patient who presents with diarrhea requires an understanding of the definition, pathophysiology, differential diagnoses, testing algorithms, and management strategies.

Diarrhea can be defined in various ways (see Table 18.1), but generally is considered to represent an increase in frequency and/or fluidity of stool. Since stool weight is proportionally related to fiber intake, stool weight in excess of 200 g daily should be used with caution as the sole defining criteria of "diarrhea." Chronic diarrhea has been defined as diarrhea lasting in excess of 4 weeks, whereas acute diarrhea typically lasts less than 2 weeks and is often self-limited.

Establishing the chronicity of diarrhea can help narrow the diagnostic considerations and facilitate testing strategies. Given the broad differential diagnosis that needs to be considered in a patient with chronic diarrhea (see Table 18.2), a thorough history is one of the most important parts of the diagnostic evaluation and allows the provider to approach the work-up in a stepwise, high-value, cost-conscious approach.

Epidemiology

The prevalence of chronic diarrhea is directly related to hygiene and sanitation practices and, therefore, varies widely throughout the world. The prevalence of chronic diarrhea in developed countries is 3–5 % but has been reported in up to 18 %

Table 18.1 Definitions of diarrhea

Stool frequency	>3 bowel movements daily
Stool weight	>200 g of stool daily
Stool form	Bristol stool type 6 (mushy) or 7 (watery)
Functional diarrhea	Loose (mushy) or watery stools without pain occurring in at least 75 % of stools[a]
Irritable bowel syndrome	Recurrent abdominal pain or discomfort at least 3 days/month associated with 2 or more of the following:[a] • Improvement with defecation • Onset associated with a change in stool frequency • Onset associated with a change in form (appearance) of stool

[a]Criterion fulfilled for the last 3 months with symptom onset at least 6 months prior to diagnosis

Table 18.2 Differential diagnosis of chronic diarrhea

Category	Conditions[a]
Functional bowel disorders	Functional diarrhea
	Diarrhea-predominant IBS
	Mixed-type IBS
Medications	Antibiotics
	Metformin
	NSAIDs
	Proton pump inhibitors
	Colchicine
	Chemotherapeutic agents
	Others
Infection	Giardiasis
	Strongyloides
	Yersinia
	Mycobacteria
	Clostridium difficile
	Other parasites and bacteria
	Human immunodeficiency virus
Carbohydrate malabsorption	Lactose
	Fructose
	Sucrose
Other osmotic etiologies	Magnesium-containing antacids
	Sorbitol-containing elixirs
	Artificial sweeteners (xylitol, mannitol, others)
	Others (phosphates, sulfates)
	Iatrogenic (lactulose, polyethylene glycol)
Pancreatic insufficiency	Chronic pancreatitis
	Cystic fibrosis
Small bowel mucosal disorders	Celiac disease
	Collagenous sprue
	Tropical sprue
	Small intestinal bacterial overgrowth
	Autoimmune enteropathy
	Eosinophilic gastroenteritis
Inflammatory bowel disease	Ulcerative colitis
	Crohn's disease
	Microscopic colitis
Infiltrative disorders	Amyloid
	Whipple's disease
Bile salt abnormalities	Postcholecystectomy
	Terminal ileal resection
	Biliary obstruction

(continued)

Table 18.2 (continued)

Category	Conditions[a]
Protein-losing enteropathies	Menetrier's disease
	Lymphangiectasia (primary/secondary)
	Retroperitoneal fibrosis
	Lymphoma
Endocrine disorders	Hyperthyroidism
	Adrenal insufficiency
	Diabetes mellitus
Motility disorders	Scleroderma
	Paraneoplastic syndrome
	Idiopathic
Neuroendocrine tumors	Gastrinoma
	Carcinoid
	VIPoma
	Glucagonoma
	Thyroid medullary carcinoma (calcitonin)
Other	Short bowel syndrome
	Laxative abuse
	Radiation enteritis/colitis/proctitis
	Chronic mesenteric ischemia
	Graft-versus-host disease
	Idiopathic

IBS irritable bowel syndrome, *NSAIDs* nonsteroidal anti-inflammatory drugs, *VIP* vasoactive intestinal peptide

[a]Some conditions may belong in more than one category

of the population when "diarrhea" was more loosely defined. According to the World Health Organization, diarrhea affects 17 billion people annually and is the second leading cause of death worldwide in children less than 5 years of age. Within industrialized countries, chronic diarrhea is not associated with high mortality rates but is associated with decreased quality of life and significantly increased work and activity impairment compared to population norms. The economic impact of chronic diarrhea is difficult to measure; however, data from 1994 suggested that $350 million was lost annually due to time away from work. This amount is much greater today, especially if one adds the financial loss associated with diagnostic testing and management. The indication of "diarrhea" or "malabsorption" accounts for approximately 3 % of upper endoscopies, 7 % of colonoscopies, and 15 % of flexible sigmoidoscopies performed in the United States, not including those performed for a "change in bowel habits." In 2009, the symptom of diarrhea accounted for over four million outpatient visits in the United States, second only to abdominal pain as a gastrointestinal complaint, and was the leading gastrointestinal symptom used as a search term by Internet users.

Pathophysiology

Stool weight and fluidity are directly related to the amount of water in the stool. The underlying pathophysiology in chronic diarrhea is either due to an increase in intestinal secretion of water or a decrease in net absorption of water. The amount of intestinal fluid is also inversely proportional to intestinal transit time, so any alteration that decreases intestinal transit time will increase stool frequency and fluidity.

Diarrhea is commonly divided into osmotic and secretory types based upon the pathophysiology. Osmotic diarrhea results from either the ingestion of nonabsorbable, osmotically active substances or the lack of small bowel mucosal disaccharidases that aid in carbohydrate absorption. Since the small bowel works to maintain an iso-osmolar state (290 mOsm/kg), any osmotically active substance within the small bowel creates an efflux of water into the intestinal lumen resulting in diarrhea. Osmotic diarrhea improves with fasting or discontinuation of the offending agent. Secretory diarrhea can be caused from many things, but in the case of infectious etiologies with toxin production (a common phenomenon), stimulation of cAMP, cGMP, or calcium-mediated pathways results in a transition from net absorption to net secretion within the small bowel. This results in a large volume of liquid stool reaching the colon, overwhelming its absorptive capacity. In secretory diarrhea, stool volume tends to be high and is not affected by fasting.

Diarrhea can also be characterized on the basis of its underlying pathophysiology. Inflammatory causes of diarrhea typically cause either macroscopic or microscopic damage to the intestinal mucosa surface, decreasing the overall absorptive surface area of the bowel. Carbohydrate malabsorption causes an osmotically mediated diarrhea. Bacterial fermentation of undigested carbohydrates also causes an increase in intestinal gas production. Fat malabsorption can result from pancreatic lipase deficiency (e.g., chronic pancreatitis), inactivation of pancreatic enzymes as occurs with Zollinger–Ellison syndrome, small bowel mucosal diseases, or impairment in the enterohepatic circulation of bile (e.g., hepatic dysfunction, biliary obstruction, extensive terminal ileal resection or disease). With resection of <100 cm of terminal ileum, excess bile spills into the colon causing a secretory diarrhea, with subsequent liver upregulation of bile production to counteract intestinal loss and maintain an adequate bile salt pool. In contrast, as alluded to previously, with >100 cm of resected terminal ileum, the hepatic production of bile is inadequate to compensate for the degree of intestinal loss, resulting in bile salt deficiency and fat malabsorption from impaired micelle production, which is required for intestinal transport of long-chain triglycerides. Protein malabsorption rarely occurs in isolation, but can be seen with mucosal erosive diseases (e.g., inflammatory bowel disease [IBD], ischemia, graft-versus-host disease), nonerosive diseases with increased permeability (e.g., eosinophilic gastroenteritis, and celiac, Whipple's, and Menetrier's disease), or conditions with altered lymphatic drainage (e.g., right heart failure, constrictive pericarditis, lymphoma, retroperitoneal fibrosis, lymphangiectasia).

Despite the ability to characterize diarrhea based on pathophysiology, this characterization is rarely pure, and many conditions will often have more than one mechanism involved in causing diarrhea.

Diagnosis and Evaluation

The diagnostic approach to the patient with chronic diarrhea (see Fig. 18.1) begins with a detailed clinical history, noting the timing and features at onset, and the relationship to other events (e.g., surgery, new medications, self-limited illness, ingestion of specific foods). The frequency and pattern (e.g., postprandial, nocturnal) of bowel movements should be obtained. Details on stool characteristics should be reviewed including the presence of blood, which may indicate an infectious or inflammatory condition, or an oily appearance, which may be evidence of fat malabsorption. Small, low-volume frequent stools may imply a distal colonic or rectal disorder, while large-volume watery stools imply a small bowel disorder. Patients should be asked about the presence of fecal incontinence, although it should be noted that not all patients with fecal incontinence have a primary diarrheal condition, as spinal cord injuries and anal sphincter defects may also cause incontinence. The presence of associated gastrointestinal and systemic symptoms should be noted. The patient's past medical history should be reviewed for evidence of autoimmune diseases (e.g., celiac disease, thyroid dysfunction, diabetes mellitus, adrenal insufficiency, microscopic colitis), immunosuppression (e.g., human immunodeficiency virus, chemotherapy, medication-induced), abdominopelvic radiation (e.g., colorectal,

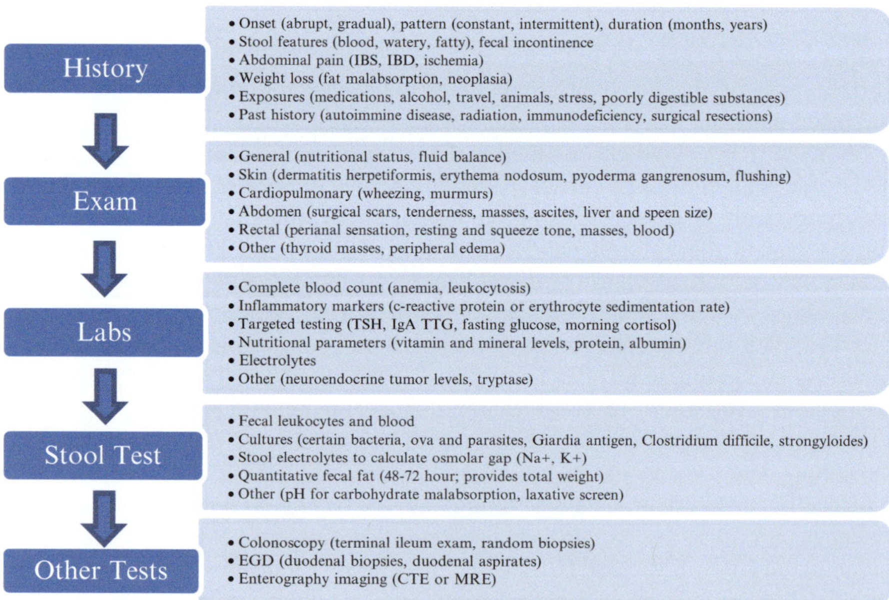

Fig. 18.1 Algorithmic approach in the evaluation of the patient with chronic diarrhea. Adapted from Schiller LR. Chronic diarrhea. Gastroenterology. 2004;127:287–93. *IBS* irritable bowel syndrome, *IBD* inflammatory bowel disease, *TSH* thyroid-stimulating hormone, *TTG* tissue transglutaminase, *Na+* sodium, *K+* potassium, *CTE* computed tomography enterography, *MRE* magnetic resonance enterography

cervical, or prostate cancer), and psychiatric conditions. Medications should be scrutinized, paying attention to timing of medication initiation, antibiotic use, and over-the-counter products (e.g., magnesium-containing antacids, herbal products containing laxatives, nonsteroidal anti-inflammatory drugs [NSAIDs]). The patient's surgical history should be reviewed for prior intestinal resections (including bowel segment and length removed), creation of blind loops of bowel (a risk factor for SIBO (small intestinal bacterial overgrowth)), and pancreaticobiliary surgeries. A family history of gastrointestinal and other relevant disorders should be obtained. Social history should focus on excessive alcohol consumption (pancreatic insufficiency), infectious exposures (e.g., daycare setting, animals, water sources), travel history, sexual preference, and dietary behavior patterns (e.g., excessive caffeine intake or gum chewing, ingestion of sugar-free foods or sugar substitutes). Review of systems should include asking about fever, which may indicate an inflammatory or infectious condition; weight loss; extraintestinal manifestations of IBD (e.g., pyoderma gangrenosum, erythema nodosum, ankylosing spondylitis, sacroiliitis, uveitis, or episcleritis); and celiac disease (e.g., dermatitis herpetiformis, infertility, premature metabolic bone disease, iron deficiency anemia).

The examination of a patient with chronic diarrhea is useful in assessing the nutritional status of the patient (e.g., muscle wasting, low body mass index) and evaluating for evidence of dehydration (e.g., orthostasis, dry mucous membranes, skin tenting). Occasionally, clues to a specific diagnosis can be found on examination of the skin. On abdominal examination, tenderness, fullness, and hepatomegaly should be noted as these may be signs of neoplasia, Crohn's disease, a neuroendocrine tumor, amyloid, or other infiltrative disorders. Perianal examination is important to assess for intact sensation and tone, presence of fissures or fistulae, and to rule out mass lesions or stool impaction.

The diagnostic evaluation of a patient with chronic diarrhea needs to be tailored based on the historical details obtained and the conditions that are most likely (see Table 18.3). Irritable bowel syndrome (IBS) is the most common cause of chronic diarrhea in Western societies. The diagnosis of IBS can be made in patients with abdominal pain and altered bowel movements in the absence of alarm features with little exclusionary testing (see Fig. 18.2). Given that the prevalence of celiac disease is 0.41–1.0 % and many of these patients fulfill the Rome criteria for IBS, many experts suggest that all patients with diarrhea-predominant IBS (or those with a mixed bowel pattern) be serologically tested for celiac disease, although prospective studies to validate this practice have not been performed. Similarly, some patients with microscopic colitis fulfill the Rome criteria, a fact that must be considered in patients who do not respond to antidiarrheal therapy, and in those with more recent onset of diarrhea, especially in older patients.

Laboratory testing for patients with chronic diarrhea needs to be logical and individually tailored and may include one or more of the following: complete blood count (to assess for anemia or leukocytosis), serum electrolytes (to evaluate for metabolic acidosis, hypokalemia, hyponatremia), IgA tissue transglutaminase antibody (to screen for celiac disease), C-reactive protein, endocrine testing (e.g., sensitive thyroid-stimulating hormone, fasting glucose, morning cortisol), serum protein

Table 18.3 Diagnostic testing in chronic diarrhea

Categories	Associated conditions	Diagnostic tests
Functional	Irritable bowel syndrome (diarrhea, mixed) Functional diarrhea	Clinical diagnoses; consider excluding celiac disease (see below)
Osmotic	Carbohydrate malabsorption Sugar alcohol consumption Magnesium-containing products	Breath testing (lactose, fructose, sucrose); stool pH <6 Avoidance trial after careful history (sugar-free substances, elixirs) Avoidance of offending medication; stool magnesium (factitious)
Secretory	Infections Bile-acid induced diarrhea Neuroendocrine tumors Motility disorders	Stool cultures (including parasites); often negative Trial of cholestyramine Gastrin, VIP, calcitonin, urine 5-HIAA Transit tests; fasting glucose (diabetes); anti-scl70 (scleroderma)
Inflammatory	Inflammatory bowel disease • Ulcerative colitis • Crohn's disease • Microscopic colitis Chronic mesenteric ischemia Infection	Combination of clinical, endoscopic, histologic, and radiographic • Colonoscopy (biopsies) • Colonoscopy (biopsies) and enterography imaging (CTE or MRE) • Flexible sigmoidoscopy or colonoscopy (biopsies) Mesenteric ultrasound; CTA; MRA; angiography Stool cultures
Malabsorptive	Fat malabsorption • Pancreatic insufficiency • Celiac disease • Small intestinal bacterial overgrowth Carbohydrate malabsorption Protein malabsorption	Quantitative fecal fat (48–72 h) • Imaging (CT, EUS); pancreas function tests; empiric enzymes • Celiac serology (TTG) and duodenal biopsies • Small bowel aspirates; hydrogen breath test; empiric antibiotics Breath testing (lactose, fructose, sucrose); stool pH <6 Alpha-1 antitrypsin stool clearance

VIP vasoactive intestinal peptide, *5-HIAA* 5-hydroxyindolacetic acid, *CTE* computed tomography enterography, *MRE* magnetic resonance enterography, *CTA* computed tomography angiography, *MRA* magnetic resonance angiography, *CT* computed tomography, *EUS* endoscopic ultrasound, *TTG* tissue transglutaminase

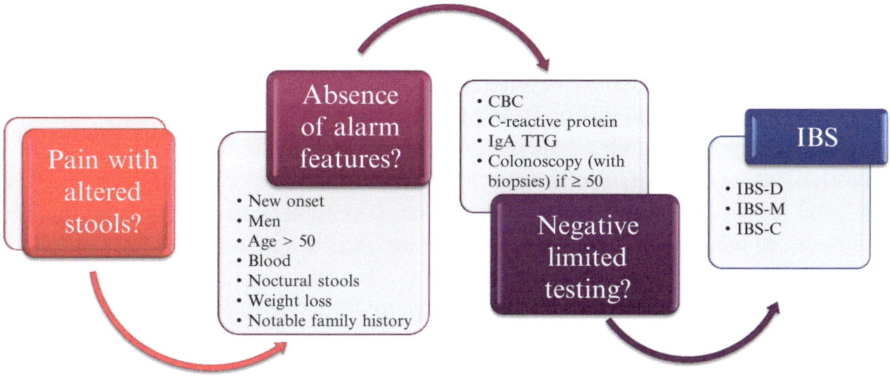

Fig. 18.2 Algorithmic approach in the diagnosis of irritable bowel syndrome. Adapted from: Spiller RC, Thompson WG. Bowel disorders. Am J Gastroenterol. 2010;105:775–85. *CBC* complete blood count, *TTG* tissue transglutaminase, *IBS* irritable bowel syndrome, *IBS-D* diarrhea-predominant, *IBS-M* mixed type, *IBS-C* constipation-predominant

electrophoresis, and, occasionally, an assessment of micronutrients (e.g., vitamin B12, vitamin D, iron, folate). The pattern of low vitamin B12 and elevated serum folate may be seen in SIBO. While a number of other laboratory studies can be considered, they should only be performed when the clinical suspicion of the associated disease states is high—such as serum tryptase (mastocytosis), gastrin (gastrinoma), vasoactive intestinal peptide (VIPoma), calcitonin (medullary carcinoma of the thyroid), urinary 5-hydroxyindolacetic acid (carcinoid), and plasma and urinary metanephrines (pheochromocytoma). It is important to recognize that because these conditions are rare, if these tests are performed indiscriminately, a positive test is more likely to be false positive than true positive.

During the evaluation for chronic diarrhea, a number of stool tests can be considered. Stool tests for inflammation including fecal leukocytes, calprotectin, or lactoferrin are easily performed. Stool cultures are usually sent to check for general enteric pathogens; however, atypical organisms including *Yersinia*, *Aeromonas*, *Plesiomonas*, and mycobacteria should be considered as well in the appropriate setting. Testing for *Clostridium difficile*, ideally with polymerase chain reaction, should be performed. Testing the stool for parasites such as *Giardia* and *Strongyloides* should be considered; in immunocompromised patients, additional parasitic studies should include those for cryptosporidia, *Cyclospora*, microspora, and *Cystoisospora*. Although uncommonly performed, a stool pH <6 suggests carbohydrate malabsorption. Stool sodium and potassium may be useful to calculate the stool osmotic gap with the calculation as follows: 290 − 2[stool sodium + stool potassium]. A stool osmotic gap of ≥ 100 indicates an osmotic cause of diarrhea, whereas a gap ≤ 50 suggests a secretory cause of diarrhea. The gold standard test to document fat malabsorption is a quantitative fecal fat, often collected over 48–72 h while consuming a standardized high fat diet (e.g., 100 g daily) both before and during the collection. Fecal fat is considered normal if <7 g/daily, indeterminate if 7–14 g/daily, and abnormal if >14 g/daily.

An esophagogastroduodenoscopy (EGD) with small bowel biopsies should be considered in all patients with positive celiac serologies (see Fig. 18.3). Small bowel biopsies can also be used to diagnose Whipple's disease (positive periodic acid Schiff stain, negative acid fast stain, and positive polymerase chain reaction), amyloid (positive Congo red stain), autoimmune enteropathy (a celiac disease mimic), infectious conditions (*Giardia*, cryptosporidia), and other infiltrative processes. An EGD should, therefore, be considered in any patient with diarrhea and clinical or laboratory features of malabsorption. A colonoscopy with terminal ileal examination and random colonic biopsies should also be considered in all patients with chronic unexplained diarrhea, particularly where there is concern of IBD. Random colonic biopsies are essential in the diagnosis of microscopic colitis, which includes both lymphocytic and collagenous colitis types (see Fig. 18.4).

Small intestinal bacterial overgrowth can be diagnosed by quantitative culture of small bowel aspirates obtained during EGD ($>10^5$ colony-forming units/mL), by hydrogen breath tests (glucose or lactulose) or by evaluating response to an empiric antibiotic trial. Specific hydrogen breath tests (lactose, fructose, sucrose) can be performed to assess for specific carbohydrate malabsorption; a positive test is suggested by a rise usually greater than 10–20 parts per million in breath hydrogen due to colonic bacterial fermentation of the malabsorbed substance. Many factors can cause both false-positive and false-negative breath test results, however (see Chap. 11).

Abdominal imaging is typically reserved for patients where there is strong concern over a small bowel process (e.g., Crohn's disease, radiation enteritis) or complications thereof and also enables the assessment of altered small bowel fold patterns (seen in celiac disease) and other anatomic abnormalities (such as small bowel diverticula, which is a risk factor for SIBO). Additionally, cross-sectional abdominal imaging allows the pancreas to be viewed and assessed for pancreatic atrophy or calcifications (chronic pancreatitis) and tumors (neuroendocrine tumors). Small bowel barium radiography has largely been replaced by enterography imaging, either with computed tomography or magnetic resonance.

Treatment

The management of chronic diarrhea is directed at the underlying diagnosis uncovered during the course of the evaluation (see Table 18.4). For patients with functional diarrhea or IBS, reassurance should be provided, invasive or excessive testing should be avoided, and symptomatic treatment recommended. In cases where there is an exposure causing the diarrhea (e.g., lactose, medications), avoidance of the offending agent is recommended. Other patients will require disease-directed therapy (e.g., amyloid, IBD, celiac disease), while some may require surgery (neoplasia).

a

b

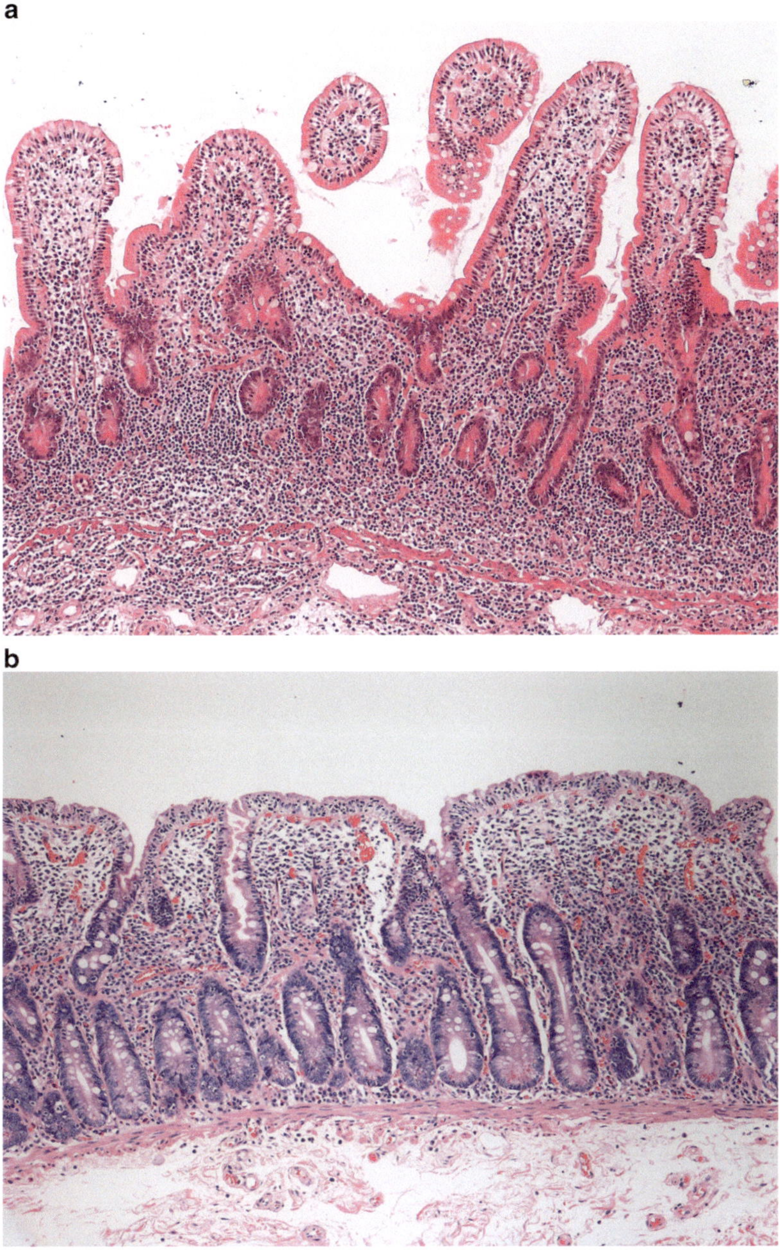

Fig. 18.3 Small bowel histology in celiac disease. Duodenal biopsy specimens showing: (**a**) partial villous atrophy, with a villous/crypt ratio of 1:1 and increased intraepithelial lymphocytes (40/100 surface epithelial cells); (**b**) total villous atrophy with markedly increased intraepithelial lymphocytes (>100/100 surface epithelial cells) (hematoxylin and eosin staining: original magnification ×100)

a

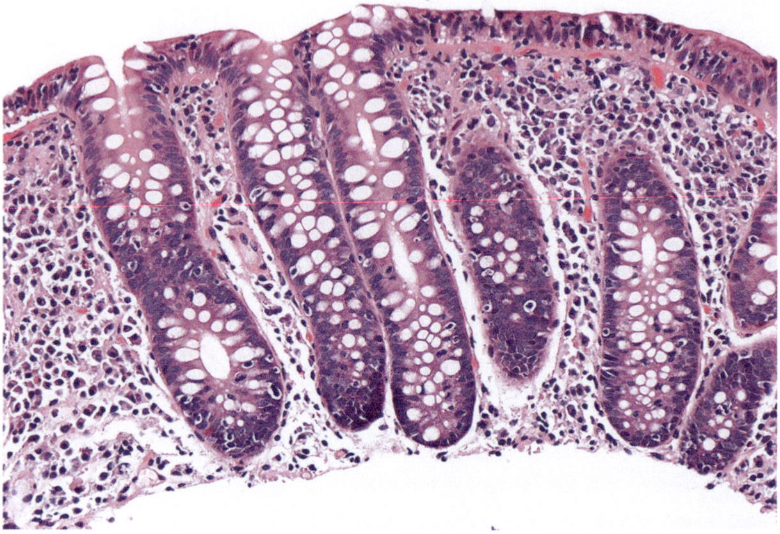

b

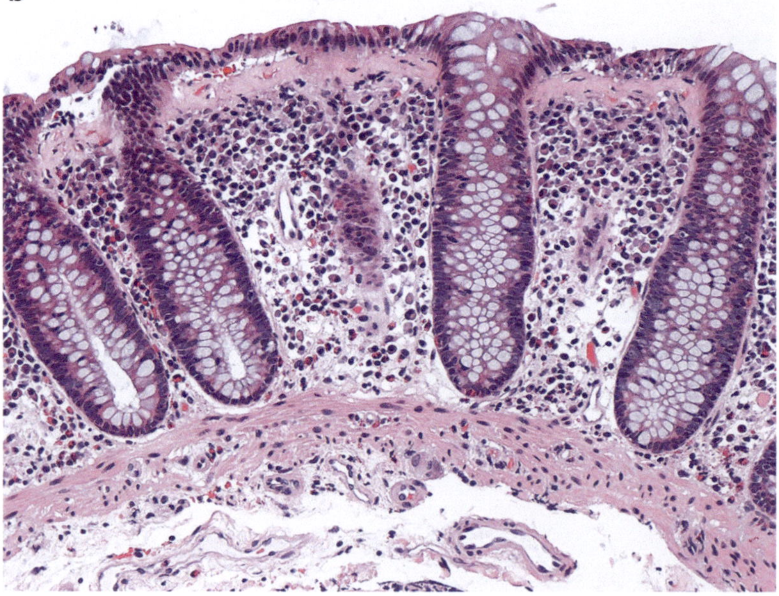

Fig. 18.4 Colonic histology in microscopic colitis. Colonic biopsy specimens showing: (**a**) lymphocytic colitis, with an inflamed lamina propria and increased intraepithelial lymphocytes within the surface and crypt epithelium; (**b**) collagenous colitis, with the surface epithelium containing increased intraepithelial lymphocytes and a thickened subepithelial collagen band measuring 40–50 μm (normal is 5 μm) (hematoxylin and eosin staining: original magnification ×200)

Table 18.4 Management options for chronic diarrhea

Diagnosis	Management
Irritable bowel syndrome	Fiber
	Loperamide
	Tricyclic antidepressants (low-dose)
	Rifaximin (non-FDA approved for IBS)
	Alosetron
Celiac disease	Gluten-free diet
	Vitamin and mineral replacement
	Assessment of bone mineral density
Small intestinal bacterial overgrowth	Rotating antibiotics
	Manage secondary lactose malabsorption
Microscopic colitis	Discontinue offending medications
	Loperamide
	Bismuth subsalicylate
	Budesonide
Ulcerative colitis	Mesalamine
	Immunomodulators (AZA, 6-MP)
	Biologic agents
Crohn's disease	Immunomodulators (AZA, 6-MP, MTX)
	Biologic agent
Pancreatic insufficiency	Modified fat diet
	Pancreatic enzyme replacement
Infectious	Antimicrobial therapy as indicated
	Manage postinfectious lactose malabsorption
	Manage postinfectious IBS
Medication-induced diarrhea	Discontinue or use lowest effective dose
	Loperamide as needed
Carbohydrate malabsorption	Reduce ingestion of offending agent
Bile salt-induced diarrhea	Cholestyramine
Bile salt deficiency	Medium-chain triglyceride-based diet
Others	Target treatment toward specific condition

IBS irritable bowel syndrome, *AZA* azathioprine, *6-MP* 6-mercaptopurine, *MTX* methotrexate

Case Resolution

The clinical presentation and diagnostic evaluation demonstrate typical features of collagenous colitis, a form of microscopic colitis. While the patient's age and underlying autoimmune thyroid disease are clues to the diagnosis, this condition is also associated with certain medication use. In this case, fluoxetine and nonsteroidal anti-inflammatory drug use has previously been implicated. Assessing the temporal association and the underlying necessity of each would be important. She was treated with a 2-month course of bismuth subsalicylate (three tablets three times daily) with a rapid return of her normal bowel pattern.

Key Clinical Teaching Points

- A careful clinical history is essential in the evaluation of the patient with chronic diarrhea in order to categorize features and approach the testing in an organized, cost-effective approach.
- Irritable bowel syndrome is the most common cause of chronic diarrhea and is a clinical diagnosis; minimal testing is required in the absence of alarm features.
- The evaluation of a patient with chronic diarrhea is individualized and stepwise and may include blood and stool testing, upper and lower endoscopy with histologic assessment, and radiographic imaging. Additional testing is reserved for those with negative first-line testing and targeted toward clinical features.

Teaching Questions

1. A 28-year-old woman presents to the clinic for an evaluation of diarrhea that has been present for more than 2 years. She reports 4–5 bowel movements daily without blood. She describes cramping abdominal pain that is relieved after a bowel movement. She complains of mild bloating but no nausea or vomiting. Her weight has been stable and she denies nocturnal diarrhea. Past medical history is notable for depression and chronic headaches. She has been on sertraline for 5 years and takes acetaminophen as needed. There is no family history of gastrointestinal diseases or neoplasia. She has not responded to simple dietary interventions such as excluding caffeine, lactose, fructose, or extra fiber from her diet. Her examination is normal.

   Which one of the following is the next best step in management of this patient?

   (A) Reassurance
   (B) IgA tissue transglutaminase antibody
   (C) Colonoscopy
   (D) Stool bacterial cultures
   (E) Trial of nortriptyline

2. A 52-year-old woman presents to the clinic for an evaluation of diarrhea that has been present for the past 3 months. She reports a history of travel to Mexico immediately prior to symptom onset. During her vacation, she had several days of diarrhea that was self-limited in nature. Symptoms recurred shortly after her return home. She reports 3–5 bowel movements daily associated with increased bloating and flatus. She denies fever, hematochezia, weight loss, or nocturnal stools. Her past medical history is significant for hypothyroidism and a cholecystectomy 3 years ago. Her only medication is levothyroxine. Examination is normal. Stool for bacteria (including *Clostridium difficile*) and ova and parasites is negative. Stool sodium is 40 mmol/L and stool potassium is 20 mmol/L.

Which one of the following is the most likely diagnosis?

(A) Postinfectious irritable bowel syndrome
(B) Microscopic colitis
(C) *Vibrio cholera* infection
(D) Lactose malabsorption
(E) Bile salt-induced diarrhea

3. A 72-year-old man presents to the clinic for evaluation of diarrhea that has been present for 6 months. He describes 6–8 stools daily that are small in volume and associated with blood and mucous. He also describes bothersome tenesmus. He denies abdominal pain, fever, or weight loss. Past medical history is significant for hypertension, hyperlipidemia, and prostate cancer, for which he underwent prostatectomy and external beam radiation 4 years ago. Medications include hydrochlorothiazide, olmesartan, and atorvastatin. His last colonoscopy was at age 70.

   Which one of the following is the most likely diagnosis?

   (A) Colorectal cancer
   (B) Ischemic colitis
   (C) Radiation proctitis
   (D) Ulcerative proctitis
   (E) Medication-induced colitis

Key References

1. Dukowicz AC, Lacy BE, Levine GM. Small intestinal bacterial overgrowth: a comprehensive review. Gastroenterol Hepatol. 2007;3:112–22. A review on the etiology, pathophysiology and treatment of SIBO.
2. Kaiser L, Surawicz CM. Infectious causes of chronic diarrhoea. Best Pract Res Clin Gastroenterol. 2012;26:563–71. A recent review article that provides a nice overview on infectious diarrheas.
3. Pardi DS, Kelly CP. Microscopic colitis. Gastroenterology. 2011;140:1155–65. A recent review on the pathophysiology and management of microscopic colitis.
4. Peery AF, Dellon ES, Lund J, Crockett SD, McGowan CE, Bulsiewicz WJ, et al. Burden of gastrointestinal disease in the United States: 2012 update. Gastroenterology. 2012;143:1179–87. This update chronicles the burden and importance of diarrhea, and compares it to that seen with other gastrointestinal conditions.
5. Rubio-Tapia A, Hill ID, Kelly CP, Calderwood AH, Murray JA. ACG clinical guidelines: diagnosis and management of celiac disease. Am J Gastroenterol. 2013;108:656–76. A state of the art overview on managing celiac disease.
6. Schiller LR. Definitions, pathophysiology, and evaluation of chronic diarrhoea. Best Pract Res Clin Gastroenterol. 2012;26:551–62. This is an excellent overview of chronic diarrhea, detailing the pathophysiology and evaluation in greater detail than is reviewed here.
7. Spiller RC, Thompson WG. Bowel disorders. Am J Gastroenterol. 2010;105:775–85. This is an excellent algorithmic approach to the evaluation of bowel disorders, including functional diarrhea and irritable bowel syndrome.

Part VI
Anorectal Disorders

Chapter 19
Fecal Incontinence

Vanessa C. Costilla and Amy E. Foxx-Orenstein

Case Study

A 66-year-old woman presents with symptoms of diarrhea and bowel incontinence for the last 6 months. In contrast to her usual pattern of one formed stool daily, she now reports soft or watery bowel movements twice daily. She wears pads when leaving her home. Fecal loss occurs with 50 % of bowel movements; she estimates that episodes of incontinence are associated with largest volume loss of approximately 1 tablespoon. There are no symptoms of abdominal pain, nausea, or vomiting. Stools are not bloody or black. She denies fevers, weight loss, or recent travel. Colonoscopy 2 years ago revealed one hyperplastic polyp. Medical history includes diabetes mellitus type 2 and depression. She had two vaginal deliveries and sustained a grade 2 tear with her first child. Medications include metformin and citalopram.

Physical examination reveals an overweight woman with normal cognitive function and gait. Visual inspection is notable for slight peri-anal moisture, healthy tissue, and no evidence of feces. Perineal sensation is intact. Digital rectal exam does not elicit pain; a small internal hemorrhoid is noted. Rectal tone is weak to modest (2/5, with 3 being normal), with a slight asymmetric, 2 cm long sphincter. She recently retired and hoped to travel but fear of fecal loss is limiting her activity. What diagnostic tests, if any, are required in this patient, and what treatment options are available?

V.C. Costilla, M.D.
Department of Internal Medicine, Mayo Clinic, Scottsdale, AZ USA

A.E. Foxx-Orenstein, D.O. (✉)
Division of Gastroenterology and Hepatology, Mayo Clinic,
13400 E Shea Blvd, Scottsdale, AZ 85259, USA
e-mail: foxx-orenstein.amy@mayo.edu

B.E. Lacy et al. (eds.), *Functional and Motility Disorders of the Gastrointestinal Tract*, DOI 10.1007/978-1-4939-1498-2_19

Introduction

Fecal incontinence (FI) is a socially and emotionally devastating disorder. The prevalence of FI among institutionalized persons reaches 45 %. Prevalence rates are similar between men and women, 7.7 % and 8.9 %, respectively, and increase with age, reaching 15.3 % in those 70 years of age or older. Due to social perception, many patients do not seek treatment, which likely leads to an underestimation of prevalence. Thirty-six percent of primary care patients reported episodes of FI but only 2.7 % of these patients had a documented diagnosis. Healthcare costs are 55 % higher in FI than continent patients, amounting to an estimated $11 billion annually. Most patients achieve significant improvement in symptoms through proper treatment. Early diagnosis may prevent complications that reduce quality of life.

Pathophysiology

Evacuation of fecal material involves a complex interaction of structural and sensory components within the anorectal unit and pelvic floor musculature. The anal sphincter is composed of three muscular components: the internal anal sphincter (IAS), the external anal sphincter (EAS), and the puborectalis muscle (PRM). The IAS comprises the smooth muscle component and provides up to 70–80 % of the resting anal canal pressure. It is under involuntary neural control and is responsible for tonic activity that maintains the anal barrier at rest. Voluntary contraction of the striated muscles of the EAS helps to further maintain continence. The PRM forms a sling around the rectum, further supplementing these barriers. It is contracted at rest and maintains the anorectal angle at approximately 90 degrees. During defecation this angle becomes more obtuse thereby allowing stool passage. The angle becomes more acute with a voluntary squeeze thus ensuring continence. Stool arriving in the rectum causes rectal distension, a reflexive decrease in anal resting pressure, and feculent sampling by the sensitive anoderm. If the urge to defecate occurs at a socially unsuitable time, sympathetically mediated inhibition of rectal smooth muscle with voluntary contraction of the EAS and PR then occurs. Adequate rectal compliance is required for deferred defecation as the rectal contents are propelled back into the rectal reservoir to await a more suitable time for defecation.

Fecal incontinence results when continence mechanisms are compromised. Disorders that reduce stool consistency, weaken striated pelvic floor muscles or the internal anal sphincter, impair sensation, alter colonic transit time, increase stool volume and/or reduce cognitive function may all contribute to FI. FI subtypes include passive incontinence, urge incontinence, and fecal seepage (see Table 19.1). Functional FI is defined in Table 19.1.

Table 19.1 Fecal incontinence

Functional fecal incontinence	Diagnostic criteria: 1. Recurrent uncontrolled passage of fecal material in an individual with a development age of at least 4 years and one or more of the following: (a) Abnormal functioning of normally innervated and structurally intact muscles (b) Minor abnormalities of sphincter structure and/or innervation (c) Normal or disordered bowel habits (i.e., fecal retention or diarrhea) (d) Psychological causes 2. Exclusion of all the following: (a) Abnormal innervation caused by lesion(s) within the brain, spinal cord, or sacral nerve roots, or mixed lesions, or as part of a generalized peripheral or autonomic neuropathy (b) Anal sphincter abnormalities associated with a multisystem disease (c) Structural or neurogenic abnormalities believed to be the major or primary cause of fecal incontinence
Subtypes	Mechanism
Passive incontinence	Loss of rectosigmoid perception and/or impaired rectoanal reflexes. Internal sphincter weakness or tear
Urge incontinence	Disruption of the external sphincter function. Altered rectal capacity
Fecal seepage	Incomplete evacuation of stool, and/or impaired rectal sensation. Normal sphincter function

Reference [7]

Risk Factors

Many factors (see Table 19.2) contribute to impaired continence, including liquid stool consistency, female gender, advanced age, and multiple childbirths. Diarrhea is by far the greatest risk factor for FI. Rectal urgency is a primary risk factor. The incidence of FI increases significantly with age, mostly due to weak pelvic floor musculature and decreased anal resting tone. Parity is associated with frequent sphincter defects due to trauma during delivery. Fecal incontinence and operative or traumatic vaginal delivery are associated, but the literature does not support a benefit of cesarean delivery over nontraumatic vaginal delivery for preserving pelvic floor health or continence.

Obesity is a risk factor for FI. While bariatric surgery is an effective treatment for morbid obesity, post-bariatric surgery patients frequently have increased FI due to changes in stool consistency.

Table 19.2 Risk factors for fecal incontinence

• Advanced age
• Female gender
• Pregnancy
• Birth trauma
• Perianal surgery or trauma
• Neurologic dysfunction
• Inflammation
• Hemorrhoids
• Pelvic organ prolapse
• Congenital anorectal abnormality
• Obesity
• Post-bariatric surgery
• Limited mobility
• Urinary incontinence
• Smoking
• COPD

In younger women, FI is strongly associated with functional bowel disorders, including irritable bowel syndrome. Causes of FI are manifold and may overlap. A sphincter injury may remain asymptomatic for years until age- or hormone-related changes, such as muscle or tissue atrophy, prevent continued compensation.

Clinical Evaluation

A detailed history and focused rectal exam are important to diagnose and determine FI contributing causes. The history should include an evaluation of medications and dietary habits that may alter bowel frequency and stool consistency. A bowel diary can be helpful. It should include the number of episodes of FI, the type of incontinence (gas, liquid, solid), the volume of incontinence, the ability to sense stool, and symptoms of urgency, straining, and feelings of constipation. Table 19.3 outlines information that should be gathered for a thorough FI evaluation.

A careful physical examination includes inspecting the perineum for moisture, irritation, feces, scars, anal asymmetry, fissures, and laxity of the sphincter. Confirm the presence of an anal wink and demonstrate that perineal sensation is intact. Note the degree of perineal descent, bulging or prolapse of the rectum with bearing down, and the presence of prolapsed or thrombosed hemorrhoids. Digital rectal examination is critical for identifying anatomic abnormalities. Sharp, knifelike pain suggests active mucosal injury such as an acute or chronic fissure, ulcer, or infection. Lax or intense anal tone at rest and with bearing down provides clues to pelvic floor disorders. A neurological evaluation should assess cognition, strength, and gait.

Table 19.3 Fecal incontinence history checklist
Medical history
☐ Diabetes mellitus ☐ Cognitive impairment ☐ Neurological disorder—such as stroke, spinal cord disease, Parkinson's ☐ Inflammatory bowel disease ☐ Colitis—infectious, ischemic, microscopic ☐ Celiac sprue ☐ Irritable bowel syndrome ☐ Radiation history to perianal area ☐ Connective tissue disease
Surgical history
☐ Anorectal surgery ☐ Bariatric surgery
Obstetric history
☐ Pregnancy ☐ Parity ☐ Prolonged delivery ☐ Delivery trauma—episiotomy, tear, forceps
Functional status
☐ Limited mobility—use of wheelchair, walker ☐ Institutional living
Medication list (not all inclusive)
☐ Diarrhea provoking: Laxatives, orlistat, metformin, donepezil, rivastigmine, antibiotics, magnesium, selective serotonin reuptake inhibitors
☐ Constipation provoking: Loperamide, diphenoxylate/atropine, opioids, tricyclic antidepressants, calcium channel blockers (verapamil), memantine, calcium
Diet (diarrhea provoking)
☐ Prunes, plums, beans, alcohol, artificial sweeteners, lactose-containing foods, caffeine
Bowel pattern and stool consistency
☐ Normal bowel pattern—frequency of bowel movements
☐ Consistency of stool
☐ Variability in stool consistency
☐ Urgency—able to arrive to the toilet in time
☐ Ability to control the passage of gas or flatus
☐ Passage of stool without awareness
☐ Volume of stool during episodes of incontinence
☐ Need to strain or self-digitate to have a bowel movement
☐ Exacerbating or relieving factors

Diagnostic Studies

Specific guidelines delineating when testing should be done do not exist. Clinicians should weigh the risk, benefit, cost, and burden of testing against empiric treatment. Consider a patients' ability to participate in testing, comorbidities, and potential diagnostic yield of the study. Diagnostic testing can aid in the following clinical scenarios: (1) presumed sphincter injury, (2) overflow incontinence, (3) pelvic floor dysfunction, (4) rapid colonic transit as a cause of diarrhea, (5) significant discrepancy between the history and the physical examination, and (5) elimination of other etiologies.

Endoanal ultrasound is the standard for identifying anal sphincter injuries. It provides excellent resolution of the internal sphincter but is less accurate with the external sphincter. Anal sphincter MRI provides superior spatial resolution of the internal and external sphincter.

Anorectal manometry quantifies internal and external anal sphincter function, rectal sensation, and compliance. Anal resting and squeeze pressures are often low in FI, suggesting weak internal and external sphincters. Patients with normal anal pressures may have other factors, including loose stool, fecal seepage, or altered sensation contributing to FI. The rectal balloon distension test measures rectal sensation and compliance by assessing sensory-motor responses to incremental volumes of air or water. Sensation may be normal, reduced, or increased in FI patients.

The balloon expulsion test requires a patient to expel a water-filled balloon while seated on a commode. Expulsion within 60 s is normal. This test is often used to screen chronic constipation patients for evidence of pelvic floor dyssynergia.

Standard defecography provides dynamic evaluation of the pelvic floor and can identify the presence of rectal prolapse and rectocele. Barium paste is inserted into the rectosigmoid colon and then dynamic anatomy and pelvic floor motion images are recorded with the patient at rest and while coughing, squeezing, and straining. Defecography is not standardized across institutions and is not widely available. Dynamic pelvic MRI is the only imaging modality that can evaluate global pelvic floor anatomy as well as the anal sphincter without radiation exposure.

Anal electromyography may identify sphincter denervation, myopathic damage, neurogenic damage, or a mixed injury. Pudendal nerve terminal motor latency (PNTML) measures the integrity between the terminal pudendal nerve and the anal sphincter, helping to determine if sphincter weakness is due to pudendal nerve injury, sphincter injury, or both. The American Gastroenterological Association recommends against routine PNTML testing for FI evaluation due to lack of data demonstrating its clinical utility.

Stool tests and intestinal transit studies may be used to explain the cause of a patient's underlying diarrhea or constipation. Endoscopy may be necessary to diagnose diseases that exacerbate FI such as inflammatory bowel disease, celiac disease, or microscopic colitis. Discovering the cause(s) of a patient's FI is necessary because it can direct treatment strategies and affect clinical outcomes.

Management

All types of fecal incontinence are initially managed the same, with lifestyle modifications to bulk stool, improve bowel derangements, and access to toileting.

Lifestyle Modifications

Medication and Dietary Changes

Polypharmacy is common in older adults. Diarrhea is a frequent side effect of medications. Adjust medications that exacerbate FI, including over-the-counter herbs and vitamins. Determine if a patient's diet includes FI exacerbating factors, including artificial sugars, excess fructose, fructans, or galactans and caffeine. A high-fiber diet may improve stool consistency and decrease episodes of FI.

Absorbent Products and Containment Devices

Few products are designed to absorb fecal material. Patients report using pads, panty liners, and pull up briefs all originally designed for urine or menstruation. Utilization of pads to contain anal leakage results in odor and skin irritation. Anal plugs come in different designs and sizes, all aimed at blocking loss of stool before it occurs. Patient intolerance of the anal plug limits its usefulness.

Toilet Access and Bowel Training

Limited mobility contributes to FI, especially in the elderly and physically impaired. Scheduled toileting and changes within the home to allow better toilet access include moving a patient's sleeping area closer to a bathroom, providing a bedside commode, and easy access to assist devices. Physical therapy and exercise to improve mobility may improve accessibility, though studies are contradictory on whether this reduces FI episodes.

Pharmacologic Therapy Based on Type of Fecal Incontinence

Fecal Incontinence with Diarrhea

Initial efforts should focus on modifying stool form because formed stool is much easier to control than loose stool. The addition of supplemental fiber is often effective. Pharmacotherapy for diarrhea with agents that slow the bowel or bind stool is usually reserved for patients with refractory symptoms that do not respond to conservative therapies. Table 19.4 provides a guideline for the use of common antidiarrheal medications in FI.

Patients with IBS-D require special consideration because fiber therapy may exacerbate abdominal pain and bloating, contributing to poor compliance. If these symptoms do not abate, initiation of other pharmacotherapy including loperamide,

Table 19.4 Antidiarrheal medications in fecal incontinence

Medical therapy for FI	Potential side effects
Fiber supplementation	Flatulence, bloating, abdominal pain, anorexia May interfere with absorption of other medications May reduce insulin requirements
Loperamide	Paralytic ileus, rash, fatigue, cramping, constipation, nausea and vomiting May increase resting anal sphincter tone Cautious use with active inflammatory disease of the colon or with infectious diarrhea
Diphenoxylate/atropine	Toxic megacolon, CNS effects Atropine may cause anticholinergics effects Cautious use with active inflammatory disease of the colon or with infectious diarrhea
Colesevelam hydrochloride	Constipation, nausea, nasopharyngitis, pancreatitis Cautious use with history of bowel obstruction. May interfere with absorption of other medications
Cholestyramine	Flatulence, nausea, dyspepsia, abdominal pain, anorexia, sour taste, headache, rash, hematuria, fatigue, bleeding of gums, weight loss May interfere with absorption of other medications
Colestipol	GI bleeding, abdominal pain, bloating, flatulence, dyspepsia, liver dysfunction, musculoskeletal pain, rash, headache, anorexia, dry skin May interfere with vitamin and medication absorption
Clonidine	Rebound hypertension, dry mouth, sedation, CNS effects, constipation, headache, rash, nausea, anorexia Wean off medication slowly if ineffective
Tincture of opium	Sedation, nausea, dry mouth, anorexia, urinary retention, weakness, flushing, pruritus, headache, rash, CNS depression, hypotension, bradycardia, respiratory depression, dependency, euphoria
Alosetron	Constipation, severe ischemic colitis Discontinue if no improvement at 1 mg twice daily for 4 weeks

a tricyclic antidepressant, probiotics, or alosetron may provide more effective relief for this subset of patients.

Fecal Incontinence with Constipation

Chronic constipation may lead to rectal distension resulting in a chronically enlarged rectum and altered rectal sensation. Increased rectal capacity and decreased rectal sensitivity can increase a patient's risk of overflow incontinence. Overflow incontinence is particularly prevalent among elderly patients. An empiric trial of fiber therapy is first-line therapy for overflow incontinence, followed by scheduled laxatives.

Fecal Seepage

Fecal seepage is different from FI in that it usually involves the loss of small liquid or soft stool after a normal bowel movement. Patients may report perianal moisture an abnormal bowel habit or symptoms more consistent with anal sphincter dysfunction, which may not be appreciated as a physiologic abnormality on objective anorectal testing. Seepage, more common in men with preserved anal sphincter function, may be caused by hemorrhoids, poor hygiene, anal fistula, rectal prolapse, and hypo- or hypersensitivity of the rectum. In patients with fecal seepage, assessment and treatment of a specific cause may resolve symptoms. If symptoms persist, clearance of the rectal vault with enemas or suppositories should be performed at scheduled times each day, regardless of urge to defecate. Tap water enemas are preferred for chronic usage as repeated application of sodium phosphate or glycerin may precipitate mucosal damage and result in rectal bleeding. The preferred designated time for routine clearance of the rectal vault should be within 30 min after a meal to maximize normal postprandial colonic reflexes.

Injectable Bulking Agents

Several agents have been used to bulk the anal sphincter to provide a barrier including silicone, carbon-coated beads, and recently dextranomer in hyaluronic acid (Solesta®). A 2010 Cochrane systematic review was unable to draw definitive conclusions on the efficacy of injectable bulking agents due to the limited number of trials available. However, it continues to hold great promise as an effective therapy with the introduction of newer agents. Adverse events include pain, bleeding, or rarely rectal abscesses.

Non-pharmacologic Options

Biofeedback

Biofeedback is a form of operant conditioning in which information about a physiological process, which might otherwise be subconscious, is presented to a subject with the aim of having the subject modify that process consciously. The process involves physiologic monitoring of the striated pelvic floor muscles to facilitate directed strengthening exercises, and may combine strengthening exercises with sensory discrimination training. Most experts agree the appropriate patient for referral should have mild-moderate symptoms, have physiological evidence of anal dysfunction, be able to cooperate, be well-motivated, possess some degree of perception of rectal distension, and have the ability to contract the external anal sphincter.

Sacral Nerve Stimulation

Originally investigated as a method for paraplegic rehabilitation, sacral nerve stimulation (SNS) was instead found to improve voiding. Subsequently SNS was noted to have a promising effect on FI with early reports showing high success rates that led to broad popularity and rapid deployment.

Long-term outcomes regarding the success of SNS are beginning to emerge with much lower success rates. Postoperative complications reach 30 % in elderly patients and include pain at the site of implant, pouch infection, sensations of an electric shock, and rarely lead displacement or battery failure requiring reoperation.

Surgery

Surgery is indicated for those with a severe anatomical defect as the cause of their FI. Sphincteroplasty using an overlapping sphincter repair technique is the most common surgery. Wound disruption leading to delayed healing occurs frequently. Up to 60 % of patients report benefit, but long-term efficacy of overlapping sphincteroplasty is poor. Graciloplasty and gluteus maximus transposition are options for patients with severe sphincter damage in which sphincteroplasty will not suffice. In graciloplasty, the gracilis muscle is mobilized, the distal tendon divided, and the muscle is wrapped around the anal canal. In dynamic graciloplasty, electrodes are attached to the muscle and connected to a neurostimulator which is implanted in the lower abdominal wall. Complications include infection, fecal evacuation problems, leg pain, bowel injury, perineal pain, and neoanal strictures.

Artificial anal sphincters may be considered when other options are limited. The artificial sphincter is placed around the native sphincter *via* perianal tunnels and remains inflated until the patient wishes to defecate, at which time the device is deactivated (i.e., deflated). Overall success rates are approximately 47–53 % in the patients who retained their device. Most patients require operative revisions and 33 % require device explantation. Complications included infection, device erosion or malfunction, chronic pain, and obstructed defecation. Colostomy or permanent stoma for FI is considered a reasonable option for patients who have failed or had poor response to multiple alternative treatments.

Case Resolution

Mrs. WB started citalopram about 3 months prior. You inform her that she is on two medications that promote diarrhea. You ask her to consider an alternative to citalopram or metformin. In addition, you advise her to increase her total fiber intake to 25 g daily and to have scheduled bathroom time after the morning meal to take advantage of the natural gastrocolic reflex. At follow-up 12 weeks later she reports that stool is more solid and episodes of incontinence are now rare.

Key Clinical Teaching Points

- Fecal incontinence is a disabling disorder resulting in reduced quality of life.
- A detailed evacuation history and anorectal exam are critical to devising a focused diagnostic and effective treatment strategy.
- All types of fecal incontinence are initially managed with lifestyle modifications to bulk stool, improve bowel derangements, and improve access to toileting.
- Injectable agents and sacral nerve stimulation have been shown to reduce episodes of fecal incontinence.
- Surgical interventions should be reserved for the rare patient that cannot be managed with more conservative approaches, such as those with clear anatomic defects.

Teaching Questions

1. A G3P3 41-year-old woman states she is having "accidents" at work. She has started to use pads for her bowel "leakage." She reports having watery stools but no melena or hematochezia. Past medical history includes three c-sections twice, obesity with a BMI of 30, and hyperlipidemia.

   What is her greatest risk factor for fecal incontinence?

   (A) Multiple traumatic deliveries
   (B) Age
   (C) Obesity
   (D) Diarrhea

2. A 26-year-old man with twice daily, loose bowel movements is referred for bothersome perianal moisture. An anal plug was not tolerated. He wipes excessively after bowel movements without a sustained drying effect. On visual inspection there is minor hemorrhoid irritation, perianal moisture, and hemorrhoids. Flexible sigmoidoscopy was notable for hemorrhoids. Anorectal manometry and defecography studies were normal.

   If conservative methods are not effective, what treatment is recommended to treat persistent fecal seepage?

   (A) Anal sphincter botulinum toxin
   (B) Dynamic graciloplasty sphincteroplasty
   (C) Tap water enemas
   (D) Fleet enema or glycerin suppository prn

3. A 73-year-old woman with Alzheimer's dementia presents for evaluation of diarrhea. She has had diarrhea more frequently and now is soiling herself intermittently. This is adding significant stress to her daughter and caregiver. The patient

ambulates slowly with a front-wheel walker. She senses the urge to defecation, but cannot always get to the bathroom in time.

Which of the following would you advise?

(A) Decrease intake sugary foods, drinks, and caffeine
(B) Increase fiber intake
(C) Decrease fiber intake
(D) A and C
(E) A and B

Key References

1. Bharucha AE, Zinsmeister AR, Schleck CD, Melton 3rd LJ. Bowel disturbances are the most important risk factors for late onset fecal incontinence: a population-based case-control study in women. Gastroenterology. 2010;139(5):1559–66. A nice study that evaluates risk factors for FI.
2. Madoff RD. Surgical treatment options for fecal incontinence. Gastroenterology. 2004; 126(1 Suppl 1):S48–54. A nice summary of treatment options for FI.
3. Rao SS. Advances in diagnostic assessment of fecal incontinence and dyssynergic defecation. Clin Gastroenterol Hepatol. 2010;8(11):910–9.e2. This paper details the diagnostic testing that may be done in fecal incontinence patients.
4. Rao SS. Diagnosis and management of fecal incontinence. American College of Gastroenterology Practice Parameters Committee. Am J Gastroenterol. 2004;99(8):1585–604. An older but still valuable article on the diagnosis of FI.
5. Rao SS. Pathophysiology of adult fecal incontinence. Gastroenterology. 2004;126(1 Suppl 1): S14–22. Reviews the pathophysiology of fecal incontinence.
6. Shah BJ, Chokhavatia S, Rose S. Fecal incontinence in the elderly: FAQ. Am J Gastroenterol. 2012;107(11):1635–46. Nice review with focus on the elderly.

Recommended Reading

7. Drossman DA, Dumistrascu DL. Rome III: New standard for functional gastrointestinal disorders. J Gastrointestin Liver Dis 2006;15:237–41

Chapter 20
Rectal Pain

Zilla H. Hussain, Brian E. Lacy, and Stefan D. Holubar

Case Study

RH is a 41-year-old man sent for a second opinion regarding persistent, daily rectal pain. The pain started approximately 2 years ago. He cannot recall any specific precipitating event, although he admits that he's been under a lot of stress at work for quite some time. RH describes an ache or pressure in his rectum; this pain negatively affects his quality of life on a daily basis. It is worse on his left side, and more intense with prolonged sitting. The pain is relieved somewhat with standing. There does not appear to be any relationship to urination or defecation. He typically has a bowel movement every day. A colonoscopy 2 years ago was normal. A CT scan of the abdomen and pelvis 1 year ago was normal. Blood work (CBC, LFTs, ESR, and PSA) in addition to a urinalysis on two separate occasions has been normal. His weight has been stable. No first-degree family member has similar symptoms; there's no family history of celiac disease, IBD, diverticular disease, or any type of GI malignancy. Prior trials of stool softeners, glycolax, and smooth muscle antispasmodics have not provided any relief of pain. Physical examination of the anorectal area does not show any gross abnormality. A normal anocutaneous reflex was present.

Z.H. Hussain, M.D. (✉)
Division of Gastroenterology and Hepatology, Dartmouth-Hitchcock Medical Center, Lebanon, NH 03756, USA
e-mail: Zilla.H.Hussain@hitchcock.org

B.E. Lacy, M.D., Ph.D.
Division of Gastroenterology and Hepatology, Dartmouth-Hitchcock Medical Center, Lebanon, NH 03756, USA

Geisel School of Medicine at Dartmouth, Lebanon, NH, USA

S.D. Holubar, M.D., M.S., FACS, FASCRS
Division of Colon & Rectal Surgery, Department of Surgery, Dartmouth-Hitchcock Medical Center, Lebanon, NH, USA

B.E. Lacy et al. (eds.), *Functional and Motility Disorders of the Gastrointestinal Tract*, DOI 10.1007/978-1-4939-1498-2_20

Table 20.1 Rome III diagnostic criteria (2006)

Chronic proctalgia
Diagnostic criteria[a] *must include all of the following*:
• Chronic or recurrent rectal pain or aching
• Episodes last minutes or longer
• Exclusion of other causes of rectal pain such as ischemia, inflammatory bowel disease, cryptitis, intramuscular abscess, anal fissure, hemorrhoids, prostatitis, and coccydynia
Chronic proctalgia may be further characterized into levator ani syndrome or unspecified anorectal pain based on digital rectal examination
Levator ani syndrome
• Symptom criteria for chronic proctalgia and tenderness during posterior traction on the puborectalis

Adapted from Appendix A Rome III diagnostic criteria for functional gastrointestinal disorders. McLean, VA: Dagnon

[a]Criteria fulfilled for the last 3 months with symptom onset at least 6 months prior to diagnosis

Good external anal sphincter tone was noted. No masses were noted in the rectal vault, although there was tenderness to palpation along the left rectal wall. What is the diagnosis, and what treatment options are available?

Introduction

Anorectal pain (proctalgia) is a common symptom affecting 6.6 % of the population. It may develop due to a variety of organic disorders or, more commonly, due to an underlying functional etiology (see Table 20.1). Patients often suffer significant impairment, decreased quality of life, and psychological distress with little relief of symptoms, as many physicians view these complaints as insignificant and fail to fully evaluate and treat the disabling symptom. This chapter will discuss common anorectal disorders with rectal pain as the main presenting symptom.

Anal Fissure

An anal fissure is an elliptical laceration or split in the epithelial lining of the anal canal inferior (distal) to the dentate line. The evacuation of stool causes severe anal pain and bleeding, the latter of which is characterized by small amounts of bright red blood on the stool or on tissue paper. The pain starts during, and continues after, defecation and is described as sharp or knifelike. In one study of over 15,000 consecutive outpatient proctology clinic visits, the prevalence of anal fissures was nearly 10 %, with men and women being equally affected. Children and geriatric patients are less likely to be affected than younger and middle-aged adults.

Fissures are characterized into acute (up to 6 weeks in duration) or chronic. Many acute anal fissures are small and heal without medical assistance.

With respect to pathophysiology, fissures were traditionally thought to occur secondary to constipation, straining, and passage of hard stool (high-pressure fissure) or IBD/diarrheal conditions from overuse (low-pressure fissure). Recent studies, however, have demonstrated that fissures may develop due to reduced blood flow in the anal canal (especially in the posterior midline) and elevated anal canal pressures (of the internal anal sphincter (IAS) in particular). These events may cause localized ischemia, predisposing to ulcer formation that may tear with minimal trauma. Once a fissure develops, spasm of the IAS pulls the wound edges further apart, preventing or delaying healing.

Physical examination of the perianal region can be difficult in patients with fissures since the anal sphincter is often in spasm, and an internal rectal examination is impossible in some patients due to severe pain but may be mitigated in some by the use of a topical local anesthetic gel. However, a complete rectal examination, including anoscopy, often has to be performed in the setting of exam under anesthesia (EUA). The majority of fissures (90 %) develop in the posterior midline or the anterior midline especially in women; a skin tag (a "sentinel" tag or pile) is often seen at the inferior (distal) edge, while a hypertrophied papilla may be seen at the superior edge. Acute fissures characteristically have clean edges, while chronic fissures have indurated, heaped-up edges. Fissures located in the lateral position are unusual and typically associated with Crohn's disease or other less common etiologies such as acquired immunodeficiency syndrome (AIDS) or tuberculosis (TB). Younger patients (<40 years of age) without warning signs (e.g., anemia, a family history of colorectal cancer, a family history of IBD) can be treated without any additional diagnostic testing. Patients >50 years of age should undergo a screening colonoscopy prior to treatment if not previously performed.

We recommend that chronic anal fissures be treated in a stepwise manner focusing on relaxing the internal sphincter, promoting atraumatic stool passage, and providing pain relief. First, patients should undergo lifestyle modification that assure adequate fiber in their diets (25–30 g/day) to avoid constipation and straining, as placebo-controlled studies have demonstrated that fiber improves fissure healing. Another key component of lifestyle modification is sitz baths which keep the perianal area clean and help relax the anal sphincter and which have been shown to increase local perfusion to speed healing. Medical therapy is the second line of treatment, and several options are available. Topical anesthetics (e.g., lidocaine) improve pain but do not improve healing; narcotics are contraindicated. Chemical sphincterotomy is the gold standard of medical therapy. A recent Cochrane meta-analysis reported that topical nitroglycerin (NTG, 0.2–0.3 % ointment applied twice daily for 4–6 weeks) improved healing in 48.6 % of patients, and other studies have reported healing rates as high as 88 %. Physiologically, topical nitrates are an excellent treatment choice, since nitrates relax smooth muscle, allow wound edges to closely appose, and improve blood flow to the anoderm. Unfortunately, headaches (in up to 70 % of patients), hypotension, and nausea are common side effects, thus limiting their use. Calcium channel blockers (CCBs, e.g., nifedipine and diltiazem, either topical or oral) relax the anal canal and promote healing of fissures in up to two-thirds of patients. Botulinum toxin A (Botox) injection improves wound healing in approximately 65 % of patients. The dose of Botox (60–100 U) used does not seem to affect healing rates. Side effects include transient incontinence in up to 3 % of patients. A recent meta-analysis noted that both Botox (described below) and topical NTG were slightly better at healing chronic fissures than CCB, although these differences were not significant. A second meta-analysis of three randomized controlled studies involving 180 patients found that Botox was as effective as NTG with fewer side effects. Both of these agents are less likely to cause side effects than NTG.

If medical therapy does not result in healing, surgery is the next step. Lateral internal sphincterotomy (LIS) is the gold standard, with healing rates of 90–95 %. Tailored division of the IAS allows the wound edges to appose and heal. The most significant complication is incontinence, which occurs in approximately 10 % of patients, although it usually involves only flatus and is minor in nature. A recent meta-analysis of four studies involving 279 patients found that LIS was more effective than Botox (relative ratio [RR] 1.31, $p<0.0001$) for the treatment of the chronic anal fissures.

Pruritus Ani

Pruritus ani, another benign condition which may cause anorectal pain, affects 1–5 % of the US population with a male to female ratio of nearly 4:1. Symptoms of intense perianal itching and burning are not relieved by having a bowel movement, and pruritus is not typically associated with bleeding. However, if there is associated excoriation, post-defecatory pain and bleeding may be present. Symptoms resolve spontaneously in some patients (acute pruritus ani), and the culprits in this group may be a medication side effect or dietary factors.

In terms of pathophysiology, symptoms of pruritus ani develop secondary to localized irritation. An inflammatory response then develops which may be limited to the superficial layers of the perianal skin or may extend deeper. For example, fecal soiling may lead to maceration of tissue that can then become infected with *Candida*, leading to chronic symptoms of itching and burning. Skin tags and fissures may interfere with proper hygiene, thus causing skin irritation, while excessive cleansing of the perianal area can further irritate the inflamed area. Regardless of the initiating event, irritation causes the patient to itch or scratch the affected area, resulting in trauma and excoriation/ulcer formation, further exacerbating the localized inflammatory response and symptoms.

The differential diagnosis for pruritus is shown in Table 20.2. A good history is essential in order to accurately diagnose the root cause of the pruritus ani. Examination of the perianal area reveals reddened, irritated skin in the acute setting. Linear or deep, punched out excoriations may be present. A careful examination should be performed, with the patient asked to strain to determine the presence of

Table 20.2 Etiology of pruritus ani

Letter name
Topical irritants
Soaps
Deodorants
Perfumes
Dry cleaning solutions
Allergies to dyes, fabric softeners
Tight fitting clothes (lack of air circulation; pressure)
Mechanical factors
Fissures
Fistula
Abscess
Fecal incontinence/fecal soiling
Hemorrhoids
Rectal prolapse and/or intussusceptions
Infections
Candida albicans
Herpes simplex
Papillomavirus (condyloma acuminata)
Staphylococcus aureus
Group A beta-hemolytic streptococcus
Corynebacterium (erythrasma)
Pinworms
Scabies
Syphilis
Gonorrhea
HIV
Dermatologic disorders
Psoriasis
Seborrhea
Lichen planus
Lichen sclerosis
Atopic dermatitis
Systemic disorders
Diabetes
Lymphoma
Leukemia
Aplastic anemia
Malignancies
Bowen's disease
Extramammary Paget's
Squamous cell carcinoma
Miscellaneous
Sensitivities to foods (tomatoes, citrus, beer, coffee, tea, cola)
Medications (mineral oil, quinidine, colchicines, neomycin)

rectal prolapse or prolapsing hemorrhoids. Patients with chronic symptoms may develop thick, whitened skin in this area consistent with lichenification. Contrary to current popular opinion, pinworms (*Enterobius vermicularis*) are an unlikely cause of pruritus in the United States. In the absence of warning signs (unintentional weight loss, anemia, rectal bleeding, family history of colon cancer), no other evaluation is required during the initial visit, although anoscopy should be considered.

Ideally, treatment should be directed at the underlying cause. Unfortunately, in many cases, the etiology is never identified. The first step is to educate the patient and encourage lifestyle modifications, so that he or she understands that persistent scratching and itching only further irritates the area and creates a cycle of recurrent inflammation due to histamine release. Antihistamines, especially when used at night, can reduce nocturnal itching. Incontinence and chronic diarrhea should be treated using dietary modifications, Kegel exercises, and loperamide or diphenoxylate–atropine. The area should be kept dry at all times, and the patient should avoid excessive wiping and cleansing. Only fragrance-free soaps and detergents should be used. Sitz baths can be used to keep the area clean, while witch hazel pads or tucks can improve hygiene and minimize irritation. Zinc oxide applied before defecation, peri-bottles, bidets, avoiding wiping, and drying with a hair drier can all help break the cycle of irritation.

If conservative measures fail, hydrocortisone cream (1 %) may be used. Topical steroids should not be used longer than 2 weeks due to the potential to cause pathologic thinning of the perianal skin. Tricyclic antidepressants improve sleep in many patients and may minimize nocturnal itching and scratching. Finally, a randomized, placebo-controlled trial of 44 patients found that a 4-week course of topical capsaicin (0.006 %) improved symptoms in 31 patients compared to placebo ($p<0.0001$). Patients who responded continued to require daily topical therapy in order to maintain symptom remission. Refractory cases should be referred to colon and rectal surgery for consideration of anal skin tattooing with methylene blue which may be efficacious in up to 80 % of patients.

Proctalgia Fugax

Proctalgia fugax (Latin for fleeting) affects approximately 3–14 % of the general population (see Table 20.3). There appears to be a slight female predominance. The defining symptom of proctalgia is the sudden, unpredictable onset of deep anorectal pain, which is described as sharp, stabbing, twisting, or lancinating in nature. Episodes occur unpredictably at anytime, although nocturnal episodes are more frequently recalled due to awakening. Pain typically remains localized, although it may occasionally radiate to the gluteal or perineal region. Episodes are generally brief in nature (seconds to minutes), with each episode resolving spontaneously. The majority of patients (85 %) have fewer than 1–2 episodes per month.

The exact etiology of proctalgia in these cases is unknown. Pathophysiologically, the proctalgia is thought to represent a spastic disorder of the smooth muscle of

Table 20.3 Rome III diagnostic criteria (2006)

Proctalgia fugax
Diagnostic criteria[a] *must include all of the following*:
• Recurrent episodes of pain localized to the anus or lower rectum
• Episodes last from seconds to minutes
• There is no anorectal pain between episodes

[a] For research purposes, criteria must be fulfilled for 3 months; however, clinical diagnosis and evaluation may be made prior to 3 months
Adapted from Appendix A Rome III diagnostic criteria for functional gastrointestinal disorders. McLean, VA: Dagnon

the anal canal. One study demonstrated an increase both in anal canal pressures and the frequency of anal canal slow waves during episodes of pain, while another study demonstrated high-amplitude, high-frequency myoelectrical activity of the anus that was temporally related to proctalgia symptoms.

Proctalgia fugax can be readily diagnosed from the patient's history without the need for expensive laboratory tests or diagnostic imaging. Physical examination is usually unremarkable without evidence of a fissure, prolapse, mass, or thrombosed hemorrhoid(s). In the current medicolegal climate, we recommend that flexible sigmoidoscopy with careful retroflexion in the rectum be performed. Anorectal manometry has little clinical value in the evaluation of rectal pain, but if performed typically shows a pattern diagnostic of pelvic floor dyssynergia (PFD).

Treatment begins by reassuring the patient of the benign nature of the disease. Medical treatment is difficult because episodes resolve quickly, usually before the patient can initiate medical therapy, and well before oral medications can be absorbed and reach peak effect. We recommend conservative therapy beginning with a warm sitz bath or even a warm water enema at the start of the attack. Longer lasting episodes generally respond to sublingual NTG (0.3 mg) or topical (perianal) NTG (0.1 %). Persistent symptoms can be treated with short-acting anxiolytics, smooth muscle relaxants (i.e., hyoscyamine or dicyclomine), or a topical CBB (i.e., diltiazem cream). One prospective, double-blind study demonstrated that an inhaled beta-agonist, salbutamol, shortened the length of each episode of pain. Patients with frequent disabling episodes may benefit from Botox injection into the anal canal, although only small series are available and well-controlled studies are lacking.

Levator Ani Syndrome

The levator ani consists of three muscles which form the pelvic floor: the iliococcygeus, pubococcygeus, and puborectalis. These muscles surround the anus to form a sling supporting the rectum. These are easily palpated during a digital rectal exam. Chronic spasm and tension of the levator muscle is thought to cause the pain characterized in levator ani syndrome. It is estimated that 6 % of the US population suffers from levator ani syndrome, with a slightly higher prevalence among women and a decline in prevalence after the age of 45. The pain associated with this syndrome is often described as a dull aching or pressure-like discomfort in the rectum, which may last for hours. Factors precipitating symptoms include prolonged sitting and defecation. Other patients have reported difficulty defecating or feeling of incomplete evacuation. An important clinical finding on examination is palpable tenderness of the overly contracted levator ani muscles as the finger moves from the coccyx posteriorly to the pubis anteriorly. Often, tenderness is asymmetric and found on the left more than the right. This syndrome has also been referred to as puborectalis syndrome, chronic proctalgia, piriformis syndrome, and pelvic tension myalgia.

Diagnosis is suggested primarily by clinical history, physical examination, and exclusion of other anorectal disorders as discussed above. An international committee proposed diagnostic criteria of "chronic or recurrent episodes of rectal pain lasting greater than 20 min for at least 3 months in the absence of ischemia, inflammatory bowel disease, cryptitis, abscess, fissure, hemorrhoids, or coccydynia." A positive diagnosis is highly likely if posterior traction of the puborectalis muscle reveals contracted levator ani muscles and elicits tenderness. The role of anorectal manometry in evaluation is not well established to date but again is likely to reveal of pattern of pelvic floor dyssynergia.

All treatment modalities are targeted to reduce anal canal pressures or levator ani muscle tension with variable success. Digital massage 3–4 times a week and sitz baths, or formal pelvic floor retraining, may improve symptoms. Muscle relaxants, such as diazepam, methocarbamol, baclofen, and cyclobenzaprine, are widely used. Local Botox injection into the puborectalis musculature, which may result in gross incontinence, has been poorly studied to date but may benefit severe refractory cases, and internal pudendal nerve block or ablation may help the occasional patient resistant to medical treatment. Surgery, such as pudendal nerve release, is not recommended due to unsubstantiated evidence and risk of incontinence.

Solitary Rectal Ulcer Syndrome

Solitary rectal ulcer syndrome (SRUS), a functional defecatory disorder associated with pelvic floor dysfunction and internal prolapse, is generally a disorder of young adults (third to fourth decade of life), with an incidence of 1–3 in 100,000 persons per year. Women are somewhat more prone to develop SRUS than men. Similar to many other functional gastrointestinal disorders psychiatric comorbid conditions are more common in patients with SRUS than in the general population, although SRUS is not the direct result of either anxiety or depression. Symptoms of SRUS are nonspecific; rectal bleeding and the passage of mucus are the two most commonly reported symptoms. Straining at stool, feeling of incomplete evacuation, rectal discomfort, and urgency are other common symptoms. The name is a misnomer, since only 25–30 % of patients have a solitary ulcer. The majority of patients have multiple ulcers (30–40 %), hyperemic mucosa (15–20 %), or polypoid lesions.

The lesions are usually on the anterior rectal wall, 4–10 cm from the anal verge. Lesions range from 0.5 to 6 cm in diameter, although most are between 1 and 1.5 cm. Some ulcers have rolled edges, are indurated, bleed, or cause a localized mass effect, which means that they can be confused with a malignant process.

The pathophysiology of SRUS is poorly understood, although a recent study found that anorectal redundancy and impaired rectosacral fixation, similar to full-thickness rectal prolapse, may play a role in its development. This results in rectal intussusception (internal prolapse), which then produces localized trauma and ischemia with subsequent ulcer development. Persistent straining, especially in patients with pelvic floor dyssynergia, may also reduce blood flow and lead to ischemia. This theory is supported by studies showing an improvement in rectal blood flow and ulcer healing with biofeedback.

The variable lesions of SRUS should be biopsied in order to exclude malignancy. Pathognomonic histologic features of SRUS include smooth muscle hyperplasia of the lamina propria with infiltration of collagen (aka "fibromuscular obliteration"), distortion of crypt architecture, disorientation and thickening of the muscularis mucosa, and an increase in mucus cells with gland dilation. Anorectal manometry and lack of balloon expulsion can identify patients with pelvic floor dyssynergia; if present, patients should be enrolled in a pelvic floor retraining program. Traditional or magnetic resonance defecography may identify intussusceptions and associated enterocele and cystocele. Barium enemas are not clinically useful, while endorectal ultrasound (ERUS) with needle biopsies should be reserved for those patients where malignancy remains in the differential diagnosis.

Treatment begins by educating the patient about the disorder, lifestyle modifications including advising patients to avoid straining and ensuring adequate fiber intake, and referral to physical therapy for a pelvic floor retraining program to restore proper evacuation techniques. Steroids and 5-ASA agents are unlikely to improve symptoms. Carafate retention enemas may reduce bleeding. Surgery is an option for those who fail standard therapy, those with persistent bleeding, or when biopsies raise the definite possibility of malignancy. Anterior resection with rectopexy, which does not address the underlying functional disorder, has been recommended in the past; however, some colon and rectal surgeons now recommend stapled transanal rectal resection (STARR). Head-to-head trials comparing surgical therapies are lacking.

Case Resolution

Focusing on RH's clinical history, one can extrapolate many clues towards a diagnosis (see Table 20.4). This patient had been suffering from chronic rectal pain/pressure described as an ache, worse on the left side, with an exacerbating factor of prolonged sitting. Reassuring findings in his medical history include a stable weight, a noncontributory family history, no evidence of anemia, and a normal anoscopy and colonoscopy. The absence of pain with defecation, constipation, rectal bleeding,

Table 20.4 Common anorectal pain disorders

Differential	Symptoms	Diagnosis	Treatment
Anal fissure	Rectal pain, bleeding	Perianal exam may require EUA, tear at the anal canal on parting the buttocks, a "sentinel pile" (skin tag) may be present	>90 % heal with high-fiber diet, sitz bath, stool softeners, chronic anal fissures (>6 weeks) not healed: topical NTG, topical or oral CCB, Botox injection, lateral internal sphincterotomy
Proctalgia fugax	Sudden brief stabbing pain (lasting seconds to minutes), unpredictable, no anal pain between episodes	History, normal perianal exam	Reassurance, conservative treatment (sitz bath, warm water enema), long episodes (SL NTG, topical NTG), and persistent symptoms (anxiolytics, smooth muscle relaxants, topical CCB, Botox injection)
Pruritus ani	Intense perianal itching, burning not relieved with defecation	History, exam reveals reddened perianal area, irritated skin, scratch marks, chronic lichenification	Treat underlying cause, educate on hygiene, antihistamines, topical steroids
SRUS	Nonspecific, rectal bleeding, passage of mucosa	Multiple ulcers (1–3 cm), anterior wall, histology smooth muscle hyperplasia of the lamina propria with infiltration of collagen, crypt distortion, disorientation/thickening of muscularis mucosa, increased mucosal cells	Fiber intake, education in avoidance of straining, biofeedback program to restore proper evacuation, surgery for those that fail conservative treatment
Hemorrhoids	Bleeding, pain, itching	Proctoscopy/anoscopy: internal occurs above pectinate line, external below pectinate line, mixed	Increase dietary fiber, topical steroids, sclerotherapy, rubber band ligation, bipolar cautery, direct-current electrotherapy, cryotherapy, infrared photocoagulation, surgery
Levator ani syndrome	Dull ache or pressure, worse with sitting	History, exam with palpable tenderness of overly contracted levator ani m. (left>right)	Reassurance, digital massage, sitz bath, skeletal muscle relaxants, anxiolytics, Botox injection

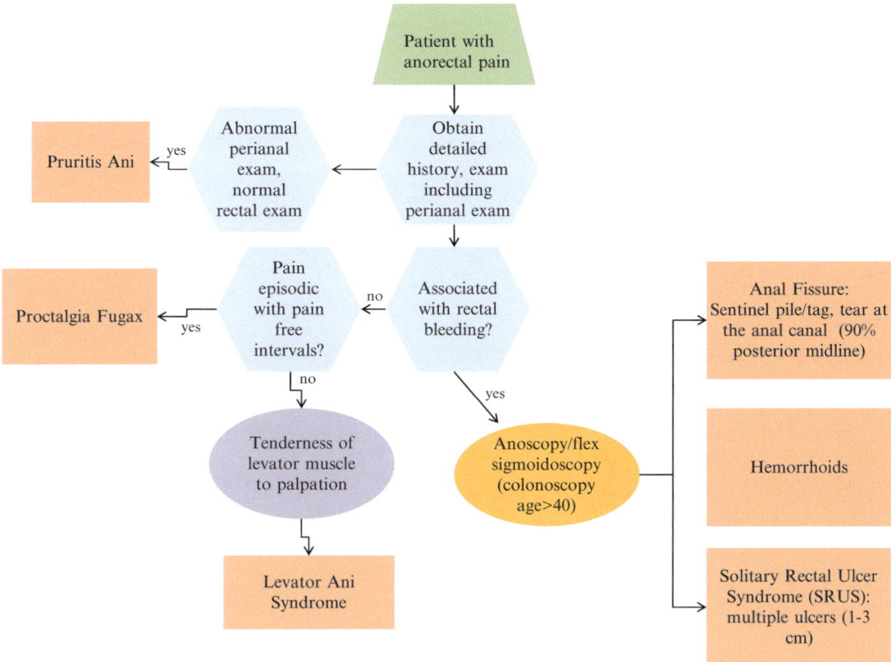

Fig. 20.1 Diagnosis of anorectal pain

and abnormal findings on anal exam makes the diagnosis of SRUS and anal fissure unlikely (see Fig. 20.1). Prostatitis is unlikely in this case due to a normal CBC, PSA, and urinalysis. Proctalgia fugax can be excluded since RH does not describe acute episodes of stabbing, fleeting pain. Physical examination revealed a tender band of muscles along the left pelvic sidewall consistent with levator ani syndrome.

Treatment for RH began with a description of the diagnosis and reassurance of its benign nature. Subsequent trials of tramadol, pregabalin, and amitriptyline were not helpful. Nightly B&O (belladonna and opium) suppositories dramatically improved his symptoms when combined with a course of physical therapy involving rectal massage.

Teaching Questions

1. What two symptoms are classic for an anal fissure?

   (A) Urgency and bleeding
   (B) Perianal pain and urgency
   (C) Perianal pain and bleeding
   (D) Perianal pain and difficult evacuation

2. What is the typical endoscopic finding in patients with SRUS (solitary rectal ulcer syndrome)?
   (A) Small (<1 cm), solitary ulcer on posterior wall
   (B) Multiple ulcers, medium in size (1–3 cm) on anterior wall
   (C) Single, large (>5 cm) ulcer on anterior wall
   (D) Single, large (>5 cm) on posterior wall
3. What is the clinical utility of anorectal manometry in a patient with rectal pain?
   (A) The clinical utility is low
   (B) The clinical utility is high
   (C) The clinical utility is high if combined with a normal sigmoidoscopic exam
   (D) The clinical utility is high if combined with normal defecography
4. What treatment options are available for patients with levator syndrome?
   (A) Serotonin reuptake inhibitors and topical nitroglycerin
   (B) Smooth muscle antispasmodics and tricyclic antidepressants
   (C) Rectal massage, smooth muscle relaxants, and benzodiazepines
   (D) Rectal massage, skeletal muscle relaxants, and benzodiazepines

Key References

1. Billingham RP, Isler JT, Kimmins MH, Nelson JM, Schweitzer J, Murphy MM. The diagnosis and management of common anorectal disorders. Curr Prob Surg. 2004;41:586–645. Provides a detailed explanation of proper examination techniques for patients presenting with rectal pain. In addition a nice brief review of less common etiologies of anorectal disorders.
2. Schubert M, Sridhar S, Schade RR, Wexner SD. What every gastroenterologist needs to know about common anorectal disorders. World J Gastroenterol. 2009;15:3201–9. A review of the current literature for diagnosis and initial management of common presenting anorectal disorders.
3. Wald A, Barucha AE, Enck P, et al. Functional anorectal disorders. In: Drossman DA, Corazziari E, Delvaux M, editors. Rome III: The functional gastrointestinal disorders. McLean, VA: Dagnon; 2006. p. 639–86. Guidelines for clinicians to define, understand, study, diagnose, and treat functional anorectal disorders.

Part VII
The Functional GI Patient

Chapter 21
Complementary and Alternative Management Strategies in Irritable Bowel Syndrome

Andrea Bollom and Anthony Lembo

Case Study

A 23-year-old woman, recently graduated from college and previously diagnosed with IBS-C, presents with symptoms of pelvic cramps, hard infrequent stools, and bloating. Her symptoms began while a freshman at college and have progressively worsened. She denies weight loss, nocturnal awakening from pain, fevers, and vomiting. She has been evaluated by several different gastroenterologists and primary care providers with a number of tests including colonoscopy, multiple CT scans, and laboratory studies including tissue transglutaminase (tTG) antibody, sedimentation rate, and complete blood count. All of these tests were normal. Because her sister has celiac disease, she also underwent upper endoscopy with biopsies of her duodenum, which were normal while on a diet containing gluten. She has altered her diet, using both gluten-free and low-FODMAP diets, with limited success. Increasing the fiber in her diet to 25 g of soluble fiber and regularly exercising have also produced minimal symptom improvement. Over the years, she has tried a variety of laxatives, including polyethylene glycol, which improved stool frequency and consistency but provided no significant benefit with respect to her bloating and abdominal pain. Lubiprostone and linaclotide also resulted in limited improvement. Most recently, she was found to have small intestinal bacterial overgrowth and was treated with several courses of antibiotics with only transient improvement in her bloating. She inquires about the use and utility of complementary medications to treat her symptoms.

A. Bollom, B.S. (✉) • A. Lembo, M.D. (✉)
Division of Gastroenterology, Beth Israel Deaconess Medical Center,
330 Brookline Avenue, Boston, MA 02215, USA
e-mail: abollom@bidmc.harvard.edu; alembo@bidmc.harvard.edu

B.E. Lacy et al. (eds.), *Functional and Motility Disorders of the Gastrointestinal Tract*, DOI 10.1007/978-1-4939-1498-2_21

Introduction

Due to the limited number of conventional treatments available for functional gastrointestinal disorders (FGIDs), the use of complementary and alternative medicine (CAM) therapies in this population is common. Studies of CAM use for FGIDs have focused primarily on irritable bowel syndrome (IBS) and functional dyspepsia (FD), while there are limited data on their use in other functional disorders. CAM is frequently used together with conventional medicine and more often in patients who have chronic conditions that are particularly difficult to treat. In the treatment of IBS, commonly used CAM therapies include probiotics, prebiotics, acupuncture, cognitive-behavioral therapy, hypnotherapy, and herbal products such as peppermint oil.

Epidemiology

CAM approaches are widely used in the United States. The 2007 National Health Interview Survey found that over 17 % of adults in the United States had used "natural" products in the previous year, including herbals and non-botanical supplements. Similarly, patients with FGIDs, including IBS, frequently use CAM therapies. An Australian study found that approximately 21 % of patients with IBS had seen a CAM provider, while in the United Kingdom, approximately 50 % of IBS patients reported using CAM. A prospective 6-month study from the United States found that in a large health maintenance organization, CAM use in patients with FGIDs was 35 %, costing each patient approximately $200 in out-of-pocket costs each year. The most frequent users of CAM tend to be women and those with higher education and incomes.

Treatment

Since most studies of CAM use in FGIDs have involved patients with IBS, this section will focus on several of the more common CAM therapies in IBS (see Table 21.1). It is important to recognize that, in general, there is a lack of high-quality controlled clinical trials evaluating the efficacy and safety of CAM when used in IBS. Indeed, most studies involving use of CAM in IBS have included small patient populations, involved a single center only, and contained a number of other methodological limitations precluding definitive recommendations regarding their use.

Table 21.1 Potential CAM therapies for IBS

Commonly used
Probiotics
Prebiotics
Acupuncture
Cognitive-behavioral therapy
Hypnotherapy
Peppermint oil
Others
Herbal medicines
– Turmeric extract
– Artichoke leaf extract
– Iberogast (combination of 9 herbal extracts)
– Padma Lax (Tibetan preparation of 12 botanicals)
– TXYF (Chinese preparation of 4 herbs)
– Other traditional Chinese herbal medicine
– Ginger root or tea
– Senna tea
– Evening primrose oil
Yoga
Biofeedback
Aromatherapy
Massage therapy

Probiotics and Prebiotics

Probiotics are live microorganisms that when administered in adequate amounts confer a health benefit on the host. The gut microbiota is thought to be involved in the pathogenesis of multiple gastrointestinal disorders, including IBS. The goal of using probiotics in IBS is to modify the microbiota and, in doing so, alter fermentation, gas production, and absorption. In general, studies involving probiotics have been of low methodological quality due to small numbers of patients, a variety of probiotic agents used, and short follow-up periods. In a systematic review of 19 studies evaluating a variety of individual and combination probiotic products in patients with IBS, the conclusion was that probiotic use generally results in modest improvement in overall symptom burden. A second systematic review found evidence for use of *Bifidobacterium infantis* 35624 in providing benefit in the composite symptom score of IBS patients on the basis of two appropriately designed clinical trials. In one study, 362 women were randomly assigned to groups that received doses of *B. infantis* at 1×10^6, 1×10^8, or 1×10^{10} colony-forming units (CFUs) per day or placebo for 4 weeks. Only the 1×10^8 CFU dose was found to provide benefit compared to placebo, significantly improving abdominal pain and secondary measures. Randomized studies of *B. animalis* and *B. lactis* in conjunction with yogurt starters have found significant reductions in abdominal distention and IBS symptoms. A probiotic product containing a combination of seven different probiotic organisms (VSL#3; three bifidobacteria, three lactobacilli, and one streptococcus) has been shown to significantly improve bloating compared with placebo. Further studies are needed to confirm these findings and establish optimal doses and duration of therapy.

Prebiotics are distinct from probiotics in that they are nondigestible food ingredients that beneficially affect the host by selectively stimulating the growth and/or activity of one of a limited number of potentially health-promoting bacteria in the colon. Prebiotics are thought to act by stimulating the growth of beneficial commensal microbes, resulting in an increase in vitamin and mineral absorption, improved digestion, and increased protection against viruses, fungi, and damaging bacteria. They may also act by increasing the amount of short-chain fatty acids and lactic acid-producing bacteria and activating carbohydrate receptor immune cells. A randomized, placebo-controlled clinical trial of the prebiotic trans-galacto-oligosaccharide (GOS) in IBS found that, compared with those receiving placebo, patients taking the prebiotic had improvements in stool consistency, bloating, and flatulence. A dose of 3.5 g/day was most successful in this study. Another study focusing on optimal dose of prebiotics found that patients ingesting 10 g/day of short-chain fructo-oligosaccharide (scFOS) for 7 days exhibited the greatest increase in fecal bifidobacteria counts while minimizing side effects, such as abdominal cramps, excess flatus, and bloating.

Acupuncture

Acupuncture is part of traditional Chinese medicine that has been practiced for thousands of years. In contrast, its use in Western society has only recently become more common and better accepted. In traditional Chinese medicine, acupuncture is believed to rebalance the "qi," the energy or life force in the body that runs through meridians, by penetrating the skin with solid, thin, metallic needles at specified acupoints, manipulated by hand or electric stimulation. While the exact mechanism whereby acupuncture may improve gastrointestinal symptoms is not known, acupuncture has been shown to influence visceral reflex activity, gastric emptying, and gastroesophageal reflux. Specifically, in IBS, acupuncture has been suggested to alter visceral sensation and motility by stimulating the somatic nervous system and the vagus nerve. Several high-quality, randomized, controlled studies have evaluated the efficacy of acupuncture in IBS. Schneider and colleagues randomized 43 patients with IBS to either acupuncture or sham acupuncture (i.e., a non-penetrating needle). There was no significant difference in quality of life ratings between subjects in each group; however, there was a significant improvement from baseline symptoms in both groups. Another recent study by Lembo and colleagues compared the effects of acupuncture, sham acupuncture, and no treatment (control) in relieving patients' IBS symptoms. No significant difference in global IBS symptoms was found between the acupuncture and sham groups; however, both of those groups demonstrated a significant effect on overall improvement in IBS compared to the waitlist control group. The results of these studies suggest that both acupuncture and sham acupuncture are effective in alleviating IBS symptoms compared to a waitlist control. These studies do not exclude the possibility that it is the ritual of acupuncture that is responsible for this positive effect.

Cognitive-Behavioral Therapy

Cognitive-behavioral therapy (CBT) is a combination of therapies that include identifying and correcting distorted, maladaptive beliefs, education, relaxation exercises, and coping skills, among others. CBT is most effective in highly motivated individuals. A recent systematic review of CBT in IBS found that a number of different techniques were used to guide patients to challenge their unhelpful beliefs and behaviors in order to decrease psychological distress and physiological symptoms. There was considerable variety in the amount of time spent with a therapist between studies. The majority of the studies found significant improvement in IBS symptom severity and quality of life measurements compared with waitlisted participants and participants receiving standard treatment. Three studies by Ljótsson and colleagues used an Internet-based intervention and compared Internet-based CBT to standard Internet stress management therapy for IBS patients. The patients in the Internet-based CBT group reported greater improvements in IBS symptom severity, anxiety, and quality of life than the group receiving generic stress management therapy. The researchers concluded that specific components of the CBT therapy contributed to IBS symptom reduction when compared to the more generic stress management strategies.

Hypnotherapy

Through hypnosis, patients with IBS are believed to gain control of their gut function, thereby changing the way the brain modulates their gut activity. Success rates have been reported to be as high as 70 % in clinical practice, though few controlled clinical trials have been published. A study by Forbes and colleagues used scripted recordings of gut-based hypnotic suggestions. Because the study included non-hypnosis components to their intervention, it is difficult to distinguish treatment results due solely from hypnosis. Regardless, no significant effects of treatment were found. Palsson and colleagues used a "pure" form of hypnosis that was individualized to the patients, using gut-related suggestions and imagery to produce relaxations and reduce pain and attention to gut symptoms. They found that hypnosis led to a significant improvement in IBS symptom severity and quality of life compared with standard medical care. A Cochrane meta-analysis published in 2007 identified four studies investigating hypnotherapy including a total of 147 patients with IBS. In the short term, in patients who failed standard medical therapy, hypnotherapy was found to be superior to that of a waiting list control or usual medical management for both abdominal pain and a composite of IBS symptoms. The quality of most trials, however, was inadequate to allow any definitive conclusion about the efficacy of hypnotherapy for IBS.

Peppermint Oil

Peppermint oil is a major component of several over-the-counter remedies for IBS symptoms. Its active ingredient, menthol, has known calcium channel-blocking activity, with a mechanism similar to dihydropyridine calcium channel antagonists. In vitro studies have shown a relaxing effect of peppermint oil on smooth muscle in the GI tract, including the lower esophageal sphincter (LES). To avoid this effect on the LES, enteric-coated peppermint oil preparations have been developed to better isolate effects in the lower GI tract. Peppermint oil has been used as an antispasmodic due to its relaxing effect on gut smooth muscle. A meta-analysis of five double-blind, placebo-controlled trials found a significant beneficial effect of peppermint oil compared to placebo in alleviation of IBS symptoms. Studies done in both adults and children have found significant reductions in the severity of abdominal pain, stool frequency, and distension.

Case Resolution

The use of CAM was discussed with the patient who was receptive to their use. She was subsequently started on the probiotic, *B. infantis*, and a yogurt containing *B. animalis*, while intermittently taking peppermint oil for abdominal pain. In addition, she consulted with a psychologist who performed CBT. At her most recent clinic visit, she reported an improvement in her symptoms and less overall interference in her daily functioning.

Key Clinical Teaching Points

- Due to the limited conventional treatment options for FGIDs, many patients seek out CAM therapies.
- The most commonly used CAM therapies for IBS include probiotics, prebiotics, acupuncture, cognitive-behavioral therapy, hypnotherapy, and peppermint oil.
- Many of the CAM therapies require further evaluation and testing in high-quality, randomized, controlled clinical studies.

Teaching Questions

1. Which one of the probiotic agents below has been studied in a dose-ranging, multicenter trial in patients with IBS?

   (A) *Bifidobacterium infantis*
   (B) *Bifidobacterium animalis*
   (C) *Streptococcus thermophilus*
   (D) *Lactobacillus bulgaricus*

2. Recent evidence supports the use of an Internet-based cognitive-behavioral therapy program for IBS.

   (A) True
   (B) False

3. Which one of the following CAM therapies has been shown in a meta-analysis to reduce abdominal spasms through inhibition of calcium influx?

   (A) Hypnotherapy
   (B) Acupuncture
   (C) Peppermint oil

Key References

1. Hungin AP, Mulligan C, Pot B, Whorwell P, Agréus L, Fracasso P, et al. Systematic review: probiotics in the management of lower gastrointestinal symptoms in clinical practice - an evidence-based international guide. Aliment Pharmacol Ther. 2013;38:784–93. This recent review synthesizes the general outcomes of studies with probiotics and IBS, providing a reference guide for clinicians.
2. Kligler B, Chaudhary S. Peppermint oil. Am Fam Physician. 2007;75:1027–30. This paper discusses recent evidence for the use of peppermint oil in IBS and functional dyspepsia.
3. Magge S, Lembo A. Complementary and alternative medicine for the irritable bowel syndrome. Gastroenterol Clin North Am. 2011;40:245–53. The review paper discussing recent studies and efficacy for select CAM therapies for IBS, including peppermint oil, acupuncture, probiotics and prebiotics.
4. Pajak R, Lackner J, Kamboj SK. A systematic review of minimal-contact psychological treatments for symptom management in Irritable Bowel Syndrome. J Psychosom Res. 2013;75:103–12. This review covers the studies of cognitive-behavioral therapy and hypnotherapy as treatment for IBS.
5. van Tilburg MA, Palsson OS, Levy RL, Feld AD, Turner MJ, Drossman DA, Whitehead WE. Complementary and alternative medicine use and cost in functional bowel disorders: a six month prospective study in a large HMO. BMC Complement Altern Med. 2008;8:46. This study collected information about CAM use from over 1,000 patients with functional bowel disorders at a large HMO.
6. Yoon SL, Grundmann O, Koepp L, Farrell L. Management of irritable bowel syndrome (IBS) in adults: conventional and complementary/alternative approaches. Altern Med Rev. 2011;16:134–51. This review examines recent evidence of CAM use for IBS, as well as a more extensive review of herbal therapies.

Appendix: Answers to Teaching Questions

Chapter 1

1. (B) Choices A, C, and D are all part of the Rome III diagnostic criteria for globus. Choice B is incorrect; a patient must deny symptoms of dysphagia and odynophagia in order to be classified as having globus.
2. (D) Studies have shown a benefit to a trial of options A, B, and C; however, no data are available regarding a benefit with the use of baclofen in the treatment of globus.
3. (D) Choices A, B, and C are all reasonable tests to perform to evaluate globus in appropriately selected patients. There is no role for endoscopic ultrasound in the evaluation of globus sensation.

Chapter 2

1. (D) Barium esophagography. The clinical history is suggestive of a Zenker's diverticulum or hypopharyngeal pouch. Answer D, barium esophagography, is the correct initial diagnostic study to identify a Zenker's diverticulum. Answer A is incorrect since upper endoscopy may not identify a Zenker's diverticulum and is associated with an increased risk of perforation. Cautious upper endoscopy may be required after diagnosis for therapeutic intervention; however, it is not the first diagnostic test of choice. Answer B, esophageal manometry, may demonstrate the underlying cause of the diverticulum (i.e., UES dysfunction) which may have predisposed to its formation, but manometry alone will not confirm the diagnosis. Answer C, CT scan of the neck, is incorrect since it is unlikely that the Zenker's diverticulum will be visualized unless very large.
2. (B) Diltiazem. Pharmacologic therapy with a smooth muscle relaxant, such as the calcium channel blocker diltiazem, is the initial treatment of choice for

B.E. Lacy et al. (eds.), *Functional and Motility Disorders of the Gastrointestinal Tract*, DOI 10.1007/978-1-4939-1498-2

diffuse esophageal spasm (DES). Calcium channel blockers and phosphodiesterase inhibitors have been shown to alleviate symptoms associated with DES. There is also observational evidence to support the use of oral nitrate therapy. Answer A, long esophagomyotomy, is an aggressive management strategy and should only be considered in severe cases refractory to other less invasive management option and with a clear delay in esophageal emptying. Answer C, botulinum toxin injection, has been shown to decrease or alleviate chest pain in DES patients; however, the results are usually only temporary. This therapy should only be considered if the patient fails pharmacologic therapy. Answer D, pneumatic dilation, has only limited evidence supporting its use in treatment of DES and should only be considered after failure of pharmacologic therapy.

3. (C) Swallowed topical steroid for 8 weeks. The first-line pharmacologic therapy for eosinophilic esophagitis (EoE) is an 8-week course of swallowed topical steroid such as fluticasone or budesonide. Systemic steroids should only be used if the patient fails topical therapy or in cases where the eosinophilia also involves the stomach or small bowel. Answer A, proton pump inhibitor for 8 weeks followed by repeat endoscopy with biopsies, is not correct due to the fact GERD has been ruled out by pH monitoring. A trial of PPI therapy would be warranted if endoscopic or pH monitoring findings were consistent with GERD. To establish the diagnosis of EoE, GERD must be excluded as a cause of esophageal eosinophilia. Although food antigens appear to be a trigger for EoE, answer B, skin-prick allergy testing with subsequent avoidance of positive reacting food antigens, is incorrect due to lack of correlation between positive skin allergen testing and EoE antigen response. Consuming an elemental or elimination diet has been shown to be an effective treatment for some EoE patients; however, the antigens eliminated are not based on skin allergen or RAST testing. Answer D, esophageal dilatation, can be used to treat symptomatic patients with strictures; however, this is usually done only if the patient fails medical or dietary therapy.
4. (B) False. If a patient is diagnosed with achalasia based upon barium esophagram, esophageal manometry should be performed to confirm the diagnosis and an upper endoscopy is required to rule out malignancy involving the gastroesophageal junction which can mimic primary achalasia.
5. (A) The most likely cause of intermittent solid food dysphagia in a patient with GERD is a peptic stricture due to chronic acid exposure. Answer B, eosinophilic esophagitis, is incorrect due to the known history of GERD. Although eosinophilic esophagitis can present in patients with a history of GERD, it is not the most likely etiology of her symptoms. Answer C, achalasia, is incorrect since it usually presents with both solid and liquid food dysphagia and regurgitation of old food. Answer D, Zenker's diverticulum, is incorrect since it usually will produce discomfort in the cervical region instead of substernal discomfort, will be associated with halitosis, and may be accompanied by a "gurgling" sensation in the cervical region.

Chapter 3

1. (D) The most common cause of noncardiac chest pain (NCCP) is GERD. An empirical PPI trial or esophageal pH testing is justified as the initial approach. Reassurance alone that the pain is not cardiac does not result in decreased pain frequency and is not appropriate at this stage. Esophageal motility testing at this point may not provide a therapeutic option and is an uncomfortable test; however, for patients who fail PPI therapy or do not have GERD and continue to have pain, it is a reasonable test. Initial treatment with nitrates may result in worsening undetected GERD. Thus, GERD should be excluded first in the initial evaluation of this patient.
2. (C) Switching to another PPI or doing a pH study has a low diagnostic yield at this point since the initial PPI trial failed to obtain response. PPI trials lead to chest pain improvement in approximately 80 % of GERD-related NCCP patients. Given the complete absence of a response, it seems unlikely GERD is playing a significant role in this patient's chest pain. Of course, compliance with correct intake, dosing, and timing should be verified prior to considering the PPI trial nonresponsive. Botulinum toxin injection has been used to treat non-GERD-related NCCP, but as this is premature, an esophageal motility disorder, particularly achalasia, should be excluded first.
3. (D) Psychiatric referral may be a future consideration since many patients with recurrent NCCP may suffer from anxiety, depression, or somatoform disorders. Calcium blockers may be tried, especially for patients with spastic esophageal motility, but her esophageal motility test was normal. Hypnosis has been used effectively for treatment of NCCP in small trials; however, it is not widely available and other alternatives are available. Specifically, visceral analgesics (e.g., tricyclic antidepressants or serotonin modulators) have been used with beneficial results in this setting.

Chapter 4

1. (D) Answer D is correct as all of the answer choices are associated with gastroesophageal reflux disease. A hiatal hernia is associated with GERD due to loss of the crural diaphragm and the augmentation it normally provides to the LES as well as to lowering of the threshold for eliciting tLESRs. Scleroderma is associated with GERD due to the absence of normal peristalsis and an incompetent hypotensive LES. Obesity is associated with GERD by an incompletely understood mechanism which may include an increased frequency of tLESRs.
2. (A) A presumptive diagnosis of GERD can be made in a patient with typical symptoms of GERD such as heartburn and regurgitation followed by empiric treatment as long as alarm symptoms are absent.

3. (B) B is correct as this is a high-risk patient with a chronic history of GERD and presence of an alarm symptom who should first receive evaluation with an upper endoscopy. Complications of GERD are thought to be more common in males, whites, and advanced age. Answers 1 and 3 are incorrect as lifestyle modification and medical therapy would be inappropriate without first performing an upper endoscopy to evaluate for a complication. Answer 4 is incorrect as an upper endoscopy should be performed to rule out a structural abnormality (e.g., malignancy) prior to performing an evaluation for esophageal dysmotility.

Chapter 5

1. (C) Aerophagia can be diagnosed based on a clinical history of troublesome, repetitive belching that occurs several times each week in addition to direct observation of the patient swallowing air. Specialized testing is not required.
2. (E) Large, randomized, prospective trials to guide therapy in adults with aerophagia are not available. We recommend starting with education and reassurance. Many patients can break the habit of gulping air inappropriately once it is pointed out to them. Some patients note improvement in symptoms with simple dietary interventions such as avoiding carbonated beverages, eating more slowly, not talking while eating or drinking, and not eating on the run. The occasional patient swallows air excessively due to occult acid reflux; empiric therapy for 6–8 weeks with a single dose proton pump inhibitor is reasonable. Finally, the occasional patient may fail all of these interventions and referral to a behavioral therapist knowledgeable in the field of functional bowel disorders can be quite useful.
3. (B) False. Transient lower esophageal sphincter relaxations are the primary physiologic event leading to gastroesophageal reflux, not rumination. Although effortless regurgitation occurs in both gastroesophageal reflux and rumination syndrome, rumination occurs due to the voluntary, although often unintentional, act of contracting abdominal wall muscles, which pushes gastric contents up into the esophagus and mouth. During this process the lower esophageal sphincter and upper esophageal sphincter typically relax. A careful history can distinguish rumination from GERD as reflux of gastric contents (GERD) is typically acidic in nature, while food that is ruminated is usually not acidic in nature.
4. (D) Impedance-pH monitoring with esophageal manometry.
   Rumination syndrome is characterized by the effortless and often repetitive regurgitation of recently ingested food into the mouth. Rumination syndrome can usually be diagnosed by history alone. However, some patients require diagnostic testing to either make or confirm the diagnosis. In these patients impedance-pH monitoring with manometry may demonstrate a rise in intragastric which precedes retrograde intra-esophageal flow on impedance. Both the lower esophageal and the upper esophageal sphincter should relax to accommodate the retrograde movement of material.

Chapter 6

1. (D) 70 %. Many clinicians are surprised to learn that 70 % of patients with dyspeptic symptoms have a normal EGD and thus are accurately categorized as having FD.
2. (B) Impaired fundic accommodation and a mild delay in gastric emptying.
   All of the individual answers listed are correct; however, since impaired accommodation accounts for approximately 40 % of FD cases and a mild delay in gastric emptying accounts for another 30 %, answer B is the best choice.
3. (D) Delayed gastric emptying and *H. pylori* infection.
   In a young patient with symptoms of dyspepsia and no warning signs on history or examination, empiric treatment can be safely initiated without any testing.
4. (B) False. Although 30–40 % of FD patients may have a mild delay in gastric emptying, prokinetics rarely improve global symptoms of FD. PPIs improve symptoms in some FD patients, although the number needed to treat is approximately 10. TCAs are effective at improving symptoms of visceral pain in many patients.

Chapter 7

1. (B) False. The differential diagnosis of chronic nausea is quite extensive and encompasses more than the gastrointestinal tract. Exploring the broad set of etiologies for patients presenting with nausea is part of a comprehensive, thoughtful evaluation.
2. (A) History. A diagnostic approach to patients with nausea needs to be based on the details of their presentation. Answer A, a comprehensive history, is the correct answer, as the history provides the framework on which to build the diagnostic approach. Although upper endoscopy (answer B) is the most sensitive tool to exclude mucosal disease, it does not address many of the important aspects in patients presenting with nausea. Answer C, a gastric emptying test, may be considered for patients with meal-related symptoms, but its utility is uncertain. Answer D should be considered in a patient with neurological symptoms, but is not part of a routine nausea evaluation.
3. (C) Meclizine. As meclizine mediates its antiemetic effects by competing for the histamine and cholinergic receptors involved in vestibular dysfunction, answer C is the best option for this patient with vertigo. Answers A and B are not the best initial choice in this situation as ondansetron (a 5-HT_3 antagonist) and aprepitant (a NK-1 antagonist) have different mechanisms of action. Answer D, omeprazole, is not the best choice, as a proton pump inhibitor would be more appropriate for presumed GERD.

Chapter 8

1. (C) EGD. While the patient has symptoms suggestive of gastroparesis, this can be diagnosed only after mechanical obstruction has been ruled out with either upper endoscopy or an upper GI series with small bowel follow through. Given the symptoms of pain, nausea, and vomiting, an upper endoscopy is most cost-effective (since the mucosa will be visualized).
2. (D) In all patients evaluated for gastroparesis a comprehensive evaluation of medications should be obtained as many medications delay gastric emptying and can produce false-positive results on gastric emptying tests. In this question both vicodin, as an opioid agonist, and exenatide, as a GLP-1 analogue, have been implicated as classes of medications which delay gastric emptying. Answer C is incorrect because metformin and glipizide have not been shown to influence gastric emptying. Metformin is a cause of drug-induced nausea. It is important to remember that if the patient's blood glucose is elevated (>270 mg/dl) at the time of the gastric emptying test, then a false-positive test may occur, as hyperglycemia delays gastric emptying. We recommend that if the blood glucose is greater than 275 mg/dl at the time of the study, it be canceled and rescheduled when the blood sugar is in better control, in order to avoid a false-positive test.
3. (A) The patient is symptomatic despite being prescribed an antiemetic, but she continues to eat normal sized meals, including fast foods with high fat content which delay gastric emptying. Answer A would likely improve her symptoms of nausea and vomiting and is safe. Answers B, C, and D all require invasive medical procedures which put the patient at risk for complications and are not indicated at this point given her dietary habits have not been addressed and pharmacotherapy has not been exhausted.
4. (A) Metoclopramide 5 mg QAC & QHS.
   Metoclopramide is FDA approved for treatment of nausea and vomiting associated with gastroparesis and is the most reasonable choice of those listed. Metoclopramide should be prescribed at the lowest dose required to ameliorate symptoms and patients should be educated regarding side effects. Patient follow-up is critical given the small risk of irreversible tardive dyskinesia associated with chronic use. Choice B is frequently prescribed in the treatment of irritable bowel syndrome in the setting of abdominal pain and may be used empirically in patients with gastroparesis who experience pain, which this patient did not report. Dicyclomine has anticholinergic properties and should generally be avoided in patients with gastroparesis. Choice C would not be the best choice because the patient does not report abdominal pain. Tricyclic antidepressants have anticholinergic activity and as a side effect can often cause worsening constipation and nausea in gastroparesis.

Chapter 9

1. (B) False. Chronic cannabis use can cause symptoms of abdominal pain, nausea, and vomiting. These symptoms may mimic CVS. Cessation of cannabis results in resolution of symptoms. However, CVS is a separate entity from cannabis hyperemesis.
2. (C) Multifactorial in nature. The etiology of CVS is multifactorial and varies from patient to patient. Putative etiologies include post-infectious syndromes, metabolic syndromes, hypothalamic–pituitary axis dysfunction, autonomic dysregulation, and an association with migraine headaches.
3. (B) False. Although CVS is more common in children it can develop de novo in adults.
4. (E) All of the above. Research studies have demonstrated that a number of therapeutic options may be effective at treating CVS. These options range from dietary interventions (a low amine diet), to medications directed at concomitant migraine headaches (Triptans) to medications for visceral pain (TCAs), among others.

Chapter 10

1. (B) Females are more likely to report an increase in abdominal girth (i.e., distension) accompanying a sensation of bloating than males. Indeed they often report feeling "6 months pregnant" by the end of the day. Why this is the case is unclear. Option "A" and "C" are not correct, as not only do some individuals not distend when feeling bloated, but distension is less prevalent in IBS-D patients than IBS-C patients. Interestingly patients with functional constipation report bloating alone more often than distension, but no objective measures of distension have been made in this group. Option "D" is incorrect. Though patients with bloating are frequently seen in both Primary Care and Gastroenterology clinics, epidemiological studies suggest that these patients tend to seek medical care for other symptoms (e.g., abdominal pain or changes in bowel habit) and bloating alone is rarely the main reason leading to consultation.
2. (D) Distension is associated with increased colonic transit time.
   Studies have shown that colonic transit time is delayed in IBS-C patients with distension, and that accelerating transit therapeutically results in an improvement in abdominal distension. Option "A" is incorrect, as numerous studies have shown FGID patients have no more abdominal gas than healthy controls. Indeed infusion of 2 l of gas into a patient's gut only leads to a less than 2 cm change in abdominal girth, which is significantly less than the average (approximately 3 cm) you see in these patients, and the 10–12 cm you sometimes record in patients

with IBS-C. Option "B" is incorrect as while patients with intestinal dysmotility disorders distend via a similar mechanism to healthy volunteers but just more excessively because of greater retention of abdominal contents (solids, liquids, gases), IBS patients show a disproportionate increase in girth because of impaired contraction of the lower rectus and external oblique abdominal muscles, and paradoxical "relaxation" of the internal oblique muscle and "contraction" (descent) of the diaphragm. Option "C" is incorrect, as increased visceral sensitivity appears to be associated with the sensation of bloating alone or gas. IBS-C patients with the greatest diurnal changes in girth (i.e., over 8 cm) appear to be viscerally hyposensitive, the reason for which is still unknown.

3. (D) Rifaximin. While rifaximin is a nonabsorbable antibiotic that might reduce the symptoms of gaseousness and bloating in some patients with IBS, a recent meta-analysis suggests that its benefit is modest with a number needed to treat of 10 in unselected IBS patients. This together with the possibility that antibiotic use can contribute to the development of further antibiotic resistance makes rifaximin unsuitable as a first-line treatment. Dietary changes, mild exercise, and certain tested probiotics, such as *Bifidobacterium* and *Lactobacillus*, may help bloating and, importantly, are exempt from side effects. Thus, answers A, B, and C are reasonable first-line treatment options in patients with bloating and distension and should be considered.

Chapter 11

1. (E) Nonspecific symptoms without a predisposing factor.
   Traditionally, SIBO presented as malabsorption with an underlying predisposing factor such as intestinal dysmotility or anatomic abnormality. Recently, however, evidence supports that SIBO usually manifests with nonspecific symptoms like bloating, flatulence, and abdominal discomfort in the absence of any predisposing factor. SIBO may be asymptomatic in the elderly.
2. (B) Although the culture of a proximal small bowel aspirate is considered to be the gold standard for the diagnosis of SIBO, there is evidence to the contrary. Moreover, it is invasive, costly, and not widely utilized. The lactulose or glucose breath test is currently the most commonly used test in clinical practice because of its simplicity and non-invasiveness. When combined with a therapeutic trial, it provides the "test, treat, and outcome" assessment which has been recommended in the absence of any true gold standard test for SIBO. Endoscopy and histology are usually normal in SIBO, imaging provides evidence only for underlying anatomic abnormalities, and laboratory findings are nonspecific and are usually absent.
3. (D) Antibiotics. While the aim of SIBO treatment should be correction of the predisposing factor, this is not usually feasible. Nutritional support is given when malabsorption is present. The cornerstone of SIBO treatment is the use of antibiotics. Since SIBO usually recurs, the majority of the sufferers will require a rotating cycle of antibiotic treatment to maintain symptom resolution.

Chapter 12

1. (D) MR enterography.
   Answer D is correct as the next step in diagnosis of CIP as enterography will generally exclude mechanical obstruction as the cause of the small bowel dilation. Celiac disease would be unlikely to cause small bowel dilation in the absence of a small bowel mass (i.e., lymphoma). Upper endoscopy may demonstrate retained food secondary to gastroparesis, but would not exclude a distal mechanical obstruction.
2. (C) Trial of nasojejunal feeding.
   Answer C is correct as the next step in nutrition management. As the patient has gastroparesis associated with CIP, she would be less likely to tolerate feeding through a gastrostomy tube (answer B) and may require jejunostomy for feeding. Answer A is incorrect as enteral feeding is preferred to parenteral nutrition. While there are case reports of partial gastrectomy to treat gastroparesis, this approach has not been studied in patients with gastroparesis and CIP.
3. (B) Colonoscopy.
   B is the correct answer as colonoscopy would not be required before transplant evaluation. A is incorrect as patients with CIP are at risk of urologic abnormalities such as megacystis. Hepatic function testing is needed as the patient has been on chronic PN and is at risk of liver disease which, if severe, may require a combined intestine-liver transplant or multi-visceral transplant. A patient with compromised gastric emptying may also require a multi-visceral transplant.

Chapter 13

1. (D) This patient needs to have initial testing to determine whether or not she has structural biliary disease. Liver and pancreatic enzymes and abdominal ultrasound will assess for the presence of inflammation in the gallbladder or pancreas and gallstones. An EGD will assess for peptic ulcer disease. At this time, a CT scan of the abdomen and pelvis is not necessary.
2. (C) Functional sphincter of Oddi disorder.
   A low gallbladder ejection fraction (GBEF) is suggestive of functional gallbladder disorder, but it is not specific for the disorder. Other conditions and medications including celiac disease, narcotic use, anticholinergic agents, oral contraceptive agents, and diabetes have all been associated with a low GBEF. Studies have not consistently found an association between functional sphincter of Oddi disorder and low GBEF.
3. (B) A 50-year-old female with severe intermittent right quadrant pain and a GBEF of 21 %.
   Only patients with classic biliary type pain and a GBEF<38 % should be considered for cholecystectomy. Bloating, epigastric fullness, and constant pain are considered atypical symptoms. Patients with atypical symptoms are less likely to

experience symptom improvement following a cholecystectomy. Narcotic agents can impair gallbladder emptying. If possible, agents known to cause a low GBEF should be discontinued prior to CCK-CS testing.

Chapter 14

1. (B) Retained common bile duct stone.
   Although bile duct injury is one of the causes of postcholecystectomy syndrome (PCS), the clinical presentation is dependent on the type of injury. Bile leak is usually detected during the first 3 days after cholecystectomy. Bile duct strictures without bile leak have a longer symptom-free interval after cholecystectomy and frequently present with symptoms of biliary obstruction. Retained common bile duct stones are the most common cause of PCS, especially in a patient with choledocholithiasis at cholecystectomy. Spillage of stones into the abdomen is a rare cause and usually presents with abscess and fever. SOD only may be a consideration after the exclusion of structural diseases.
2. (C) Magnetic resonance cholangiopancreatography (MRCP). ERCP should be reserved for therapeutic purposes. Abdominal ultrasonography has a lower sensitivity (<50 %) for detecting common bile duct stones. MRCP has high sensitivity and specificity to detect stones in common bile duct; however, EUS is considered a better option to detect small stones (<6 mm). MRCP has also the advantage of providing anatomic images of biliary tree when planning an ERCP for removal of stones. Given the elevation in liver tests, upper endoscopy would not be considered initially.
3. (B) ERCP with biliary sphincterotomy.
   The patient described has type I SOD. Patients with type I SOD usually have a fibrotic cause for sphincter dysfunction (true papillary stenosis). As the majority of type I SOD patients have abnormal SO manometry and biliary sphincterotomy results in a near uniform long-term response, manometry is not considered necessary. Nifedipine and other agents administered to reduce SO pressure are not considered first-line options for the treatment of type I SOD. Surgical therapy is reserved for patients with restenosis following endoscopic therapy that is refractory to endoscopic management.

Chapter 15

1. (D) Overflow incontinence.
   The elderly are at risk for constipation. Neurologic conditions and institutionalization are associated with decreased mobility and limited toileting access. Polypharmacy is also a risk factor for constipation, and medication lists should

be regularly reviewed for offending agents. Fecal incontinence in this case is most likely caused by fecal stasis/impaction in the rectum, resulting in overflow incontinence. Treatment would be improved mobility, access to toileting, and laxatives to prevent retention. Excessive perineal descent can cause constipation, not incontinence. Bacterial overgrowth may cause diarrhea, but not usually in a background of constipation.
2. (C) Colonoscopy. He has alarm symptoms of a recent change in the appearance and consistency of stool, rectal bleeding, and anemia. This should be evaluated by colonoscopy or by flexible sigmoidoscopy if colonoscopy is not feasible. Defecography evaluates pelvic floor and recto-sigmoid bowel function during evacuation; it would not be adequate to define a mass, inflammation, or fissure. Anoscopy examines the anal sphincter and distal rectum only; it is not an adequate test to evaluate alarm symptoms.
3. (B) Transit tests objectively measure the speed of digesting contents through the intestine. WMC measures transit time of the stomach, small intestine, and colon, which can aid in diagnosing a number of intestinal motility disorders including slow transit constipation, gastroparesis, and pseudo-obstruction. Sitzmark provides a measure of colon motility only. As her symptoms suggest generalized dysmotility, measuring complete intestinal transit times would be important. MRI defecography is the only imaging modality that can evaluate global pelvic floor anatomy and the anal sphincter without radiation exposure, while anal manometry quantifies internal and external anal sphincter function; neither test would add significant information about her intestinal function.

Chapter 16

1. (C) Nocturnal bowel symptoms.
   As per the Rome Criteria definition of IBS, all of the above are part of the definition except nocturnal bowel movements. Also not mentioned above is that symptoms are generally partially or fully relieved by having a bowel movement. Further, nocturnal bowel movements are more commonly seen with organic disorders like inflammatory bowel disease.
2. (E) Immunoglobulin deficiency. Immunoglobulin deficiency to date has not been postulated as a possible pathophysiologic mechanism for IBS. In post-infectious IBS there may be immunological changes; e.g., rectal biopsies have demonstrated increased mast cells. In addition to the other mechanisms mentioned the role of genetics and environment is still being studied.
3. (A) Lubiprostone.
   Lubiprostone is a chloride channel activator used in the treatment of constipation-predominant IBS. Linaclotide is a guanylate-cyclase agonist also used for the treatment of IBS-C. When using medications for the treatment of IBS it is particularly important that one treat the predominant bowel habit and be very clear

on whether the medication is being used to treat diarrhea or constipation. Historically one of the reasons that alosetron had an increased incidence of side effects when it was initially approved was that the medication which is for IBS-D was being incorrectly prescribed to IBS patients with constipation.

4. (B) FODMAP diet.
   In recent studies the FODMAP foods (fermentable oligosaccharides, disaccharides, monosaccharides, and polyols) have been found to be the cause of many IBS symptoms, particularly bloating and diarrhea. One of the most common substances in these groups of carbohydrates is fructose and fructans which are found in many fruits and vegetables. Some fruits and vegetables such as pears, watermelon, onions, and asparagus are higher in these carbohydrates than others. A full discussion of this is beyond the scope of this chapter, but further information can be found in **The Complete Low-FODMAP Diet: A Revolutionary Plan for Managing IBS and Other Digestive Disorders by** Sue Shepherd PhD and Peter Gibson MD.

Chapter 17

1. (A) Colonic motility study (with manometry and/or a barostat) is necessary to diagnose colonic inertia.
   Answer B is not correct because a substantial proportion of patients, up to 50 % in some series, with a defecatory disorder have slow colonic transit. Therefore, the presence of delayed colonic transit does not exclude a coexisting defecatory disorder. Surgery is indicated and useful in patients with medically refractory slow transit constipation who have demonstrated colonic inertia but not a defecatory disorder. In the absence of alarm symptoms, it is not necessary to repeat a colonoscopy in this patient with long-standing symptoms; the a priori likelihood that constipation since childhood is due to a structural colonic lesion is low.
2. (D) All of the above. D is the best answer since ICC in the colon generates electrical slow waves, influences the smooth muscle membrane potential, and conveys electrical effects to smooth muscle leading to colonic smooth muscle contraction.
3. (B) A defecatory disorder.
   A defecatory disorder is the one condition essential to exclude in patients with colonic inertia being referred for possible surgery. If not identified preoperatively, patients with a significant defecatory disorder may continue to have symptoms of constipation despite having had their colon removed. Gastroesophageal reflux disease, celiac disease, and functional dyspepsia are not contraindications to surgery in patients who are refractory to medical therapy.

Chapter 18

1. (B) IgA tissue transglutaminase antibody. This patient likely has a diagnosis of diarrhea-predominant irritable bowel syndrome (IBS) based on the long-standing nature of her symptoms and the features of diarrhea with abdominal pain that is relieved after defecation. Patients with IBS require little exclusionary testing if there are no alarm features present (none in this case), but patients with diarrhea- or mixed-type IBS should undergo serologic testing for celiac disease given the prevalence of disease. Reassurance alone will be unsatisfying to the patient who has come seeking relief of symptoms, and may overlook celiac disease as a diagnosis. Colonoscopy is not recommended as the first step in the evaluation of a young patient with long-standing diarrhea, and is not indicated in this patient with IBS. Stool bacterial cultures are highly unlikely to be positive in a patient with 2 years of symptoms, especially in the absence of fever, hematochezia, or other risk factors. While a trial of nortriptyline would be very reasonable in this patient in managing her diarrhea, abdominal pain, and chronic headaches, testing for celiac disease should be done first.
2. (D) Lactose malabsorption. This patient likely has a post-infectious lactose malabsorption which results from damage to the surface microvilli where lactase resides, and is usually transient until mucosal healing occurs. Clues to the diagnosis are the post-infectious nature, features of carbohydrate malabsorption (bloating and flatus), and the stool osmotic gap of 170. None of the other conditions listed would result in a stool osmotic gap.
3. (C) Radiation proctitis. This patient likely has chronic radiation-induced proctitis, which may manifest years after external beam radiation therapy and is most common after radiation for prostate, colon, or cervical cancer. Symptoms include diarrhea with blood and mucus, and often tenesmus from the rectal inflammation. Although colorectal cancer should always be considered in an elderly patient with new-onset change in bowel habits, it is less likely in this case given symptom onset was less than 2 years after his last colonoscopy. Ischemic colitis typically causes an acute onset of abdominal pain and diarrhea, followed by bloody diarrhea; it should not cause chronic symptoms. New-onset ulcerative proctitis is possible and symptoms may mirror those of radiation proctitis; however, the history of pelvic radiation makes radiation-induced proctitis more likely in this elderly patient. Medications should always be scrutinized in patients with diarrhea. While olmesartan has been associated with a celiac-like malabsorption pattern, it is not known to cause bloody diarrhea.

Chapter 19

1. (D) Diarrhea.
   Diarrhea is by far the greatest risk factor for fecal incontinence. The other items are also risk factors, but diarrhea is the greatest. Therapy should target bulking her stools and treating her diarrhea.

2. (C) Tap water enemas.
   Clearance of the rectal vault at scheduled intervals with tap water enemas is a preferred treatment for fecal seepage. While sodium phosphate and glycerin suppositories can be tried, regular use may precipitate mucosal damage and bleeding. Botulinum toxin and sphincteroplasty are not treatments for fecal seepage.
3. (E) A and B.
   First-line treatment for fecal incontinence should include lifestyle modifications, including altering diet to increase fiber intake and decrease sugary foods and caffeine which can promote diarrhea. She should also be instructed to ensure she always has access to her walker and her bedroom is close to the bathroom. Providing a bedside toilet may also help those with very limited mobility.

Chapter 20

1. (C) Perianal pain and bleeding.
   Anal fissures are elliptical tears in the anal canal inferior to the dentate line. The prevalence of anal fissures has been estimated to be approximately 10 %; they are more common in younger and middle-aged adults and less common in children and the elderly. Classic symptoms of an anal fissure include severe anorectal pain and bleeding. Patients with proctalgia fugax and levator syndrome do not bleed; patients with hemorrhoidal bleeding do not report such significant pain, unless they have a thrombosed hemorrhoid. Physical examination may be difficult in some patients due to severe perianal pain, and some patients require anesthesia for a thorough examination. Most anal fissures are in the posterior midline; an acute fissure characteristically has sharp edges. A "sentinel" tag (a skin tag) may be seen at the inferior edge of the fissure.
2. (B) Multiple ulcers, medium in size (1–3 cm) on anterior wall. Solitary rectal ulcer syndrome (SRUS) is an uncommon disorder (1–3 in 100,000 patients) that typically affects young adults. Women are more commonly affected than men. Symptoms of SRUS are nonspecific and include rectal bleeding, passage of mucus, straining at stool, feeling of incomplete evacuation, rectal discomfort, and fecal urgency. Sigmoidoscopic examination often reveals multiple ulcers rather than a single ulcer. The lesions are usually on the anterior rectal wall and most are 1–1.5 cm in diameter. Histologic features of SRUS include smooth muscle hyperplasia of the lamina propria with infiltration of collagen (aka "fibromuscular obliteration"), distortion of the crypt architecture, disorientation and thickening of the muscularis mucosa, and an increase in mucous cells with gland dilation.
3. (A) The clinical utility is low.
   Anorectal manometry is a minimally invasive test routinely used to evaluate disorders of the pelvic floor and anorectum. Standard measurements include length of the anal canal, resting pressure of the anal canal, external anal sphincter tone, and external anal sphincter squeeze pressures. In patients with symptoms of con-

stipation, a balloon expulsion test is frequently included to look for evidence of pelvic floor dyssynergia. Anorectal manometry has been shown to be useful in the evaluation of patients with fecal incontinence and constipation; it is not thought to be clinically useful in patients with anorectal pain.

4. (D) Rectal massage, skeletal muscle relaxants, and benzodiazepines.
   Treatment begins by reassuring the patient of the benign nature of this chronic disorder. Medical treatment can be difficult because large, prospective therapeutic trials are not available to guide clinical care. Since levator syndrome is thought to represent a spastic disorder of the levator ani muscles (iliococcygeus, pubococcygeus, puborectalis) then therapies to relax these muscles seem most appropriate. If patients would like to start simply and/or avoid medications then warm sitz baths or even a warm water enema may be useful. Many patients note improvement by performing rectal massage; others note improvement by performing Kegel exercises, although this occasionally worsens symptoms in some. Long-acting anxiolytics such as diazepam are helpful in some patients, while others note improvement using a muscle relaxant such as cyclobenzaprine. Some clinicians recommend calcium channel blockers or smooth muscle relaxants; however, since these act on smooth muscle, they are unlikely to improve symptoms thought related to skeletal muscle spasm, and we do not recommend them. Finally, the occasional patient with frequent disabling episodes may benefit from botulinum toxin injection of the levator ani muscle group although well-controlled studies are lacking.

Chapter 21

1. (A) *Bifidobacterium infantis*.
   Bifidobacterium animalis, *Streptococcus thermophilus*, and *Lactobacillus bulgaricus* have not been studied in dose-ranging, multicenter clinical trials.
2. (A) True. Recent studies found that Internet-based CBT programs specifically tailored to IBS are effective in IBS symptom reduction, when compared with standard therapy and generic stress management therapy.
3. (C) Peppermint oil.
   Peppermint oil has been shown to be effective in alleviating abdominal pain. It reduces spasms in the GI tract by relaxing smooth muscle. Acupuncture is thought to work by stimulating the somatic nervous systems and altering visceral sensation. Hypnotherapy aims to change patients' symptoms through gut-related hypnotic suggestion.

Index

B.E. Lacy et al. (eds.), *Functional and Motility Disorders of the Gastrointestinal Tract*, DOI 10.1007/978-1-4939-1498-2

MIX
Papier aus verantwortungsvollen Quellen
Paper from responsible sources
FSC® C105338

If you have any concerns about our products,
you can contact us on
ProductSafety@springernature.com

In case Publisher is established outside the EU,
the EU authorized representative is:
Springer Nature Customer Service Center GmbH
Europaplatz 3, 69115 Heidelberg, Germany

Printed by Libri Plureos GmbH
in Hamburg, Germany